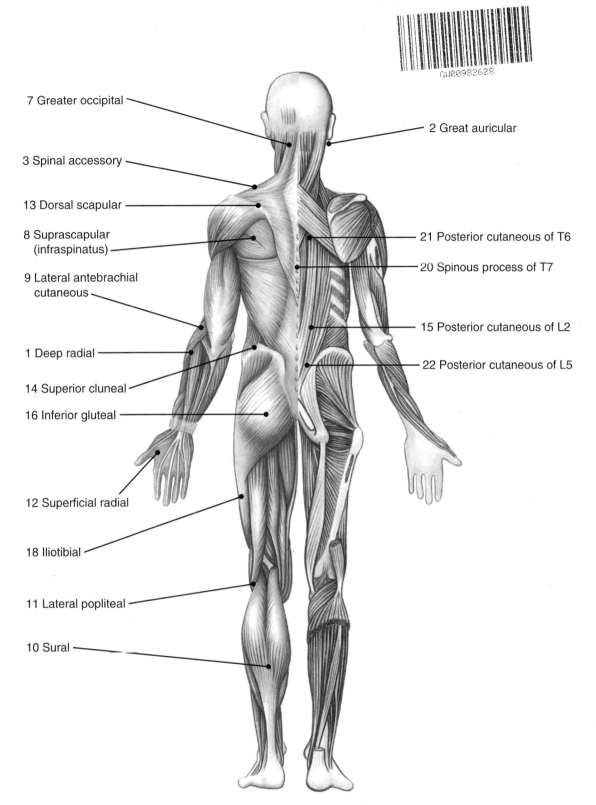

7 Greater occipital

2 Great auricular

3 Spinal accessory

13 Dorsal scapular

8 Suprascapular
(infraspinatus)

21 Posterior cutaneous of T6

20 Spinous process of T7

9 Lateral antebrachial
cutaneous

15 Posterior cutaneous of L2

22 Posterior cutaneous of L5

1 Deep radial

14 Superior cluneal

16 Inferior gluteal

12 Superficial radial

18 Iliotibial

11 Lateral popliteal

10 Sural

Twenty-four Homeostatic Acupoints (HAs)

Biomedical Acupuncture for Pain Management

AN INTEGRATIVE APPROACH

Biomedical Acupuncture for Pain Management

AN INTEGRATIVE APPROACH

Yun-tao Ma, PhD
Director of Bio Medical Acupuncture Institute
Boulder, CO

Mila Ma, LicAc
Bio Medical Acupuncture Institute
Boulder, CO

Zang Hee Cho, PhD
Professor, Radiological Sciences
University of California, Irvine
Irvine, CA

With 174 illustrations

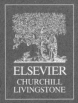

ELSEVIER
CHURCHILL
LIVINGSTONE

ELSEVIER
CHURCHILL
LIVINGSTONE

11830 Westline Industrial Drive
St. Louis, Missouri 63146

BIOMEDICAL ACUPUNCTURE FOR PAIN MANAGEMENT: AN INTEGRATIVE APPROACH

NOTICE

Acupuncture is an ever-changing field. Standard safety precautions must be followed, but as new research
and clinical experience broaden our knowledge, changes in treatment and drug therapy may become
necessary or appropriate. Readers are advised to check the most current product information provided by
the manufacturer of each drug to be administered to verify the recommended dose, the method and duration
of administration, and contraindications. It is the responsibility of the licensed prescriber, relying on
experience and knowledge of the patient, to determine dosages and the best treatment for each individual
patient. Neither the publisher nor the author assumes any liability for any injury and/or damage to persons
or property arising from this publication.

The Publisher

ISBN-13: 978-0-443-06659-7
ISBN-10: 0-443-06659-0

Publishing Director: Linda Duncan
Acquisitions Editor: Kellie White
Senior Developmental Editor: Kim Fons
Publishing Services Manager: Pat Joiner
Project Manager: David Stein
Design Project Manager: Bill Drone

Printed in the United States of America

Last digit is the print number: 9 8 7

AcuMedic CENTRE
101-105 CAMDEN HIGH STREET
LONDON NW1 7JN
Tel: 020 7388-6704/5783
info@acumedic.com   www.acumedic.com

To you, dear reader, who feel the pain of others as your own, we dedicate this book on the art of pain management.

"If I can save a person from days of torture, that is what I feel is my great and ever-new privilege."
—Albert Schweitzer, 1953

About the Authors

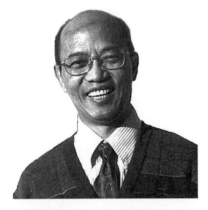

Yun-tao Ma, PhD, was trained as a neuroscientist and has conducted research on neuronal rehabilitation and pain mechanism for the past 22 years. He has also practiced acupuncture since 1970. Dr. Ma co-authored the book, *Scientific Acupuncture for Health Professionals,* which was published in China in 2000. Presently Dr. Ma is a Director of the Biomedical Acupuncture Institute (BAI). He conducts seminars and teaches biomedical acupuncture to healthcare professionals in the United States and worldwide. Dr. Ma can be contacted at **www.BioMed Acupuncture.com.**

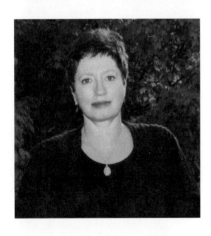

Mila Ma, LicAc, has practiced acupuncture for pain and trauma rehabilitation in Europe and the United States and has personally experienced the benefits of acupuncture after a serious rock climbing accident.

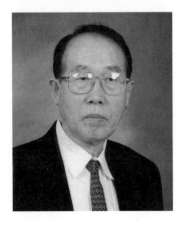

Zang Hee Cho, PhD, is a member of the National Academy of Science-Institute of Medicine and the National Advisory Council for the U.S. NIH National Center for Complementary and Alternative Medicine. Dr. Cho has worked on MRI since the late 1970s, developing numerous high-speed imaging techniques and methods essential for today's fMRI. Dr. Cho pioneered acupuncture-fMRI. This study demonstrated a correlation between acupuncture stimulation and activation of the corresponding brain cortex.

"The authors of this remarkable book have recognised that only through complete biomedicalisation can acupuncture ever be integrated into a modern, scientific healthcare practice. Their book represent the culmination of four decades of research that have led to the development of a unique and biologically plausible system of acupuncture for the management of neuromusculoskeletal pain. This text will allow contemporary healthcare professionals, who already have a deep understanding of current biomedical science and clinical issues, to incorporate biomedical acupuncture into their routine practice as an effective modality, without the difficulties of having to learn the antiquated procedures of traditional acupuncture."

Luke Rickards, Osteopath, LicAc, Australia

"Dr. Ma has changed the face of acupuncture forever and his pioneering work represents the future of acupuncture."

Zhen-ging Jin, MD, China
Director of People's Hospital

"I had an active interest in acupuncture ever since the days when I was in my pain management program. However, the mysticism and very difficult learning process always put me off learning acupuncture. When I read the book *Biomedical Acupuncture for Pain Management*, it was an eye opener - finally the mysticism associated with acupuncture was dismantled - The INMAS System was completely scientific, reproducible and made tremendous sense. It really does teach "HOW TO REMOVE ACUPUNCTURE FROM THE BOTTLE WITH A NARROW NECK"."

Sukdeb Datta, MD, USA

"*Biomedical Acupuncture for Pain Management, Integrative Approach* provides an effecitve learning system for medical professionals. It is a right step leading to integration of acupuncture into mainstream medicine."

Gen-Cheng Wu, MD, China
Chairman of Department of
Integrative Medicine
Shanghai Medical College of Fudan University

Reviewers

David A. Bray, CMD, D. Ac. & Dipl. C.H. (NCCAOM)
Guangzhou University of Traditional Medicine (PRC)
Human University of Traditional Chinese Medicine (PRC)
Toronto, Ontario, CANADA

Elizabeth Chen Christenson
Maumee, Ohio, USA

Steve Given, L.Ac.
Bastyr University
Bastyr Center for Natural Health
Kenmore, Washington, USA

James Saper, R.TCM.P. B.E.S.
Guelph, Ontario, CANADA

Foreword

Chinese acupuncture, developed thousands of years ago, has had an enduring impact on health care and has been a significant cause of the widening international appreciation of the brilliance of Chinese civilization. In the 21st century, with modern science predominating in every field, acupuncture continues to be valued for its contribution to the health and longevity of mankind.

Today many people, both Westerners and Easterners alike, are returning to a lifestyle which values nature and natural healing. Acupuncture is a treasure of Oriental medicine whose central philosophy is based on the self-healing potential of the human body, and this is how it contributes to modern medicine.

In teaching acupuncture to medical professionals in China and around the world for many years, I frequently observe that they are excited about learning acupuncture and are amazed at its therapeutic results. However, they soon feel overwhelmed by the prospect of studying the clinical procedure with its complicated meridian-acupoint system and mysterious manual techniques rooted in Taoist philosophy.

The authors of this book have developed a unique treatment protocol, the Integrative Neuromuscular Acupoint System (INMAS). This system is a result of the biomedicalization of traditional acupuncture but it also succeeds in maintaining the essence of Traditional Chinese Medicine (TCM). Biomedical terminology and concepts are used to interpret the basic mechanisms and clinical procedures of acupuncture. The most essential spirit *(Shen)* of Oriental medicine, which emphasizes "whole-person therapy" and "promoting health while treating the disease," is carefully preserved.

I recommend INMAS as an effective protocol for treating neuromuscular pain. It is applicable not only in pain management but also in treating *Zang-fu*-related diseases and promoting general health.

Being a fourth generation practitioner of TCM with 40 years of clinical experience, as well as a Master of Qigong and director of the TCM Research Institute, where my duties include teaching Chinese medicine to medical professionals world-wide, I deeply believe that this book, *Biomedical Acupuncture for Pain Management: An Integrative Approach,* is a milestone on the road towards integrating acupuncture into mainstream medicine and that it will open the door of acupuncture therapy to Western healthcare professionals.

Shanghai, China, March 10, 2004

Song Zhen-zhi, OMD, Ph.D.

Executive Secretary of the Chinese Association of Outstanding Acupuncture Techniques
Committee member of the World Traditional Medicine Organization
Director of the Kangfu Research Institute of Traditional Chinese Medicine
Faculty Member of the Doctorate Program of the Beijing International Health Institute
Laureate of "The 100 Best TCM Doctors in China"

Preface

"PEARLS AND STRINGS" IN CLASSICAL ACUPUNCTURE OR "HOW TO REMOVE ACUPUNCTURE FROM THE BOTTLE WITH A NARROW NECK"

Acupuncture has evolved for thousands of years and continues to grow vigorously. During its long history, ancient doctors formulated the "channel" ("meridian," or *Jingluo*) theory to explain the clinical discovery of specific interrelations between different parts of the human body. Their "channel" theory became the foundation of classical acupuncture.

A scientific theory or hypothesis contains two components: empirical facts and an explanation of these facts. The empirical facts can be referred to metaphorically as valuable *pearls*, with the explanation of these facts taking the role of the *string*. The basic form of scientific advancement can be seen as a continuous process of changing the string while preserving the pearls, and the "channel" theory is no exception.

In "Channel" theory, however, the pearls and string are tightly tangled together and are difficult to differentiate. This perplexity leads to the situation that no one has been able to clarify what "channels" are, despite the fact that modern research on this question has been continuing for more than four decades. One study[1] shows that students who have modern medical backgrounds, Chinese and foreign alike, are not able to understand what the "channels" really mean.

To understand the value in the "Channel" theory, it is crucial to separate the valuable pearls from the string. Above all, the "Channel" theory has conveyed the precious message that *there is specific interrelatedness between different parts of the body surface and between the body surface and viscera. The "Channels" themselves, reflecting the physiological knowledge of the ancient doctors who created them, serve only as a tentative explanation of this interrelatedness.*

The "Channel" theory has successfully accomplished its historical mission of preserving and developing acupuncture; now it has become the narrow neck of the bottle which is impeding the further development of acupuncture medicine in the 21st century.

Our research on the literature of classic acupuncture has identified the "pearls" that need to be connected with new biomedical "string." The inevitable biomedicalization of classic acupuncture will result in an increase in scientific understanding of the interrelatedness of the human body. This process will work to eliminate the demarcation between Western and Oriental medicine, and a new integrative medicine will facilitate worldwide access to the great treasure of traditional Chinese medicine.

Professor Long-xiang Huang, OMD

Vice President of the Acupuncture Research Institute of the Academy of Traditional Chinese Medicine
Vice Director of the Key Laboratory of the Channel (Jingluo) Research Center of the State Administration of TCM
Chief Editor of *Acupuncture Research* and *World Acupuncture*
Professor Huang is the author of *International Course of Acupuncture, Historical Development of Acupuncture* (published in Beijing, Taipei, and Seoul), and he has produced revised versions of seven ancient classic acupuncture textbooks.

1. Hua-xi Chen: On the "Channel" (Jingluo) concept, *Chinese acupuncture and moxibustion*, vol 4, 4/2001.

Introduction

PURPOSE

The goal of this book is to facilitate the integration of acupuncture into mainstream medicine as a complementary modality in the field of pain management.

Integrate is defined in Webster's College Dictionary as "to meld with and become part of the dominant culture."

Biomedical acupuncture results from the integration of conventional Western medicine and traditional Oriental medicine. This integration is harmonious, or as the Chinese say, like "milk dissolved in water," not "oil mixed with water."

Biomedicine is defined in the same dictionary as "the application of the natural sciences, esp. the biological and physiological sciences, to clinical medicine." This is exactly what biomedical acupuncture means: it is the application of biological and neurophysiological principles to clinical acupuncture.

The acupuncture system presented in this book allows healthcare professionals—medical doctors (MDs), doctors of osteopathy (DOs), doctors of chiropractic (DCs), dentists, podiatrists, nurses, physical therapists, and others—to learn acupuncture within the familiar framework of biomedical principles and practice it on the basis of their own previous medical training.

Contemporary healthcare professionals have a profound understanding of basic biomedical science and clinical issues as a result of their many years of school training and clinical practice. After a short period of additional training, these professionals will easily be able to incorporate biomedical acupuncture into their routine medical practice as an effective, problem-solving modality, without having to face the difficulties of learning all the ancient procedures of classical acupuncture. This is because acupuncture has the same physiological basis as mainstream biomedicine. The quantitative method introduced here will also be of great benefit to traditionally trained acupuncturists who will find it a useful addition to their practice.

BIOMEDICAL ACCULTURATION OF CLASSIC ACUPUNCTURE INTO MODERN HIGH-TECH SOCIETY IS INEVITABLE

Acupuncture has been practiced for about 5000 years in China and other Asian countries. Over the course of these millennia the ancient practitioners developed many elaborate concepts and systems that reflected the religious beliefs and the medical and sociocultural traditions of their time.

Acupuncture therapy has evolved into the twenty-first century still dragging with it a collection of empirical facts which though valuable are inextricably combined with ancient concepts and methods and all the various misinterpretations that have arisen during its long history.

As acupuncture encounters modern biomedicine in societies such as the United States and China, healthcare practitioners, Western and Eastern alike, are puzzled by its ancient character: they cannot judge from a medical perspective what is right and what is wrong in this venerable healing art nor can they understand how it works. Many healthcare practitioners decide to keep away from this bizarre modality, unable to believe that it can be justified scientifically. Others, attracted by anecdotal evidence of its efficacy, spend months or years studying acupuncture and traditional Chinese medicine (TCM), but even after years of study and practice, they may still find confusing such alien concepts as *Qi* or "fire," or "five elements," and the tangled maze of meridians and the various systems of acupoints.

Clinical evidence shows that acupuncture has its own special merits which are not the same as those of the high-tech–oriented Western medicine. It is effective for a variety of health problems, but particularly for cases in which Western medicine has little to offer, and especially in the field of pain management. It is a safe, low-cost modality which is easy to administer and has no side effects if performed by a trained practitioner; it can be effective by itself or as a complement to other medical procedures.

The integration of acupuncture into mainstream medicine, especially in pain management for neuromusculoskeletal conditions, cannot happen without biomedicalization. This inevitable process, however, is not some new and exceptional event in the history of acupuncture. During the past several thousands of years the acculturation and reacculturation of acupuncture has occurred many times as it has adapted to different cultures and geographical circumstances: in China, Japan, Korea, Vietnam, and other Southeast Asian countries. After each acculturation, acupuncture practice changed to a certain degree and usually it was enriched by new methods and ways of understanding. It has been able to survive all these changes because the underlying medical mechanisms have stayed the same, regardless of the different clinical styles of the host cultures.

Now, in the twenty-first century, an enormous amount of laboratory data and clinical evidence enable us to reach a deeper understanding than ever before of the inner workings of acupuncture, using knowledge that ranges from molecular medicine to the modern understanding of human anatomy.

HISTORICAL DEVELOPMENT OF TRADITIONAL ACUPUNCTURE: NEW DISCOVERIES

Acupuncture medicine is a rich inheritance from TCM. To successfully biomedicalize this ancient healing art, its historical origin and social evolution need to be understood.

For over 20 years Professor Long-xiang Huang of the Acupuncture Research Institute of the Academy of Traditional Chinese Medicine in Beijing has meticulously studied all of the ancient acupuncture literature available in China and Japan, from archaeological relics to Qing dynasty manuscripts. Using these documents he has painstakingly traced every possible clue leading to an understanding of how the ancient practitioners created the whole theoretical web of acupuncture and its clinical application. Now, for the first time, Professor Huang has been able to reconstruct the history of the development of acupuncture from the earliest records of its beginning.

How Acupoints Were Discovered

When examining their patients, the ancient Chinese practitioners felt pulsation at arterial loci (pulsing points). They believed that this pulse was caused by a vital force, which they called Qi. The difference between life and death was due to the presence or absence of Qi and all parts of the body were connected by a Qi channel or vessel. These ancient doctors diagnosed by palpating the arterial loci (pulsing points) all over the body and then they needled these points to treat a disease. Since they could not feel the pulsation along the entire presumed Qi channel, they postulated channels of connection between the acupoints on the loci of arteries, thus making a visible map of the unseen parts of the channel. Different practitioners in different times and places evolved their own ways to connect together the acupoints which they had identified, and this gave rise to a variety of theories to explain the channels or meridians. Even today traditional Chinese medical doctors are trained to feel this arterial pulsation, though only on the radial artery proximal to the wrist. The pulsing points of arteries were the earliest acupoints.

The Origin of Channel or Meridian Theories

Early acupuncture theories were formed from empirical experience. For example, ancient doctors found that for treating pain or other symptoms of the genitals, lower abdomen, and lumbar areas, needling certain pulsing loci on the dorsum of the foot and medial part of the lower leg was more effective than anywhere else. Thus they drew lines to connect the effective needling points with the parts of the body that were most affected by the needling, making a visible representation of the channel which connected all the points together. In this example the arterial points on the dorsum, the medial leg, the genital area, the lumbar area, and up to the tongue were joined together and thus the "liver channel," or "liver meridian," was gradually formulated. The other eleven meridians that are used today evolved in a similar way.

The theory of meridians, or channels, became one of the cornerstones of TCM. As there were many different ways to delineate the same channel there were soon many different theoretical explanations. In his reconstruction of the development of ancient acupuncture practice Professor Huang shows that the ancient Chinese used the same character "*mai*" (脉) to represent both "channels" and "blood vessels." In most Western textbooks, the character "*mai*" has been translated as "meridian" or "channel." Even today, acupuncture practitioners must learn a large and complex map of Qi channels (meridians) and other medical principles that are based on the ancient *Yellow Emperor's Canon of Internal Medicine*.

If the old practitioners had recourse to the advances of modern medicine that we now take for granted, they would not have needed to "connect the dots" to map out the unseen parts of the arterial channels.

The Historical Integration of the Various Channel Theories Into a Single System

The Yellow Emperor's Canon of Internal Medicine (Huang Di Nei Jing), which was probably compiled between 206 BC and 220 AD, stands as a unique monument of ancient medical science. It became the foundation of traditional Chinese medicine and is still used today as a textbook by acupuncturists all over the world.

The *Canon* integrated the various channel theories into one system. Inconsistencies in this book reveal that the authors had differing types of medical experience and were from different historical periods. In the years that followed the appearance of the *Canon*, acupuncture continued to evolve by incorporating more theories, and an ever-increasing number of acupoints and channels, into the existing system. Professor Huang shows that when clinical realities did not fit into an existing theory, the facts were often suppressed to ensure the continuance of the theory. New theories were forced to coexist with old ones, in a style that the Chinese call "cutting the foot to fit the shoe." Thus classical acupuncture as we know it today is made up of theories and clinical experience that are valuable, mixed with fallacious concepts and imperfect explanations. We should also bear in mind that we in the twenty-first century have great difficulty in understanding and correctly interpreting this ancient text, because we lack the scholastic mentality of the time in which it was created.

The Genuine "Pearls" of Acupuncture Theory

Scholars and scientists of the People's Republic of China conducted an intensive research program for over four decades, utilizing a national investment of enormous human power and financial resources, but no evidence was found that could support the traditional theory of acupuncture meridians. Professor Long-xiang Huang, who is currently in charge of the national program of acupuncture research, ascribes this result to the fact that researchers were not able to separate, in his words, the "pearls" (the valuable medical facts) from the "string" (the ancient explanations) that connects them. Professor Huang emphasizes that *the most valuable discovery in acupuncture theory is the interrelatedness between the parts of the body surface, and between the parts of the body surface and the internal organs. These are the immortal "pearls" of classic acupuncture.*

At the present time the situation is incongruous: scientists have been exploring the physiological and molecular mechanisms of acupuncture with high-tech facilities in laboratories for more than four decades while modern medical professionals who wish to study acupuncture are still using textbooks based on *The Yellow Emperor's Canon of Internal Medicine,* written 2500 years ago. We hope this situation will change soon.

Many healthcare practitioners have found the old system unnecessarily difficult and incompatible with their medical training but they have no modern system to turn to if they want to practice acupuncture. The authors of this book have developed the *Integrative Neuromuscular Acupoint System* (INMAS), which uses both the principles of classic acupuncture and the latest scientific explanations of the underlying mechanisms, and can be easily learned by any healthcare professional who wants to integrate acupuncture into their routine practice of pain management.

WHAT IS ACUPUNCTURE, WHAT DOES IT TREAT, AND HOW EFFECTIVE IS IT?

It is no more correct to refer to a single universal "traditional Chinese acupuncture" than it would be to speak of a single universal "traditional European medicine." For example, there are more than 80 different acupuncture styles in China alone, in addition to many Japanese, Korean, Vietnamese, European, and American styles.

What has enabled acupuncture to survive for such an incredibly long time in so many different geographical areas across different historical periods? It is important to understand that the longevity of acupuncture is not based on the exact procedures of any particular style, but on its powerful underlying biomedical mechanisms.

The common feature shared by all the different types of acupuncture is using needles to make lesions in the soft tissue (acu-puncture). Needles and needle-induced lesions activate the built-in survival mechanisms that normalize homeostasis and promote self-healing. This process consists of two parts: central and peripheral.

For the central mechanism needling and needle-induced lesions stimulate parts of the brain that activate the principal survival systems—the nervous, endocrine, immune, and cardiovascular systems—and normalize the physiological activities of the whole body (see Chapter 4).

In the case of the peripheral mechanism needling and the resulting lesions trigger physiological reactions around the needling sites that involve all four survival systems in desensitizing and repairing the damaged tissues. At the needling site, a cascade of survival reactions occurs, including the immune reaction, and we call this the local needling reaction (see Chapter 3).

Thus acupuncture can be defined as a physiological therapy coordinated by the brain which responds to the stimulation of manual or electrical needling of peripheral sensory nerves. In relation to this definition, there is one concept that cannot be overemphasized: that *acupuncture does not treat any particular pathological symptom but normalizes physiological homeostasis and promotes self-healing*. Thus acupuncture, in terms of its therapeutic mechanisms, is non-specific: acupuncture does not target any particular symptom or disease but treats the body as a whole.

Understanding this nonspecific nature of acupuncture can provide an answer to the puzzling question: what symptoms and diseases can it treat?

As a physiological therapy, the efficacy of acupuncture depends on (1) the healability of the symptom(s) or disease(s), and (2) the self-healing potential maintained by each patient.

The same symptom or disease can be completely healable in one patient but only partially healable or even not healable at all in another because the self-healing potential varies from one person to another. Therefore, acupuncture effectiveness varies from person to person. When treating the same symptom or disease, acupuncture therapy might achieve a miraculous result in patient A, partial relief in patient B, and have little or no effect in patient C. In Chapter 6, we describe our 16-point quantitative evaluation method, which is based on the discoveries of Dr H. C. Dung, for predicting the effectiveness of acupuncture treatment for each type of patient.

WHY DOES ACUPUNCTURE PRODUCE MORE PREDICTABLE RESULTS IN SOFT TISSUE PAIN MANAGEMENT?

As early as 1890 acupuncture was recommended for lower back pain by the famous Canadian doctor Sir William Osler in his classic textbook *The Principle and Practice of Medicine*. Today in Western societies acupuncture is largely used in pain management, and this analgesic function is still the most studied aspect of acupuncture. We have a better understanding of the way acupuncture works when it is used to treat symptoms of soft tissue pain, and for this reason the results can be more accurately predicted than when it is used for other kinds of symptoms.

We explained above that acupuncture involves central and peripheral mechanisms. When we treat soft tissue pain, needling makes lesions directly in the painful tissues and these lesions locally activate neuroendocrine, immune, and cardiovascular reactions around the needling sites in the painful tissues. These local "needle reactions" directly desensitize the painful nerves and repair the damaged soft tissues. The process of desensitization and tissue repair is often triggered immediately by the "needle reaction" at the needling sites.

When we treat internal disorders such as stomachache, we cannot directly create the "needle reaction" in stomach tissues, so we can only needle segmental nerves to activate the cutaneovisceral reflex, which creates a balance between sympathetic and parasympathetic nerves to promote self-healing of the stomach. This is an example of "indirect" treatment by acupuncture.

Clinical experience shows that acupuncture can be effective for both peripheral soft tissue pain and internal disorders, but in the case of peripheral soft tissue pain the result is more predictable because of the local needle reaction.

In pain management we transform the nonspecific effect of needling into a specific effect for specific symptoms by creating, or "inoculating," the lesions directly in the painful areas. The Chinese have an old saying that nine out of ten diseases produce pain, and according to statistics, 85% of the pain in our daily lives is soft tissue pain. This is why acupuncture is seen primarily as a modality for pain management in Western societies.

THE INTEGRATIVE NEUROMUSCULAR ACUPOINT SYSTEM IS A WORKING MODEL FOR PAIN MANAGEMENT

This book presents a working model, utilizing a neuroanatomically defined system of acupoints, that is based on the integration of conventional Western medicine and traditional Oriental medicine. INMAS combines laboratory research and practical clinical experience; it is derived from two great traditions—300 years of Western analytical science and 2500 years of Oriental empiricism; and it succeeds in providing both the standardized treatment protocol that Western scientific medicine demands and the adjustable personalizable approach of Oriental medicine.

Biomedical acupuncture and INMAS are easy to understand and can be safely and effectively practiced after a short training by any healthcare professional of either Western or Oriental medical background.

While modern biomedical principles are applied both in theory and in clinical practice, the major principles of Oriental medicine are also completely retained:

1. Restoring physiological homeostasis (the balance of *yin* and *yang*)
2. Maximizing self-healing without side-effects
3. Treating both *ben* (the root of the disease, the whole body) and *biao* (the symptoms of the disease)

INMAS has all the characteristics required by a clinical procedure:

1. *Simplicity:* the whole procedure from evaluation of the patient to insertion of needles can be performed in a very short time in the clinic
2. *Reproducibility:* all the procedures and therapeutic results are reliable and reproducible by any practitioner, beginner and experienced alike
3. *Predictability:* this method enables the practitioner to predict the results of the treatment as follows:
   a. Whether the patient will respond to acupuncture treatment or not
   b. If the patient is a responder, how many treatments will be needed to achieve pain relief
   c. Whether the pain will return at some time after the initial relief is achieved

ONE PROTOCOL FOR MOST PAIN PATIENTS: THE COMBINATION OF STANDARDIZED PROCEDURE WITH INDIVIDUALIZED ADJUSTMENT

The same protocol can be applied to most patients because of the nonspecific nature of acupuncture therapy: it does not target any particular symptoms or diseases but promotes self-healing by activating the built-in survival mechanisms.

It is very commonly seen that when patients come for treatment of symptom A, they experience simultaneous relief of symptoms B and C. This nonspecific nature of acupuncture, combined with laboratory research data from neurochemistry to fMRI, has enabled us to develop an INMAS protocol that is effective for most patients, regardless of their different symptoms and diseases.

With the INMAS protocol practitioners are able to adhere to the standardization of treatment procedure that is required in modern biomedicine. To individualize the treatment for each patient, as is the essence of Oriental medicine, they can use the special procedure of INMAS and also draw on their own medical experience.

INMAS is not a "magic bullet," a miraculous answer for everything, but it is a protocol containing the principles of both Western and Oriental medicine that can be easily learned and applied successfully by any practitioner, even a relative beginner.

We believe that the whole-person approach of traditional acupuncture is of great value and will find a deserved place in the modern healthcare system. Biomedical acupuncture offers an explanation of its neural mechanism, and thus opens the door of integrative medicine for Western healthcare professionals.

Acknowledgments

Our grateful acknowledgment is made to the following colleagues and friends for their support and comments: Dr. Zhen-zhi Song, OMD, PhD, faculty member of the Doctorate Program of the Beijing International Health and Medicine Institute; Professors Xiao-ding Cao, MD; Gen-cheng Wu, MD; Xian-fen Huang, MD, the Department of Integrative Medicine, the Shanghai Medical College of Fudan University.

Our heartfelt thanks go to our friends Dr. H.C. Dung, former professor of the University of Texas Health Science Center at San Antonio, and Professor Long-xiang Huang, OMD, Vice President of the Acupuncture Research Institute of the Academy of Traditional Chinese Medicine in Beijing. Their pioneer work and input were indispensable to this book.

Kellie White, the "dream come true" editor of Elsevier Publishing, and her team have provided us with a warm unwavering support through all the stages of production.

The authors would like to express their sincere gratitude to a wonderful daughter and best friend Katrine Merlushkin, JD, first reader of the book, for her thoughtful comments on the manuscript. The style of the book has been greatly improved by the expert work of our good friend and talented copyeditor Ashik Peter Lynch, MA (Oxon).

Yun-tao Ma and Mila Ma

Contents

CHAPTER 1

From Neurons to Acupoints: Basic Neuroanatomy of Acupoints

INTRODUCTION

The efficiency of acupuncture therapy is based on the selection of effective acupoints. There are 361 classic meridian acupoints, and more than 2000 new extrameridian acupoints have been recorded in the Chinese literature on acupuncture. Anatomic examination of the 361 classic meridian acupoints shows that most acupoints are associated with certain anatomic structures of the peripheral nervous system (PNS). Researchers have indicated that 309 acupoints lie on or near the nerves and that 286 acupoints are situated next to major blood vessels, which are surrounded by small nerve bundles.[1]

Modern neuromuscular medicine named some of these points *trigger points, motor points,* and *dermopoints*. Dr. Ronald Melzack[2] found that more than 70% of the classic meridian acupoints correspond to commonly used trigger points. Whatever terms are used, all these points are characterized by the ability to become painful or tender or to create other physical discomforts as a result of sensitized nerves. It is extremely important to understand that although more than 70% of the classic acupoints share the same characteristics as trigger points, acupoints and trigger points are not the same.

In their book *Muscle Pain,* Drs. Siegfried Mense and David G. Simons define trigger points as follows: "(1) A *central* trigger point is a tender, localized hardening in a skeletal muscle. Clinical characteristics include circumscribed spot tenderness in a nodule that is part of a palpably tense band of muscle fibers, patient recognition of the pain evoked by pressure on the tender spot as being familiar, pain referred in the pattern characteristic of trigger points in that muscle, a local twitch response, painful limitation of the stretch range of motion, and some weakness of that muscle. Diagnostic criteria of *active* trigger points are circumscribed spot tenderness in a nodule of a palpable taut band and patient recognition of the pain, evoked by pressure on the tender spot, as being familiar. *Latent* trigger points cause no complaint of clinical pain. (2) *Attachment* trigger points have tenderness in the region of muscle attachment caused by enthesitis or enthesopathy induced by the persistent tension of the taut band muscle fibers."[3]

These trigger points as defined clearly refer to tender spots only on the skeletal muscles. The classic acupoints are found not only in the skeletal muscles but also in other soft tissue structures such as in tendons and fascias. Thus trigger points share *some* but not *all* characteristics of acupoints, whereas acupoints include *all* the characteristics of trigger points. This means that trigger points have some inclusive but not exclusive parameters of the classic acupoints.

In laboratory and clinical experiments, acupuncture stops being effective in a region supplied by a sensory nerve when that nerve is blocked by local anesthesia, cut by surgery, numbed by ice (low temperature), or bound by a band.[4] These experiments prove that sensory nerves are vital anatomic components of acupoints. Sensory nerves are distributed all over the human body and are absent on only a few structures, such as nails and hair. Thus where there are sensory nerves there will be acupoints.

About 2500 years ago, the *Yellow Emperor's Canon of Internal Medicine* (Huang Di Nei Jing) described about 135 bilateral acupoints. In the next 2000 years, the masters of traditional Chinese medicine (TCM) gradually discovered more and more acupoints and organized them into a meridian system according to Taoist principles.

The Chinese doctors of ancient times noticed that, in addition to meridian acupoints, some nonmeridian acupoints are as effective as classic meridian points. The two types of nonmeridian acupoints are *Ashi* acupoints and *extrameridian* acupoints. Ashi acupoints appear unpredictably in relation to individual symptoms. Extrameridian acupoints are not located on any of the 14 meridians but have fixed locations on the body. Gradually more and more extrameridian acupoints were recorded and incorporated into the classic acupuncture system. The recent Chinese acupuncture literature has recorded more than 2500 "new" acupoints.

In the last three decades, an impressive number of modern studies show that acupuncture efficacy does not always depend on the precise location of acupoints as indicated on meridian charts.[5] Scientific data suggest that there is no statistical significance between needling either "sham" or "true" acupoints in treating patients with chronic pain.[6] Well-known clinician Dr. Felix Mann, after many years of observation, has concluded that acupoints, in the classic understanding, do not exist at all.[7]

From a neuroanatomic point of view, acupoints can be defined by combining the classic concepts with the results of modern research.

Tender acupoints appear on the bodies of both healthy persons and pain patients alike. Let us look at a healthy person first. Dr. H.C. Dung discovered that tender acupoints appear in a generally consistent and predictable pattern. Dr. Dung provided an anatomic explanation for why acupoints appear in such a predictable pattern (see Chapter 2). This discovery is regarded as "a turning point in acupuncture's long history."[8]

When we examine patients who have similar pain symptoms, certain tender or painful points share the same anatomic location in these patients, even though each patient may carry some different tender acupoints that reflect his or her personal symptoms. For example, almost all patients with low back pain have similar tender points located at the iliac crest and 2 inches lateral to the spinous process of the second lumbar vertebra (refer to acupoints H14 and H15 on the figure in the inside cover). The area (size) of each tender acupoint changes dynamically. In the patient with acute pain, the tender acupoints are smaller and fit into the locations defined by the classic acupoint chart, whereas in a patient with severe or chronic pain, the tender areas are significantly increased and the whole muscle mass may become tender and painful, showing that the size of acupoints will grow depending on the chronicity of the pain symptoms. Acupoints are *pathophysiologically dynamic structures*.

BASIC NEUROANATOMY FOR DEFINING ACUPOINTS

Anatomically the human nervous system consists of two subdivisions: *the central nervous system* (CNS) and the PNS. This book focuses on the PNS because it is the most important structure affecting both diagnosis and treatment in acupuncture therapy.

Functionally the nervous system is divided into two systems: the *somatic nervous system* (SNS) and the *autonomic (visceral) nervous system* (ANS). The SNS controls the muscles and carries information to the brain; the ANS operates without conscious control as the caretaker of the body. For example, the ANS controls heartbeat and respiration without our consciousness.

Neurons, or nerve cells, are the basic morphologic and functional units of the nervous system. Here we discuss these complicated structures only in relation to acupuncture medicine.

Neuron (Nerve Cell)

A neuron, or nerve cell, is the anatomic and physiologic unit of the nervous system. Neurons vary in size, shape, and complexity (Figure 1-1). All neurons share common structural and functional features. Typically a neuron has one or more processes, called *dendrites,* radiating from the cell body. The endings of the dendrites are called *receptors*.

The dendrite receptors are morphologically specialized for particular function. The neuron is a dynamically polarized cell that serves as the major signaling unit of the nervous system.

Acupuncture needles directly stimulate and activate the dendrite receptors of the sensory neurons in the skin, muscles, and other soft tissues. Figure 1-2 shows some of the sensory nerve endings (receptors), such as free nerve endings and encapsulated nerve endings.

Another *single* process, called an *axon*, extends from the cell body (see Figure 1-1). An axon of a sensory neuron sends the impulses from the cell body to the next neuron, or an axon of a motoneuron brings the impulses to the muscles. Stimulation of the receptors by acupuncture needling generates electrical signals, which travel from receptors along the dendrites to the cell body and then to the axon. Stimulation below the threshold will not generate incoming signals to the brain. When stimulation to the receptors is strong enough, it will initiate in the cell body a transient electrical signal called an *action potential,* which will propagate from the cell body along the axon to the axon terminal. The axon terminal passes the signals to the dendrites or cell body or axon of another neuron through a special structure called a *synapse*. Thus signals generated by receptors are transmitted from one neuron to another neuron and finally reach the brain (Figure 1-3).

Within the brain, the signals are processed, either suppressed or strengthened, and may continue to travel to different neurons.

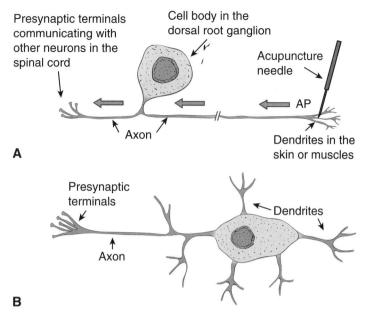

Figure 1-1   Diagram of two types of neurons. The common structure of all the neurons are dendrites, a cell body, and an axon. When dendrites are stimulated, the electrical impulses always travel unidirectionally from dendrites to presynaptic terminals. **A,** The typical form of a sensory nerve. The action potentials (AP) generated by stimulation or disturbance are conducted from dendrites in the skin and muscle to the spinal cord. The action potentials usually bypass the cell body. When the intervertebral disk is herniated and presses the dorsal root ganglion, the cell bodies of the sensory neurons also generate impulses that cause pain. **B,** The most prevalent form of neurons in the spinal cord and brain. Extensive branching of the dendrites emanates from the cell body and an axon emerges from the opposite end of the dendrites.

The Central Nervous System

A neuron is a major functional unit in the nervous system. The CNS consists of the brain and the spinal cord. Electrophysiologic[9] and neurochemical research shows that both the brain and the spinal cord actively react to acupuncture stimulation. Today, after more than three decades of research, we know more about the involvement of the CNS in acupuncture therapy, but the exact mechanism of this correlation is still unclear. We briefly discuss this mechanism in Chapters 3 and 4.

The Peripheral Nervous System

The importance of PNS in clinical acupuncture cannot be overstated. The PNS is an extension of the CNS. Acupuncture needles directly stimulate and activate the PNS to achieve the desirable therapeutic results because all the nervous structures outside the brain and the spinal cord belong to PNS. The PNS is complex, and we discuss only the parts of PNS that are directly related to clinical acupuncture.

The PNS consists of the cranial nerves from the brain and the spinal nerves from the spinal cord, a total of 12 pairs of cranial nerves and 33 pairs of spinal nerves. Traditionally Roman numerals are used to designate the cranial nerves. Among them, the *trigeminal nerve* (V), *facial nerve* (VII), and *spinal accessory nerve* (XI) are the most important in acupuncture therapy (Figure 1-4).

According to their location in relation to the spinal cord, the 33 pairs of spinal nerves are categorized into five groups: 8 cervical, 12 thoracic, 5 lumbar, 5 sacral, and 3 coccygeal. The coccygeal nerves are less important in acupuncture because of their relatively small size, although severe pain in the coccyx or tailbone may occur and will need to be attended (Figure 1-5).

The PNS also contains *ganglions,* which are groups of nerve cells outside the spinal cord. The

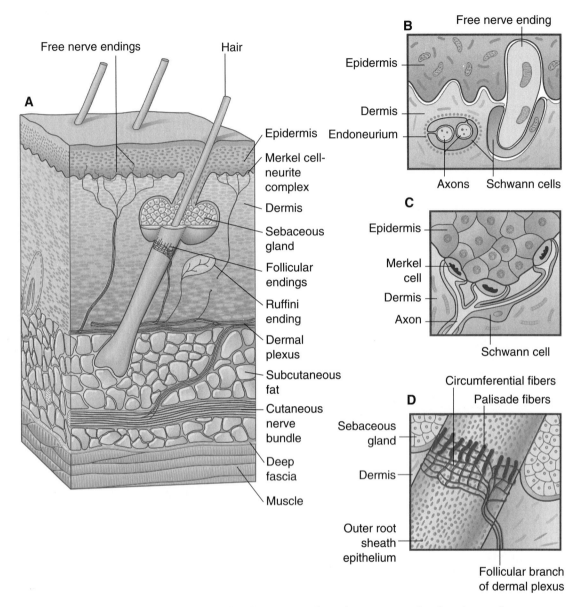

Figure 1-2   Examples of specialized sensory endings that innervate the skin: free ending (most for pain and temperature), Ruffini endings (shearing stress), follicular endings (when the hairs are being bent). (From FitzGerald M, Folan-Curran J: *Clinical neuroanatomy and related neuroscience,* ed 4, Philadelphia, 2002, WB Saunders.)

nerve fibers of the PNS are distributed to all areas of our body except the nails or hair, which is why nails and hair can be cut without pain.

Functionally the PNS comprises *sensory neurons, motor neurons,* and *sympathetic ganglion neurons.* Whenever we insert needles into the body, the needles will stimulate sensory nerve endings, which cover the body; sympathetic nerves, which control the blood vessels and glands; and motoneu-

rons if the needled location is innervated by the motoneuron fibers.

Somatic Nervous System

We classify the nervous system into the CNS and the PNS according to anatomic structure. Functionally we divide the nervous system into two groups: the SNS and the ANS. The SNS is the part

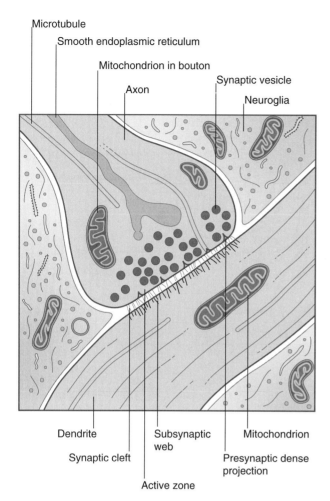

Microtubule

Smooth endoplasmic reticulum

Mitochondrion in bouton

Axon

Synaptic vesicle

Neuroglia

Dendrite

Synaptic cleft

Subsynaptic web

Active zone

Mitochondrion

Presynaptic dense projection

Figure 1-3   An ultrastructural diagram of an axon synapsing with a dendrite of another neuron. The synaptic vesicles contain the chemicals that will activate or deactivate the dendrite of another neuron. (From FitzGerald M, Folan-Curran J: *Clinical neuroanatomy and related neuroscience,* ed 4, Philadelphia, 2002, WB Saunders.)

of the nervous system that innervates the structures of the body wall: *muscles, skin, and mucous membranes.* The part of the nervous system that controls visceral organs is referred to as the ANS. From the viewpoint of acupuncture therapy, the SNS is similar to parts of the PNS.

Autonomic (Visceral) Nervous System

The ANS consists of portions of the CNS and PNS. It controls the physiologic activities of cardiac muscles, the smooth muscles in viscera (such as in the blood vessels), and the glands. The ANS also transmits sensory information from the previously mentioned target organs to the brain. The ANS includes efferent pathways (motor), afferent pathways (sensory), and groups of neurons (nuclei) in the brain and spinal cord that regulate the target organs.

Anatomically the efferent components, the outflow pathway of the ANS, are characterized by a two-neuron chain (Figure 1-6). The first neurons, or the primary neurons, are located in the CNS in the brainstem nuclei (groups of neurons in the brain are called nuclei) or in the lateral gray column of the spinal cord.

The primary neurons are named *preganglionic neurons.* The preganglionic neurons send their axons out to synapse with the *secondary* neurons. Secondary neurons are located in one of the autonomic ganglions outside the spinal cord. The secondary neurons are named *postganglionic neurons.* The axons of postganglionic neurons, named *postganglionic fibers,* travel to the target organs, such as glands in the skin, blood vessels, and organs.

Functionally the ANS is further subdivided into two divisions: *sympathetic* and *parasympathetic.*

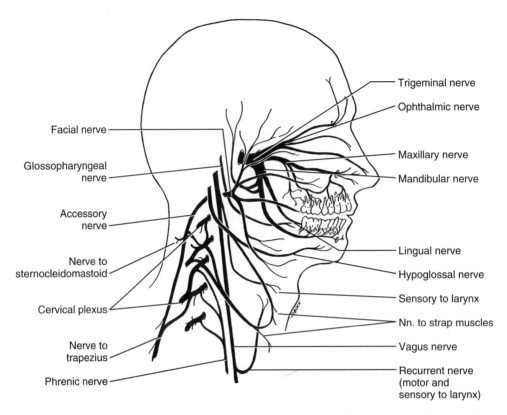

Figure 1-4   The cranial nerves accessible by acupuncture needling in the head and neck: trigeminal nerve (V, three branches: ophthalmic, maxillary, and mandibular), facial nerve (VII), and accessory nerve (XI). Also note that, activated by acupuncture stimulation, the vagus nerve plays a very important role in restoring homeostasis and antiinflammatory immune reaction (see Chapter 4 for further explanation). (From Jenkins D: *Hollinshead's functional anatomy of the limbs and back,* ed 8, Philadelphia, 2002, WB Saunders.)

The sympathetic (thoracolumbar) division (Figure 1-7) originates from neurons (*preganglionic* neurons) in the spinal cord (C8-L2).

The parasympathetic (craniosacral) division (Figure 1-8) comprises preganglionic neurons in the gray matter of the brainstem and of the middle three segments of the sacral cord (S2-4).

Sympathetic and parasympathetic nervous systems are functionally opposite to each other in the same way as the yang (active) and the yin (passive) pair in Taoist concept. The functional goal of a two-part nervous system is to balance the visceral activities.

The sympathetic system helps to maintain a constant internal body environment. To perform this function adequately, the sympathetic system is responsible for increasing adrenaline and blood sugar levels, regulating body temperature, and maintaining the contractibility of blood vessels

(vasomotor tone). Such activities are needed for surviving in life-threatening situations.

This protective or survival mechanism, which results in hyperactivity of the sympathetic nervous system, is an energy-consuming process. Sometimes the sympathetic nervous system is able to inhibit pain sensation. It is well known that some soldiers do not feel pain for hours after being injured in the battlefield. In our daily lives, if hyperactivity of the sympathetic system persists too long, we become exhausted because of consuming stored energy; our immune system becomes suppressed; we are more likely to get sick; and finally our constant body environment, *homeostasis,* starts to decline. In this event the body becomes excessively sensitive to pain (hyperalgesia).

When the sympathetic nervous system calms during rest and a period of tranquility, the parasympathetic system becomes active. The decreasing

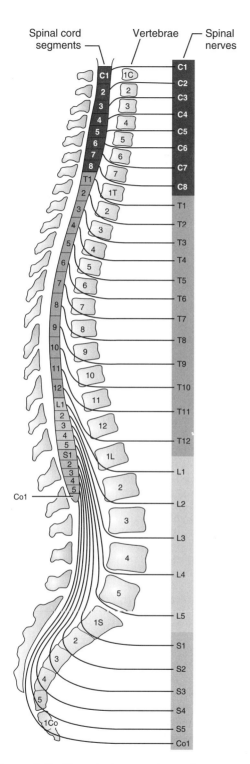

Spinal cord segments — Vertebrae — Spinal nerves

Figure 1-5 The spinal nerves that make up most of the peripheral nerves of the body. (From Jenkins D: *Hollinshead's functional anatomy of the limbs and back,* ed 8, Philadelphia, 2002, WB Saunders.)

hyperactivity of the sympathetic system ensures, for example, such functions as proper food digestion, which helps to absorb and supply energy flow to the body systems.

Clinical evidence shows that acupuncture stimulation normalizes the activities of the sympathetic and parasympathetic systems to restore optimal homeostasis, which means that acupuncture stimulation calms the sympathetic activities and activates parasympathetic functions.

Nerves and Nerve Fibers

Input signals from a peripheral nerve, carried by the dendrites of neurons, reach the cell bodies located in the ganglions, in the spinal cord, or in the brain. The processed output signals come out along the axons from the cell bodies and reach the peripheral organs, such as skin, muscles, glands, and viscera.

A nerve, also called a *nerve fiber,* may contain many dendrites and axons. The dendrites and axons existing in the same nerve fiber may convey different input or output in the form of electrical or chemical signals. A nerve or nerve fiber may carry thousands of axons and dendrites or carry just one axon or dendrite.

Different signals can travel in different directions in the same nerve. To ensure that the delivery of the functional signaling reaches the exact address, something must function like an insulating tube to cover a dendrite or axon to protect the signals. Schwann cells provide this insulating layer, called a *myelin sheath* (Figure 1-9).

As noted, all peripheral nerves are functionally categorized as either *efferent nerves* or *afferent nerves*. An efferent nerve (motor fiber) contains only axons and carries the signals from the CNS to the peripheral target organ. An afferent nerve (sensory fiber) is formed by the dendrites and carries signals to the CNS. The afferent nerve is also called a *sensory nerve*. A nerve is called a *mixed nerve* when it contains both afferent (sensory) and efferent (motor) fibers.

Efferent (Motor) Nerves Efferent nerves innervate muscles and glands and are involved in motor functions such as the contraction of muscles or the secretion of glands.

The three types of muscles are skeletal, smooth, and cardiac. In the face and head, the efferent fibers arise from the brain and innervate the muscles of mastication and the muscles of facial expression by the trigeminal nerve (V) and the facial nerve (VII), respectively. The skeletal

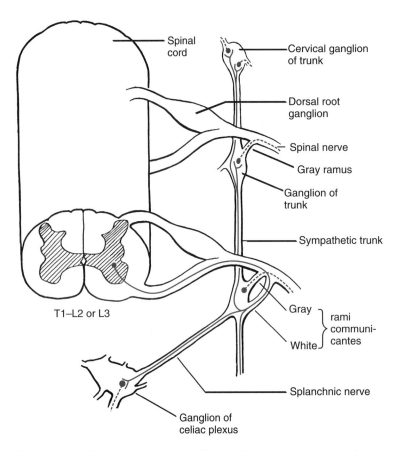

Figure 1-6   Course of sympathetic fibers. The segment shown at the cross-section of the cord is representative of the sympathetic outflow from T1 to L2 or L3. A single preganglionic fiber (solid line) is used to illustrate the possible courses that preganglionic fibers can take. They travel through the ventral root of a spinal nerve and leave the nerve to reach the sympathetic trunk. At the trunk they have one of several courses: they may synapse with the ganglion cells in the first ganglion they reach; they may run up or down the trunk to synapse in ganglia above or below the level at which they enter the trunk; or they may leave the trunk without synapsing, to end in ganglia of the celiac or other ganglia around the aorta. Postganglionic fibers (broken line) arise from cells of the trunk ganglia and return to the spinal nerves to be distributed with them, arise from the ganglia of the celiac and related plexuses to be distributed along the blood vessels to the viscera, or leave as a direct branch of a cervical ganglion to structures in the head and neck. (The association of the cervical ganglia to spinal nerves is the same as that for other ganglia of the trunk, but it is not illustrated.) Note: There are preganglion fibers that go to the medulla of the suprarenal gland to synapse directly on cells there. (From Jenkins D: *Hollinshead's functional anatomy of the limbs and back,* ed 8, Philadelphia, 2002, WB Saunders.)

muscles situated all over the body are innervated by the efferent fibers. The efferent fibers originate from the motor nerve cells in the anterior horn of the spinal cord. Smooth muscles innervated by autonomic nerve fibers are found in the blood vessels and in all visceral organs. Cardiac muscles are heart muscles that are innervated by autonomic nerve fibers. It is important to understand how the three types of muscles function during an acupuncture treatment.

Acupuncture needles directly stimulate and relax the skeletal muscles by creating tiny lesions in the muscles. The lesions created by needling stimulate the spinal cord and the brain to secrete neurobiochemicals such as endorphins, which relax the smooth muscles, cardiac muscles, and skeletal muscles. Activating this mechanism by acupuncture treatments provides temporary relief from tension of the blood vessels (such as in high blood pressure) and the smooth muscles (such as in asthma).

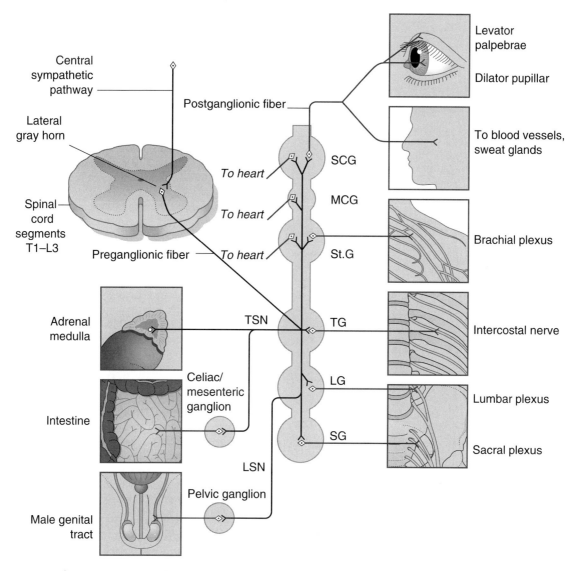

Figure 1-7 General plan of the sympathetic system. Preganglionic neurons are located in the lateral gray horn of the spinal cord. Ganglionic neurons are shown in gray. *LG,* Lumbar ganglia; *LSN,* lumbar splanchnic nerve; *MCG,* middle cervical ganglion; *SCG,* superior cervical ganglion; *SG,* sacral ganglia; *St.G,* stellate ganglion; *TG,* thoracic ganglia; *TSN,* thoracic splanchnic nerve. (From FitzGerald M, Folan-Curran J: *Clinical neuroanatomy and related neuroscience,* ed 4, Philadelphia, 2002, WB Saunders.)

Afferent Fibers and Sensory Receptors

Afferent fibers transmit the information of sensation by receptors from every part of the body to the CNS. With certain stimulation such as mechanical (piercing), chemical (acid), or physical (pressure), sensations can be generated anywhere along the afferent fibers. In acupuncture therapy this means that we may stimulate the end branch of the nerve or the middle of the nerve trunk to create input signals.

The specialized ending structure of the afferent fibers that produces sensations is called the *sensory receptor*. Different sensory receptors generate the same electrical signals, but these signals may induce different sensations in the brain, such as pain or heat.

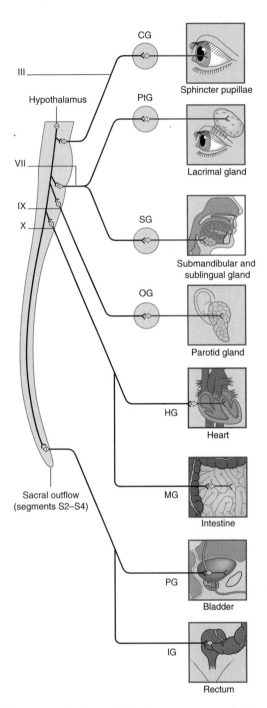

Figure 1-8   General plan of the parasympathetic system. Preganglionic neurons are located inside the brainstem and sacral segment of the spinal cord. *CG,* Ciliary ganglion; *HG,* heart ganglia; *IG,* intramural ganglia; *MG,* myenteric ganglia; *OG,* otic ganglion; *PtG,* pterygopalatine ganglion; *SG,* submandibular ganglion. (From FitzGerald M, Folan-Curran J: *Clinical neuroanatomy and related neuroscience,* ed 4, Philadelphia, 2002, WB Saunders.)

Physiologically the four types of sensations are superficial, deep, visceral, and special. *Superficial* sensation is pain, touch, temperature, and two-point discrimination (i.e., the shortest distance between two stimuli our brain can recognize as two points). *Deep* sensation is related to deep muscle pain, muscle and joint position sense (proprioception), and vibration sense. *Visceral* sensations are relayed by autonomic afferent fibers, including visceral pain, hunger, and nausea. *Special* sensations are smell, vision, hearing, taste, and equilibrium, which are transmitted by certain cranial nerves.

We also refer to the superficial, deep, and visceral sensations as the *general sensations,* in contrast to the *special sensations.* During an acupuncture treatment, needles can directly stimulate sensory receptors associated with superficial and deep sensations to achieve therapeutic results. Clinical observation shows that needling also indirectly helps visceral sensations such as visceral pain and nausea. Acupuncture has an indirect effect on disorders of special senses, such as taste, vision, and smell; some patients feel that their vision and hearing problems are improved after acupuncture treatments.

Please note that a nerve fiber can only be either *efferent* or *afferent.* A *somatic* efferent fiber supplies the skeletal muscle; an *autonomic* efferent fiber innervates smooth and cardiac muscles and glands. The three nerve fibers of most concern in clinical acupuncture are the efferent fibers to the skeletal muscles, the postganglionic sympathetic or parasympathetic nerve fibers, and the afferent fibers for the general senses.

The Nerve Bundles

Acupuncture needles stimulate nerve fiber receptors, generating sensations such as tenderness, soreness, heaviness, and sometimes pain. All these receptors are associated with nerve bundles or nerve trunks. A nerve bundle or trunk is a congregation of nerve fibers. Some nerve trunks are so fine that they are invisible to the naked eye, whereas others are thicker and distinctly identifiable, such as the sciatic nerve.

Acupuncture needling concerns two types of nerve trunks: muscular nerves and cutaneous (skin) nerves. A muscular nerve innervates skeletal muscles and consists of three types of fibers:

1. Afferent fiber, which brings the general senses to the spinal cord or the brain
2. Efferent fiber from the spinal cord or the brain to the skeletal muscles

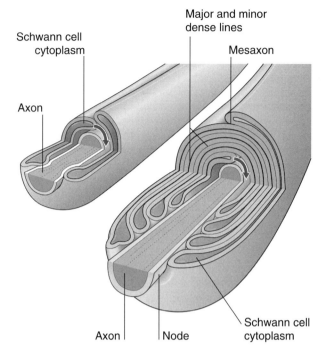

Figure 1-9   Schwann cell and myelination in peripheral nervous system. (From FitzGerald M, Folan-Curran J: *Clinical neuroanatomy and related neuroscience,* ed 4, Philadelphia, 2002, WB Saunders.)

3. Postganglionic sympathetic fibers from sympathetic ganglia that control blood vessels

A cutaneous nerve is distributed to the skin and carries afferent fibers for the general senses and postganglionic fibers for the glands (such as sweat glands) or the blood vessels in the skin.

The skin contains no skeletal muscles. Note that acupuncture needles always stimulate either cutaneous or muscular nerves. To understand the degree of therapeutic effects of needling during acupuncture treatments, it is important to pay attention to the nerve fiber components stimulated by needling.

Some nerve fibers are thicker because they are wrapped with a thick myelin sheath. Some nerve fibers are thinner because they are wrapped with a thin myelin sheath. The finest nerve fibers are not covered by any myelin sheath and are called *unmyelinated nerve fibers.*

Note that the electrical signals travel faster along thicker nerve fibers. The skin is innervated with three types of sensory fibers: A beta, A delta, and C fibers. A beta fibers are sensitive to gentle pressure and vibration, the thinner A delta fibers are sensitive to heavy pressure and temperature, and the very thin and unmyelinated C fibers are responsive to pressure, chemicals, and temperature. When needles are inserted into the skin or muscle tissue, they stimulate the two finest fibers: A delta

fibers and C fibers. A small electrical stimulus, such as that used in transcutaneous electrical nerve stimulation (TENS), preferentially excites the large A beta fibers. The physiology of these fibers is summarized in Table 1-1.

Our clinical experience shows that when needle stimulation is applied, different tissues may generate different sensations. For example, the sensation of numbness is generated mostly by the nerve trunks; the sensation of soreness is generated by the bone membrane (periosteum); soreness and the feeling of distention are generated by muscles; and the sensation of sharp pain is generated by pierced small blood vessels. Clinically it is advisable to relocate the needle slightly when a patient feels sharp, burning, or stinging pain.

C fibers have free endings that are not covered by the myelin sheath. These free endings are specifically sensitive to tissue-threatening *(noxious)* stimuli such as heavy pressure, intense heat, and strong chemicals. C fibers are called *polymodal nociceptors* in pain management. Acupuncture needling mostly stimulates C fibers by producing in the tissues a tiny lesion, which may last 2 to 5 days.

Anatomic Configuration of Acupoints

At present the exact anatomic identity of acupoints has not been clearly established. After

Table 1-1
Nerve Fibers Stimulated by Acupuncture Needling

Fiber Type	Diameter (m)	Velocity (m/s)	Function	Needling Sensation
A gamma	3-6	15-30	In muscle spindles	Numbness
A delta	2-5	12-30	Pinprick sensation, cold, pressure	Aching, distention, heaviness
C	0.4-1.2	0.5-2	Pain, itch, heat, heavy pressure	Soreness

careful clinical observation and meticulous laboratory research, Dr. H.C. Dung suggested 10 anatomic features associated with acupoints.[10] Each acupoint may contain one or more of these features.

The numeric sequence of these anatomic features is important because it is not random and is based on the anatomic features of the acupoints. To understand this subject better, the neuroanatomically defined acupoints are compared with classic meridian acupoints whenever possible.

TEN BASIC ANATOMIC FEATURES OF ACUPOINTS

1. Size of the Nerve Trunk

Acupoints are always associated with either cutaneous nerves or muscular nerves. The acupoints associated with a larger nerve trunk are more likely to become tender than those associated with a smaller nerve trunk. As stated previously the electrical signals travel faster along thicker nerve fibers. For example, in headache patients, the infraorbital nerve acupoint (H19, trigeminal V2) invariably becomes tender first and the supraorbital nerve point (H23, trigeminal V1) becomes tender later. The fact that the infraorbital nerve is larger than the supraorbital nerve explains this sensitization order of the two acupoints.

Clinically when we palpate these two acupoints, if only one acupoint is tender on a headache patient, it is usually the infraorbital nerve acupoint (H19) and it may indicate that in this case the headache is not difficult to treat. If the headache persists, the second acupoint, the supraorbital nerve acupoint (H23), becomes tender. The presence of two tender points often suggests a longer history of headache and the need for more treatments compared with a patient with only one tender point. If the third trigeminal nerve, which passes through the mental foramen on the lower jaw (trigeminal V3), also appears to be tender, the headache is a difficult case because of the exten-

sively sensitized trigeminal nerve in all three branches. When other anatomic determinants are involved, however, nerve size may not be the only factor that dictates the pathophysiologic dynamics of the acupoints.

2. Depth of the Nerve

More acupoints are formed along superficial nerve trunks than along deeper ones. The superficial nerve receptors become sensitized more easily than do the nerves located deep in tissue. For example, the sciatic nerve is the largest nerve trunk in the human body, but only a few acupoints are attributable to this nerve in the gluteal and thigh region because in this region the nerve lies deeply beneath the thick gluteal and hamstring muscles. As the sciatic nerve enters the posterior compartment of the thigh and popliteal fossa and reaches the leg, it emerges superficially and gives out branches. In this region more acupoints are found along the nerve's branches in the leg. The same principle is applicable to other nerve trunks.

The upper extremity has the same pattern of acupuncture formation as the lower extremity. Nerve trunks in the upper limbs are located either deep beneath the muscles or inside the neurovascular compartment. As a result only a few acupoints are formed in the upper arm. On their way to the forearm, nerve trunks emerge closer to the surface, and therefore more acupoints appear in this region. This is why more acupoints form below the elbows and knees.

The following is an example of how acupoint formation is affected by the depth of a nerve. The deep radial nerve is derived from the brachial plexus and courses through the upper arm without forming any important acupoints. When the deep radial nerve emerges from the deep fascia to the superficial fascia in the forearm, it forms an important acupoint in the body (H1, deep radial nerve).

The superficial acupoints become tender more often than do the deeply located acupoints because of the abundant assemblage of sensory receptors around the location where the acupoints are formed. An interesting neurologic fact is that the limbs below the elbows and knees occupy larger areas in the sensory gyrus in the brain. Therefore the acupoints below the elbows and knees also occupy a larger area in the cortical representation in the postcentral sensory gyrus in the brain. This may explain why the acupoints below the elbows and knees contain more sensory receptors and why needling stimulation to these points may induce a greater reaction and activity in the brain. This principle clearly supports the concept of using certain acupoints below the elbows and knees (the so-called five-Shu points in the classic meridian system) as diagnostic and treatment points during acupuncture treatment.

3. Penetration of Deep Fascia

The term *fascia* is rather loosely applied in anatomy. Most fascias are connective tissue layers, and they are arranged in sheets or tubes between or around anatomic structures. *Superficial* fascia is a padding connected with dermis located above the fascia. *Deep* fascia lies deep under the superficial fascia and often forms the outer connective layer or covering of the structures underneath, such as blood vessels, nerves, or muscles. Acupuncture points are formed at the locations where a nerve trunk penetrates the deep fascia and emerges close to the surface.

4. Passage Through Bone Foramina

Acupoints are found at the bone foramina, where nerve trunks emerge to distribute cutaneously. The cutaneous branches of the trigeminal nerves (V) give rise to such acupoints at the foramina as the infraorbital (H19, V2), the supraorbital (H23, V1), and the mental (V3) nerves (see Figure 5-2, p. 58).

5. Neuromuscular Attachments

Acupoints are formed at the loci where the nerve trunks enter the muscle. Muscular nerve trunks contain afferent (sensory) fibers, efferent (motor) fibers, and sympathetic fibers. Two acupoints formed this way can be found at the centers of supraspinous and infraspinous fossae, where the suprascapular nerve enters supraspinatus and infraspinatus muscles.

The preceding example one nerve forms two attachments with two muscles, but the infraspina-

tus attachment is more superficial because the muscle is thinner; so this locus (H8, infraspinatus) usually becomes tender before the supraspinatus point as the latter lies deeper below the round, thick supraspinatus muscle.

Theoretically each muscle has at least one neuromuscular attachment; however, most similar attachments do not form acupoints because the attachments are located deep in the muscle masses and do not often become sensitive.

6. Concomitant Blood Vessels

Concomitant arteries and veins course along the nerve trunks to form neurovascular bundles to reach the muscle attachments. Acupoints associated with neurovascular bundles tend to become tender more readily than do acupoints associated with only cutaneous nerves because the cutaneous nerves are not accompanied by concomitant blood vessels.

The deep radial nerve is a good example of how an acupoint is formed by concomitant blood vessels and nerves. At the lateral surface of the proximal portion of the forearm, the deep radial nerve is buried inside the intermuscular septum between the muscles of the brachioradialis and the extensor carpi radialis longus. Both nerves, the deep radial and the lateral antebrachial cutaneous nerves, are located in similar depth and have similar size except the deep radial nerves are associated with rich concomitant blood vessels. The acupoint H1 deep radial appearing in this location always becomes tender before the acupoint H9 lateral antebrachial cutaneous associated with lateral antebrachial cutaneous nerve. (Refer to the figure in the inside cover.)

The physiologic role of blood vessels in forming acupoints is unknown. Presumably more sensory receptors are formed where the nerve innervates the smooth muscles of the blood vessel.

7. Nerve Fiber Composition

As noted a cutaneous nerve contains only afferent (sensory) and postganglionic sympathetic fibers, whereas a muscular nerve contains these two types of fibers as well as efferent (motor) fibers to the skeletal muscles. Thus the cutaneous and muscular nerves differ in their nerve fiber composition. When all other anatomic features are similar, acupoints associated with nerve trunks containing more nerve fibers are more likely to become tender.

The afferent (sensory) fibers provide sensory receptors attached to the blood vessels, muscle fibers, muscle spindles, muscle tendons, and skin.

The sensory fibers collect sensory information from all these structures.

The efferent (motor) fibers innervate skeletal muscles. The postganglionic sympathetic fibers innervate glands in the skin and internal organs. The motor fibers activate the muscle contraction, whereas the sympathetic fibers control the activities of the glands and internal organs.

8. Bifurcation Points

Acupoints are found at locations where a large nerve trunk branches into two or more smaller branches. For example, acupoints are found in the distal portion of four limbs, particularly in the dorsal surfaces of the hand and foot (Figure 1-10).

9. Sensitive Ligamentous Structures

Sensitive loci can become acupoints. Sensitive ligamentous structures include ligaments, muscle tendons, bone retinacula, thick fascial sheets, joint capsules, and collateral ligaments. They are all formed by dense fibrous connective tissue and are sensitive to pressure, palpation, or stretching because of rich afferent nerve receptors in the tissues. For example, a number of tender or even painful points can be found on the collateral ligaments when the knee hurts.

10. Suture Lines of the Skull

Acupoints are formed along the suture lines of the skull. The acupoints can be palpated along the coronal suture, sagittal suture, and lambdoidal suture (see Figure 5-2, p. 58). Such acupoints appear at the nasion, fontanelle, bregma, pterion, and so on. When chronic headache is not adequately treated, eventually tender points will appear at these locations.

SUMMARY

The basic 10 neuroanatomic features of acupoints provide a solid foundation for understanding the nature of acupoint structural formation, their pathophysiologic dynamics, and their clinical meaning in evaluation and point selection during treatment procedures using our Integrative Neuromuscular Acupoint System (INMAS) (see Chapter 5).

Other structures could also contribute to the formation of acupoints. Japanese researchers, for example, suggested a close association of some acupoints with lymphatic channels.[11]

Each acupoint can have one or more of the 10 basic anatomic features. As discussed previously the 10 anatomic features are set forth in numeric order based on the anatomic features of the acupoints. Acupoints with an anatomic feature having

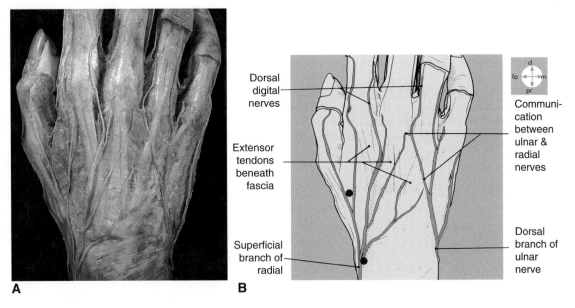

A   **B**

Figure 1-10   Acupoints are formed at the locations where a nerve trunk divides into smaller branches. (Modified From Gosling J, et al: *Human anatomy: color atlas and text,* ed 4, St Louis, 2002, Mosby.)

a lower number in the order (such as feature 1, the size of the nerve trunk) usually become tender earlier than do acupoints with an anatomic feature having a higher number in the order (such as feature 10, suture lines of the skull).

Thus deep radial nerve acupoint (H1 deep radial, with feature 1) on the forearm always becomes tender before the superficial radial nerve point does (H12, superficial radial, with feature 8) on the hand. The former will be selected first because it provides more therapeutic signals.

The preceding pathophysiologic and clinical phenomena play important roles in our INMAS for pain management and serve as a foundation for our quantitative evaluation and prognostic prediction method described in Chapter 6.

The basic 10 features of acupoints provide the following:

1. The possibility to measure objectively a patient's pain on a quantitative basis
2. Reliable information for evaluating the healing potential or homeostatic status of a patient
3. Prediction of prognosis during acupuncture therapy treatments

All tender acupoints, no matter where they appear, are invariably formed in association with sensory nerves. Sensory nerves are extensively distributed in the structures of the soft tissues like skin, muscles, ligaments, joint capsules, fascias, blood vessels, and bones.

The tenderness of acupoints arises from pathological conditions affecting either peripheral or central nerve fibers. Peripherally the sensory nerve fibers could be sensitized by the chemicals leaked from the damaged tissues to form the tender points. Centrally the neurons in the spinal cord can become sensitized by lasting stimulation of nerve impulses from peripheral receptors, such as in the case of chronic pain or cumulative trauma disorders (repetitive use of the same muscles).[12]

It is important to note that chronic pain is not prolonged acute pain because the pain mechanisms involved are different. Acute pain is the warning signal of tissue injury, which is locally restricted; chronic pain itself is a disease that sensitizes both the tissues of peripheral structures and neurons of the spinal cord.

Some tender points may indicate local damage in the affected area at the same time that local damage could produce distant pain by the mechanism of referred pain. An example of referred pain in the case of angina pectoris is the tenderness of acupoints palpated on the medial side of the left arm, on the upper back, or on the lower jaw.

Tender points may represent any type or types of damage of the tissue innervated by sensory nerves. For example, five or six tender acupoints in the lumbar area and lower limbs (H15, H14, H22, H16, H18, and H10) are usually presented in the case of lower back pain syndrome (refer to the figure in the inside cover), but the cause of the tenderness could be related to many different factors: nerve damage; infection or inflammation of the dura of the nerve roots; muscle contraction, mostly of large muscles such as the erector spinae muscles, although sometimes small muscles are involved; pathological problems with fascias, joint capsules, or ligaments; herniated disks; bone fracture; arthritis; infections; tumors; emotional disorders; and mechanical abnormalities between vertebrae.

From a neuroanatomic perspective the features of acupoints could be summarized in the following way:

1. Acupoints exist in collaboration with sensory nerves or tissues innervated by sensory nerves. Sensory nerve fibers are extensively distributed over the body, except to the nails and hair. Where there are sensory nerve fibers, there are acupoints.
2. The anatomic structure of acupoints varies according to their location on the body, but all acupoints have sensory nerve receptors as their common structural elements.
3. The neuroanatomic configuration of acupoints determines the pathophysiologic dynamics; thus some acupoints are more likely to become sensitized than others.
4. Acupoints are not discrete, static points but are dynamically changing structures. Under certain pathophysiologic conditions, they will appear tender and the size of the tender area may grow. Some points remain tender, whereas some become less tender or not tender at all after healing is completed.
5. The tenderness of acupoints may indicate injuries to peripheral tissues, such as nerves, muscles, ligaments, joint capsules, and bones; or it may indicate that the sensitized neurons in the CNS provoked peripheral tenderness.

The pathophysiologic quality of each acupoint (the sensitivity and size of tenderness) and the clinical quantity of acupoints (the total number of tender acupoints in a person) provide indispensable information for our quantitative evaluation and prognosis method described in Chapter 6 and serve as a foundation for our Integrative Neuromuscular Acupoint System for pain management, also described in Chapter 6.

References

1. Chan SH: What is being stimulated in acupuncture evaluation of the existence of a specific substrate, *Neurosci Biobehav Rev* 8:25-33, 1984.
2. Melzack R, Stillwell DM, Fox EJ: Trigger points and acupuncture points for pain: correlations and implications, *Pain* 3:3-23, 1977.
3. Mense S, Simons DG: *Muscle pain, understanding the nature, diagnosis, and treatment*, Philadelphia, 2001, Lippincott–Williams & Wilkins.
4. Chiang CY, et al: Peripheral afferent pathway for acupuncture analgesia, *Scientia Sinica* 16:210-217, 1973.
5. Taube HA, et al: Studies of acupuncture for operative dentistry, *J Am Dent Assoc* 95:555-561, 1977.
6. Pomeranz B: Acupuncture analgesia: basic research. In Stux G, Hammerschlag R, editors: *Clinical acupuncture scientific basis*, Berlin, 2001, Springer.
7. Mann F: A new system of acupuncture. In Filshie J, White A, editors: *Medical acupuncture*, Edinburgh, 1998, Churchill Livingstone.
8. Macdonald AJR: Acupuncture's non-segmental analgesic effects: the point of meridians, In Filshie J, White A, editors: *Medical acupuncture*, Edinburgh, 1998, Churchill Livingstone.
9. Ma Y-T, Sluka KA: Reduction in inflammation-induced sensitization of dorsal horn neurons by transcutaneous electrical nerve stimulation in anesthetized rats, *Exp Brain Res* 137:94-102, 2001.
10. Dung HC: Anatomical features contributing to the formation of acupuncture points, *Am J Acupuncture* 12:139, 1984.
11. Iguchi K, Sawai Y: Correlationship between the meridians and acute lymphangitis. In *Proceedings of the 3rd World Conference on Acupuncture*, Kyoto, 1993.
12. Wall P: *Pain: the science of suffering*, New York, 2000, Columbia University Press.

CHAPTER 2

Dynamic Pathophysiology of Acupoints

INTRODUCTION

Acupoints in different parts of the human body have different anatomic characteristics. All acupoints, however, have one element in common: they are able to become sensitive, tender, or even painful when exposed to a pathologic disorder. The process of sensitizing is still a puzzle to scientists and clinicians. Recent research data and clinical observations related to muscle pain[1] help to explain more clearly *some* of the characteristics of acupoints.

It is important to clarify confusion regarding the differences between acupoints and trigger points.

1. The definition of acupoints is *neurogenically* oriented, whereas the definition of trigger points is *myofascially* defined. A trigger point is classically defined as an exquisitely tender spot *in the muscle.*[2] By contrast, an acupoint can form anywhere in the body. In this book a *tender* acupoint is defined as any anatomic structure associated with sensitized sensory nerves. This neurogenic definition suggests that acupoints may appear on any part of the body where there is a sensory nerve. Sensory nerves are distributed all over the body, which means that acupoints may appear anywhere in the body, such as in the muscles, tendons, joints, at bone foramina, and in the suture lines of the skull. About 70% of classic acupoints are also trigger points because muscles constitute a large proportion of the body. Acupuncture therapy and trigger point therapy are different by both definition and clinical practice.
2. Tender acupoints gradually develop when homeostasis declines. These tender acupoints, therefore, are defined as homeostatic acupoints (HAs) in this book. As a rule, homeostatic acupoints develop symmetri-

cally in the human body because the distribution of peripheral nerves is bilaterally symmetrical. By contrast, most trigger points are activated directly by the pain symptoms and are not necessarily symmetrical. Trigger points share some, but not all, characteristics of acupoints, which means that trigger points have some inclusive but not exclusive parameters of acupoints. Acupoints share all the characteristics of trigger points. *Thus not all acupoints are trigger points, but all trigger points are acupoints*. Note that trigger points correspond to symptomatic acupoints in our Integrative Neuromuscular Acupoint System (INMAS).

One of the most important concepts of acupuncture is that acupoints are pathophysiologically dynamic entities. The degree of their sensitivity changes when homeostasis (the yin-yang balance) changes. Most acupoints show practically no sensitivity when the homeostasis is optimal. Acupoints become tender when homeostasis declines or the body is insulted by pathologic factors. Thus the number of tender HAs can be the quantitative indicator of the homeostasis status of the body. The more tender the HAs detected in the body, the more imbalanced the homeostasis is. Once the homeostasis declines, the health deteriorates.

Then the chain reaction follows: the immune function is suppressed, self-healing capability is impaired, and different pathological disorders may be developed. Patients with more tender acupoints in their bodies need more treatments than those with less tender acupoints.

An understanding of acupoint physiology is important for clinical practice because at the practical level such understanding enables a practitioner to perform quantitative acupuncture evaluation to obtain a reliable prognosis of acupuncture treatment, to predict how many treatment sessions will be needed, and to achieve maximal pain relief in more than 90% of pain patients.

DYNAMIC PHASES OF ACUPOINTS

Dr. H.C. Dung described three phases of acupoints: *latent, passive,* and *active.*[3] Generally in healthy people some acupoints are neither sensitive nor tender. These nonsensitive acupoints are referred to as *latent* acupoints.

Under the influence of pathophysiologic disturbances, such as chronic pain or disease, nonsensitive (latent) acupoints are gradually transformed into sensitive or *passive* acupoints. Almost everyone has a number of passive (tender) acupoints, but people are not consciously aware of them until an experienced practitioner palpates these acupoints with a certain amount of pressure, at which acupoint a person may feel tender or sore at the palpated locations. Most acupoints encountered in acupuncture practice are passive acupoints.

As pathologic disturbances continue to insult the body, pain becomes more intense, and finally passive acupoints become active acupoints. Patients feel painful active acupoints without any palpation and are able to show the precise location of these points and areas to their doctors.

Latent acupoints represent normal tissues. Neurologically passive acupoints have a lower mechanical threshold than normal tissues do and start to fire impulses to the spinal cord and brain under normal mechanical pressure. The same amount of pressure will not induce impulses on latent points. *Active* acupoints have the lowest mechanical threshold; they may continuously fire impulses to the brain, even without being submitted to external mechanical pressure, and may finally sensitize the neurons in the spinal cord and brain. As the mechanical threshold decreases, the physical size of a sensitized acupoint increases. The phase transition from latent to passive or from passive to active is a *continuous* process without any clear demarcation; so there is no quantitative measurement for differentiating acupoints of different phases. Table 2-1 provides some criteria, based on our clinical experience, to differentiate the three phases of acupoints. The pressure used to palpate

the acupoints is about 2 or 3 pounds. In the clinic we use the thumb to press the points. The pressure is about 2 or 3 pounds when the thumbnail turns from pinkish to whitish. The pressure used to palpate may need to be adjusted because some patients tolerate less pressure if their acupoints are very sensitive or even painful.

We postulate that because passive and active acupoints have different mechanical or pain thresholds, they have different neurophysiologic characteristics. For example, passive acupoints will increase electrical signals to the brain only on palpation or needling stimulation. Active acupoints, which continuously fire electrical signals to the brain, will reduce electrical signals to the brain on or after needling stimulation. In other words, acupuncture needling increases impulses from passive acupoints but calms signals from active acupoints. This electrophysiologic difference between passive and active acupoints has been confirmed by experimental data in rats (Y.-T. Ma, unpublished data).

We also believe that chronic pain becomes "wired" or "programmed" into the spinal cord and possibly the brain centers to build up "pain memory." This occurs partly because the active acupoints continuously fire impulses to the central nervous system (CNS), thus activating the silent synapses (connections) between the neurons in the CNS to form the "pain circuitry." This "pain memory" could explain the difficulties in treating chronic pain because the practitioner needs to erase the pain memory in the CNS in addition to healing peripheral injuries.

Clinical cases show that there are direct and indirect events that stimulate or activate the transition of acupoints from latent to passive and from passive to active phases. Acute injuries, overuse fatigues, repetitive motions, compression of nerves such as radiculopathy, and joint dysfunctions such as arthritis *directly* turn the local (symptomatic) acupoints tender. Chronic disorders, fever, cold, visceral diseases (such as those of the heart, lung, gallbladder, stomach), and emotional distress *indirectly* sensitize both homeostatic (systemic) and

Table 2-1 Three Pathophysiologic Phases of an Acupoint		
Physiologic Phase	**Physiologic Feature**	**Physical Features (Size)**
Latent	Nonsensitive	Normal tissue
Passive	Sensitive on palpation	Diameter <2 cm
Active	Painful without palpation	Diameter usually >2 cm

symptomatic (local) acupoints. In the latter cases, the tender symptomatic acupoints often appear neurosegmentally related to the disturbed organs, possibly through neural viscerocutaneous reflex.

PHYSICAL PROPERTIES OF ACUPOINTS

Physical properties of acupoints refer to the physical representation of acupoints on the body surface in terms of quality (sensitivity) and quantity (size of each tender acupoint and total number of tender acupoints in the body). Physical properties of acupoints include three parameters: *sensitivity, specificity,* and *sequence.*[3] These physical properties of acupoints indicate the severity or chronicity of pain symptoms.

Sensitivity

Passive acupoints may ache or feel tender, sore, or painful when palpated with adequate pressure (about 2 or 3 pounds at fingertip, as previously discussed). The amount of sensitive intensity is termed *sensitivity.* Some patients describe their reaction on palpation of passive acupoints as "a little bit tender," whereas others cry out with pain. The latter patients clearly feel more pain from the same palpation during examination and their symptoms are either more severe or more chronic. Thus these patients may need more treatments to achieve pain relief than patients with less sensitive acupoints. In other words the amount of sensitivity of an acupoint is proportional to the amount of pain: the more sensitive the acupoint, the more pain the patient feels.

Specificity

Specificity refers to the size and precise location of a passive acupoint. In the beginning of the passive phase, the area or surface size of a tender acupoint is relatively small, about 0.5 cm (1/5 inch) in diameter, and difficult to locate. This means the sensitized acupoint is related only to a limited tissue structure and restricted to a particular anatomic location. This condition is referred to as *higher specificity.* When symptoms become more severe, the sensitivity of the acupoint spreads to surrounding tissues, and consequently the surface size of the acupoint grows. The surface size of the acupoint may grow by up to or even more than 3 to 4 cm (1.5 inches) in diameter, and the acupoint becomes more easily palpable. This condition is referred to as *lower specificity.* Some practitioners[4] found that

careful palpation reveals large, tender regions varying from 16 to 200 cm^2 (about 1.5 to 5 inches in diameter) surrounding a tender point.

It is more difficult to locate a smaller, less sensitive acupoint than a larger, more sensitive acupoint. Therefore the smaller acupoint is defined as being more specific. An acupoint is more specific when it is limited to a small area and less specific when it is larger and covers a broader area. Specificity is inversely proportional to sensitivity: specificity decreases when sensitivity increases and vice versa.

Sequence

Acupoints appear in the human body according to two models: *systemic* or *symptomatic.*[3] A physically healthy person always has from a few to about 20 passive acupoints in the body. More passive acupoints will appear symmetrically *all over the body* when the healthy person gradually develops chronic problems, such as chronic diseases, and degenerative problems related to age, poor diet, bad posture, lack of exercise, or persisting physical or emotional stress. This phenomenon is referred to as the *systemic model* of acupoint formation, which indicates that passive acupoints appear all over the body systemically when homeostasis declines. Most important, in the systemic model all passive acupoints are formed in predictable locations and in a predictable sequence. The predictable sequence shows which acupoint becomes sensitive first and which acupoint will be sensitized next. This predictability in all people, healthy or sick, provides a quantitative basis for evaluation of a patient's health status and allows the development of a standardized treatment protocol for acupuncture therapy aimed to restore homeostasis (see Chapter 6). We call these predictable acupoints *homeostatic acupoints* because they are related to homeostatic decline. Once homeostasis is restored, some HAs are gradually desensitized and eventually the tenderness disappears.

If a healthy person sustains an acute injury, such as in vehicular accidents or sports-related injury, or is afflicted with an acute disease, such as a cold or muscle sprain, tender points will appear around the injured area or in related skin or muscle segments. These local tender points are termed *symptomatic acupoints* (SAs). An acute injury is an example of the symptomatic model of acupoint formation. The local appearance of SAs reflects the personal nature of the acute injury or disease. Each patient may present particular symptomatic acupoints.

In physically healthy bodies HAs are transformed from latent phase into passive phase following a highly predictable pattern. For example, the H1 deep radial acupoint (located on the deep radial nerve where the nerve enters the lateral side of the forearm to supply the extensor muscles of the wrist and fingers) is always first to become tender in everyone (refer to the figure on the inside cover).

The number of tender HAs in the body serves as a quantitative indicator of the patient's health status. Usually a healthier person has less tender acupoints in his or her body. If a healthy person has acute pain, a few acupuncture sessions will relieve the pain. Less healthy people have more tender acupoints, and such patients will need more acupuncture sessions to achieve relief of even minor acute pain. Thus the number of tender HAs in the body is the quantitative indicator of (1) health status, (2) self-healing capacity (healthy persons heal better and faster), and (3) the number of acupuncture treatments that may be needed to achieve pain relief. This quantitative indicator provides us with a reasonably objective method to evaluate patients and to predict the prognosis of treatments (see Chapter 6).

Suppose two patients complain about similar symptoms of low back pain, but patient A has 20 passive acupoints on the body, whereas patient B has more than 40 passive acupoints on the body. Clinically patient A is likely to need two to four treatments to achieve pain relief, whereas patient B may need eight treatments to achieve similar relief. Moreover patient A is likely to enjoy long-term or permanent relief from pain after these two to four treatments, but there is a high possibility that patient B will experience a relapse of the symptoms a few months after the initial eight treatments. Because the homeostasis of patient A indicates that the patient is healthier than patient B and has a stronger healing potential, patient A (1) will experience faster therapeutic results with fewer acupuncture treatments, (2) will enjoy longer and complete pain relief, and (3) is less likely to experience a relapse of the same pain symptom.

ELECTROPHYSIOLOGY OF ACUPOINTS

Muscles and nerves are excitable tissues that generate electrical signals when stimulated. When not disturbed, that is, in the so-called healthy state, muscles and nerves are electrically silent at rest. Dr. David G. Simmons and his colleagues investigated the electrical activity in trigger points.[1] They

found two significant components of electrical activity in trigger points:

1. Intermittent and high amplitude spike potentials
2. Continuous lower-amplitude noise-like recordings, which they named *spontaneous electrical activity* (SEA)[5]

Dr. Y.-T. Ma also discovered similar electrical activities of the neurons in the spinal cord and the midbrain (periaqueductal gray matter [PAG]) in responding to induced pain in animal experiments. In normal tissues the activities of the neurons in the spinal cord and the PAG are silent at rest. When pain or inflammation is introduced into the muscles, the spikes and SAE appear in both the spinal cord and the PAG. As the pain intensity increases, the frequency and amplitude of spikes increase and the frequency may reach more than 200 spikes a second. Electrophysiologically the pain intensity is translated into spike frequency in the nervous signaling system.

ACUPUNCTURE NEEDLING RESTORES NORMAL ENERGY METABOLISM OF ACUPOINTS

Dr. David G. Simmons has shown that muscular contraction knots are the *histopathologic characteristics* of trigger points.[5] Dr. C. Chan Gunn also suggests a similar histologic structure of the shortened muscles with palpable tender or painful bands or points (Figure 2-1).

Careful examination of pathologic activity of passive or active acupoints and the muscles harboring these tender acupoints shows that, in addition to pronounced pain symptoms, at least two other abnormal phenomena are present:

1. The surface temperature of most acupoints is a little higher than that of normal tissues
2. The affected muscles are tight and resist stretching

In 1950 medical scientist Y. Nakatani (see Chapter 1) from Japan's Kyoto University discovered that acupoints on the skin have a high level of electrical conductivity. Moreover the electrical conductivity of some acupoints increased significantly during sickness. He found 370 such points, incorporated them into the classic meridians system, and called these acupoints *Ryodoraku points,*[6] which in both Japanese and Chinese languages means meridian point with good electrical conductivity.

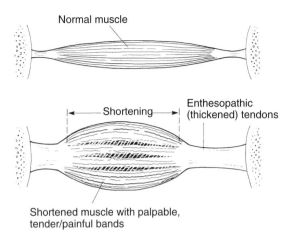

Normal muscle

|←——— Shortening ———→| Enthesopathic (thickened) tendons

Shortened muscle with palpable, tender/painful bands

Figure 2-1   A trigger point contains shortened muscle fibers, which may present as palpable tender or painful knots or bands. The entire muscle may become shortened and tight if it harbors trigger point(s) and resists stretching. The shortened muscle constantly pulls the tendons and causes tendinitis. (From Filshie J, White A: *Medical acupuncture: a Western scientific approach,* Edinburgh, 1998, Churchill Livingstone.)

In 1977 Nakatami noted that Ryodoraku points were situated on areas containing sweat glands and inferred that the higher electrical conductivity of Ryodoraku is due to the high electrical conductivity of the sweat glands. Modern Ryodoraku theory focuses on interactions between the sympathetic and somatic nervous systems.[6] There is no doubt that abnormal energy metabolism is actively involved in the formation of passive and active acupoints related to soft tissue metabolism, as discussed below.

First we briefly review the process of normal energy metabolism in the muscles. After receiving electrical signals (motor-unit action potentials) from a motor neuron in the spinal cord, a muscle cell (muscle fiber) will release calcium into its cytoplasm from its storage pool, the cellular organelle called *sarcoplasmic reticulum* (SR). This higher cytoplasmic concentration of calcium triggers cellular contractile activity

After contraction the cellular machine pumps calcium from cytoplasm back to the SR to reduce the concentration of cytoplasmic calcium. Once the concentration of cytoplasmic calcium declines, muscle fibers immediately relax, so the muscles are able to prepare for the next signal-induced contraction. Normal muscle fibers contract only when they receive a signal (motor-unit potential) from the spinal cord.

The contraction and relaxation of the muscles require energy to move calcium back and forth between cytoplasm and the SR. If muscle fibers are injured or deprived of energy supply, the cellular machine stops pumping calcium from the cytoplasm to the SR, which results in a persistent high concentration of cytoplasmic calcium. This persistent high concentration of cytoplasmic calcium leads to sustained contraction of muscle fibers.

One of the consequences of this sustained contraction of muscle fibers is the tenderness of acupoints. Note that this sustained contractile activity happens without any signals (motor-unit potentials) from the spinal cord.

The sustained contraction significantly increases the demand for energy and leads to "energy crises." Sustained muscle contraction shuts the capillary network that supplies the region with nutrition and oxygen and therefore generates a low-oxygen environment *(hypoxia)*. Without energy and oxygen, the cellular machine cannot pump calcium from cytoplasm back to its storage pool (SR), which results in sustained high calcium concentration in the cytoplasm and the consequent persistent sustained muscle contraction. Thus the vicious cycle is built and perpetuated (Figure 2-2).

Here we briefly discuss the molecular mechanism of muscle contraction. In healthy skeletal muscle fibers (cells), calcium is stored in a cellular organelle, the SR. When the motor nerve fiber sends impulses to the muscles, the impulses initiate the action potential in the membrane of the muscle fiber. This action potential spreads into the SR (whose membrane is a continuum of the muscle membrane), resulting in the release of calcium into cytoplasm. The high concentration of cytoplasmic calcium triggers the coupling between two linear proteins (actin and myosin). After coupling, these two linear proteins slide against each other, thus leading to shortening of the muscle fiber. This coupling and sliding between the two protein molecules consume a large amount of energy in the form of ATP. If there are no further impulses from the motor nerve fiber after the initial shortening, the SR will reuptake the calcium back to storage, causing the concentration of cytoplasmic calcium to drop. The low cytoplasmic calcium decouples the contractile proteins actin and myosin, resulting in the relaxing of the muscle fiber.

If a muscle fiber is damaged, SR is unable to reuptake the cytoplasmic calcium back for storage, which creates a persistent high concentration of cytoplasmic calcium. The two contractile protein molecules cannot decouple because of this high concentration of cytoplasmic calcium. This results

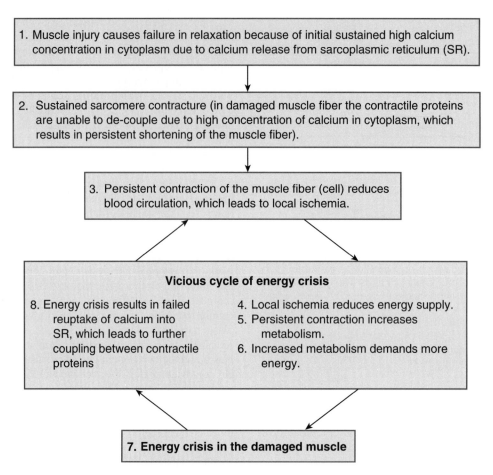

1. Muscle injury causes failure in relaxation because of initial sustained high calcium concentration in cytoplasm due to calcium release from sarcoplasmic reticulum (SR).

2. Sustained sarcomere contracture (in damaged muscle fiber the contractile proteins are unable to de-couple due to high concentration of calcium in cytoplasm, which results in persistent shortening of the muscle fiber).

3. Persistent contraction of the muscle fiber (cell) reduces blood circulation, which leads to local ischemia.

Vicious cycle of energy crisis

8. Energy crisis results in failed reuptake of calcium into SR, which leads to further coupling between contractile proteins

4. Local ischemia reduces energy supply.
5. Persistent contraction increases metabolism.
6. Increased metabolism demands more energy.

7. Energy crisis in the damaged muscle

Figure 2-2   Energy metabolism and the cellular process of muscle fiber contracture in a tender acupoint. The energy crisis hypothesis is suggested by Dr. David G. Simons. (Redrawn from Simons DG, Travell JG, Simons LS: *Travell & Simons' myofascial pain and dysfunction: the trigger point manual, vol 1, Upper half of body,* Philadelphia, 1999, Lippincott–Williams & Wilkins.)

in persistent contraction of the muscle fiber, even without any impulse from the motor nerve. If this energy-consuming process (the energy crisis) continues, tender muscle bands or acupoints will be formed and the tender bands will become a permanent contracture if the energy crisis persists a long time. Finally, this energy crisis may cause chronic inflammation in the involved soft tissues. Both energy crisis and inflammation increase the local temperature.

Acupuncture needling creates a tiny lesion and bleeding in the contractile muscle and surrounding tissues. As a result of the needling, the tight contracted muscle immediately relaxes and blood circulation improves. Thus acupuncture needling breaks the vicious cycle of energy crises in trigger points inside the muscle.

The needled lesion disturbs the surrounding tissue and generates a small electrical current of up to 500 mA/cm,[7] which we call the *lesion current*. The needle lesion causes a tiny local bleeding, which stimulates secretion of numerous growth factors, such as platelet-derived growth factors and neurotrophic factors.

The electrical current generated by the lesion and the bleeding caused by needling promote healing and regeneration of damaged tissues and induce DNA synthesis of new proteins and collagens, which repair damaged cellular organelles and restore normal functions. A needle-induced lesion may last at least 2 days or longer before the body heals it, which means that lesion-induced stimulation may last as long. During the healing period, the lesioned cells are digested and replaced by the same types of tissue cells. This explains why acupuncture needling can achieve longer-lasting results. After the needles are removed, the needle-induced lesions keep working for at least 48 hours.

Another important feature is that needling and needle-induced lesions also trigger the local and systemic immune and antiinflammatory reaction that controls the inflammation in the area of needle-induced lesions (see Chapter 4). This explains the antiinflammatory function of acupuncture therapy.

SUMMARY

Acupoints are mainly composed of sensory nerve receptors. Acupoints become tender or painful because their sensory nerve receptors are pathologically sensitized. This sensitized condition is a dynamic process: tender acupoints will appear and grow when health deteriorates, or they disappear when health is restored. Normal physiologic homeostasis will reduce the sensitivity of acupoints; acute injuries or chronic diseases will sensitize acupoints.

Pathophysiologically an acupoint evolves through three stages:

1. Latent phase (nonsensitive)
2. Passive phase (sensitive but without conscious awareness)
3. Active phase (oversensitive or painful).

The physical property of acupoints can be described as specificity, sensitivity, and sequence. Specificity of an acupoint is inversely proportional to its sensitivity. As an acupoint becomes more sensitive, the physical size of its tender area increases but its specificity decreases.

There are two types of tender acupoints related to pathophysiologic changes: HAs and SAs. The HAs are those that become sensitized symmetrically all over the body when homeostasis declines. HAs appear in a predictable pattern in terms of their locations and sequence. *Sequence* means the order in which acupoints become sensitized in the whole

acupoint system (refer to the figure in the inside cover). This predictable pattern of acupoint formation is basically the same in all human bodies. Thus the number of HAs in a person is a quantitative indicator for evaluating the homeostasis status of the person. This quantitative indicator also provides information to predict the progress and prognosis of acupuncture treatments. Clinically HAs are needled to restore healthy homeostasis.

Acute injuries or acute diseases create local tender points. These tender points are named SAs, which appear in different locations, depending on the nature of the injury or disease of each patient.

Some passive or active acupoints appear as a result of a vicious circle of metabolic energy crises. Such acupoints maintain a higher temperature than surrounding tissues because of sustained muscle contraction. Muscle contraction itself is an energy-demanding process, but the sustained contraction creates an environment of low energy and low oxygen (hypoxia) as a result of reduced blood circulation. Acupuncture needling is able to relax the muscle, which breaks the vicious circle of energy crisis and restores normal blood circulation.

References

1. Mens S, Simons DG: *Muscle pain*, Philadelphia, 2001, Lippincott–Williams & Wilkins.
2. Kellgren HJ: The distribution of pain arising from deep somatic structures with charts of segmental pain areas, *Clin Sci* 4:35-46, 1939.
3. Dung HC: *Anatomical acupuncture*, San Antonio, 1997, Antarctic Press.
4. Macdonald AJR: Acupuncture's non-segmental and segmental analgesic effects: the point of meridians. In Filshie J, White A: editors: *Medical acupuncture*. Edinburgh, 1998, Churchill Livingston.
5. Simons DG, Travell, JG, Simons LS: *Travell & Simons' myofascial pain and dysfunction: the trigger point manual, vol 1, Upper half of body*, Philadelphia, 1999, Lippincott–Williams & Wilkins.
6. Nakatani Y, Yamashita K: *Ryodoraku acupuncture*. Osaka, 1977, Ryodoraku Research Institute.
7. Jaffe LF: Extracellular current measurements with a vibrating probe, *TINS* December:517-521, 1985.

CHAPTER 3

Peripheral Mechanisms of Acupuncture

INTRODUCTION

To incorporate acupuncture as an effective medical procedure for pain management and trauma rehabilitation, health care practitioners need a basic understanding of needling mechanisms.

Unique Biomedical Mechanisms of Acupuncture Needling

Sound physiologic bases for the scientific explanation of why and how acupuncture works have been already established by distinguished scientists. A prominent researcher in the field of acupuncture analgesia, Professor Bruce Pomeranz of the University of Toronto said, "We know more about acupuncture analgesia than about many chemical drugs in routine use. For example, we know very little about the mechanisms of most anesthetic gases but still use them regularly."[1]

Acupuncture is a unique therapy because it uses fine needles to inoculate minute intrusive "traumas," or lesions into the tissues, which stimulates many of the survival mechanisms of the body. The acupuncture needling and its induced lesions activate self-healing mechanisms, including restoring homeostasis, facilitating repair mechanisms such as antiinflammatory reaction and tissue regeneration, and pain modulation. After needles are removed, the needle-induced lesions continue to stimulate the body until the lesions heal. Usually the healing of needle-induced lesions takes 2 days, although some patients feel the lesion stimulation for up to 1 week.

Four physiologic systems stand on the defense frontier in our survival mechanisms: the *nervous system,* which coordinates our responses to external and internal stimuli; the *cardiovascular system,* which provides energy, active molecules, highway transportation of endocrine molecules, and cellular cleansing; the *endocrine system,* which secretes molecules for different conditions; and the *immune system,* which defends the body from invaders. Clinically acupuncture stimulates all four systems.

Why Patients Respond Differently to the Same Acupuncture Treatment

We should keep in mind that acupuncture therapy activates the built-in survival mechanism of our body: the self-healing potential. Thus acupuncture is effective for those symptoms that can be completely or partially healed by the body.

We inherit the self-healing potential for biological survival. This inherited self-healing potential is modified by genetic makeup, medical history, lifestyle, and age. Therefore each of us has a different self-healing capacity. The self-healing potential, however, is dynamically changing. It will deteriorate if a person abuses his or her health, and will improve if a person takes good care of his or her health. The efficacy of acupuncture therapy depends on (1) the status of self-healing potential of the body (e.g., the healthier a person is, the better his or her self-healing potential) and (2) the potential healability of the symptoms (e.g., acute low back pain heals faster than chronic low back pain). This is why different patients respond differently to the same acupuncture treatment.

Using an innovative, well-defined, and reliable evaluation procedure as presented in this book (see Chapter 6), we can categorize patients into four groups of responders: excellent (Group A), good (Group B), average (Group C), and weak (Group D). Professor H.C. Dung[2] discovered these important clinical phenomena after examining and treating 15,000 patients.

Integrative Neuromuscular Acupoint System (INMAS): The User-Friendly Protocol

The modernized acupuncture treatment protocol for pain management and trauma rehabilitation presented in this book is user friendly, effective, and applicable to all pain symptoms. This protocol is based on the following:

1. Our broad clinical experiences, incorporating discoveries by Professor H.C. Dung[2] of acupoint phase transformation in relation to homeostatic changes
2. The traditional Chinese acupoint system
3. Segmental and nonsegmental mechanisms of needling as suggested by Professor Pomeranz[1]

This protocol was created by using the unique combination of selected homeostatic and symptomatic points. In fact this protocol is also applicable to nonpain symptoms because acupuncture therapy by its nature is nonspecific. The following is a summary of the scientific data that help to explain the mechanisms of acupuncture treatment. Readers interested in more detail are referred to the reference list.

Electrical Acupuncture

Electrical acupuncture (EA) stimulates peripheral nerves, especially the large A beta fibers, which send strong impulses to the spinal cord and brain. With *different* stimulating frequencies, EA can induce *different* endorphins at different levels of the central nervous system (CNS). Endorphins exert many physiologic functions. They modulate the pain mechanisms to relieve pain, relax the cardiovascular systems, and improve immune activity by reducing the physiologic stress. EA stimulation results in accelerated self-healing.

Endorphin mechanisms are nonspecific. EA and needling stimulate endorphin mechanisms, whereas chiropractic manipulation, massage, and physical exercises also lead to the secretion of endorphins. The mechanisms of EA are discussed in more detail in Chapter 15. The following discussion focuses on the unique local mechanisms of acupuncture needling.

GENERAL PRINCIPLES OF HEALING PROCESS INDUCED BY ACUPUNCTURE NEEDLING

Researchers have accumulated an impressive amount of evidence of the cellular and molecular events underlying tissue response to needling. Clinical observation shows that acupuncture needling achieves at least four therapeutic goals:

1. Release of physical and emotional stress
2. Activation and control of immune and antiinflammatory mechanisms

3. Acceleration of tissue healing
4. Pain relief

Needling reduces bodily stress by stimulating the secretion of endorphins, relaxing the cardiovascular and muscular systems, and restoring the physiologic and autonomic balance *(homeostasis),* which includes normalizing visceral functions that are impaired during stressful assault via neurohormonal pathways.

Our clinical evidence shows that acupuncture is an effective modality in controlling inflammation. Needling and needle-induced lesions are foreign invaders to our body. Needling and its lesions stimulate and increase the number and the activity of immune cells and control the inflammatory process (see Chapter 4), which reduces both acute and chronic inflammation.

Needling promotes and accelerates soft tissue healing. Soft tissue includes nerves, muscles, connective tissues (tendons, ligaments, joint capsules, fascial coating of muscles), and some functional structures like blood and lymphatic vessels. Soft tissue damage may be caused by physical activities, injuries from accidents, or inflammation from repetitively overusing the muscles. In addition, almost all internal diseases, for example, asthma, gastritis, nephritis, and especially arthritis, cause discomfort, pain, or inflammation in superficial soft tissues. After acupuncture treatments, soft tissue inflammation and pain subside. Often internal diseases are alleviated or cured along with peripheral tissue healing.

Finally pain relief is achieved by homeostatic balancing and soft tissue healing in most cases, whereas immediate pain relief frequently happens even before tissue healing is complete.

NEEDLING AND DE QI SENSATION

Modern sterile stainless steel acupuncture needles with plastic guide tubes make needling safe, technically easy, and less painful. Needling, however, always produces a certain sensation. The nonpainful sensations produced by needling are traditionally called *de qi* (deh chee) in traditional Chinese medicine (TCM).

The needling process includes the following procedures:

1. Selecting the points
2. Inserting a needle through the skin, subcutaneous connective tissue, deeper fascia, muscles, tendon, or periosteum

3. Retaining the needle at the point from a few seconds up to 20 minutes, proper manipulation of the needles such as rotation or up and down pistoning, and/or applying additional electrical stimulation
4. Removing the needle

During procedure no. 3, a needle can be manipulated by unidirectional or bidirectional (i.e., clockwise or counterclockwise) rotation or "pistoning" (up and down motion). This manipulation creates winding of connective tissue around the needle, which makes the practitioner feel the needle being grasped by body tissue.[3]

Once the needle has punctured the deeper tissues, especially the muscles, the patient will feel nonpainful sensations termed *de qi* (deh chee) in traditional Chinese acupuncture, which means that *qi* (i.e., the vital energy flow) has obtained or arrived. About 90% of needling will produce some sort of *de qi* sensation, depending on the nerve fibers encountered by needling and surrounding tissue milieu, such as tissue perfusion and inflammatory mediators.[4] Needling the points on limbs may produce a *de qi* sensation of brief electric shock running up or down along the entire length of the limb. When needling the points on the back, a *de qi* sensation could be experienced more as localized sensations, like deep aching, soreness, and heaviness.

The phenomenon of *de qi* sensations can be explained by the types of nerve fibers stimulated by the needling (Table 3-1). Types II, III, and IV muscular afferent fibers not only generate *de qi*, but they also produce pain sensation if they are injured or pathophysiologically excited; so they represent *de qi* and pain-transmission nerves. Patients should be warned that some needling sensations such as aching or soreness may last 1 or 2 days.

A needling-induced lesion stimulates the epidermis, dermis, underlying connective tissues (elastic fibers, collagen, basal lamina, deeper fascia), muscular tissues (skeletal muscles and smooth muscles of blood vessels), and nervous tissues (nerve fibers of sensory neurons and postganglionic neurons). The cells lesioned by the needling will be replaced with the same type of fresh cells without scar formation, since the lesions are very fine and tiny.

A needling activates chain reactions in both local tissues and the CNS (the spinal cord and brain). Thus we categorize needling mechanisms as peripheral and central. Both peripheral and central mechanisms, however, are physiologically inseparable. This chapter describes some of the major peripheral tissue reactions and the next chapter discusses the central mechanisms.

The following local chain reactions are started right after needling:

1. Local skin reaction and cutaneous microcurrent mechanism
2. Local interaction between needle shaft and connective tissues
3. Local relaxation of concurrent muscle shortening and contracture, which improves local blood circulation through muscular reaction and autonomic reflex
4. Neural mechanism: nociceptive and motoneuronal activation, CNS-mediated neuroendocrine activity, segmental and nonsegmental pathways
5. Blood coagulation and lymphatic circulation
6. Local immune responses
7. DNA synthesis to replace the injured tissues and repair the acupuncture lesions

LOCAL SKIN REACTION AND CUTANEOUS MICROCURRENT MECHANISM

The neurovasculoimmune function of the skin is the first line of the body's defense system. Needling stimulates the following skin tissues:

1. Afferent somatic neuron fibers (cutaneous A-delta and C fibers) and sympathetic neuron fibers (for controlling the sweat glands and fine blood vessels)

Table 3-1	
■ *De Qi* Sensation and Its Related Nerve Fibers in the Muscles	

Types of Afferent Nerve Fibers	Types of Sensation
Type II	Numbness
Type III	Heaviness, distention, pressure, compression, aching
Type IV (unmyelinated)	Soreness, tingling, pain

2. Fine arterial and venous blood vessels (nutrition supply and temperature regulation)
3. Lymphatic tissue, mast cells (immune function)
4. Connective tissues (structural and functional support)

When an acupoint transits from latent phase (normal tissue) to passive phase, it becomes tender (Chapter 2). Around a tender acupoint the skin electrical conductance increases and the resistance decreases as discussed in Chapter 2. Inserting a needle into this acupoint will provoke an acute local inflammatory defensive response from all the previously mentioned tissues. The first visible response is the flare response, resulting in the appearance of redness around the needle. This vasodilatation function of the autonomic nervous system (ANS) is mediated by substance P secreted by cutaneous nociceptive sensory nerves. Then the immune reaction is triggered by mast cells, which produce histamine, platelet activating factor (PAF), and leukotrienes. The needle-induced lesion simultaneously activates interaction between the blood coagulation system and the immune complement system.

The body surface wears a layer of electric charges because the human body bathes in the electromagnetic field of the earth. Normally, dry skin has a DC resistance in the order of 200,000 to two million ohms. At acupuncture points this resistance is down to 50,000 ohms.[5] Melzack and Katz[6] found no difference in conductance between acupuncture points and nearby control points in patients with chronic pain.

This phenomenon can be explained by the dynamic nature of the acupoints. In a healthy person, DC resistance of the acupoints is the same as that of nonacupoints. In a chronically sick person, the acupoints transit from the latent phase (healthy tissue) to the passive phase (tender or sensitized tissue) in a predictable sequence and location (see Chapter 2). The sensitive area of acupoints is getting larger in chronic conditions, which contributes to high electrical conductance and low resistance.

In acute injury, acupoints appear around injured tissue. There is 20 to 90 mV of resting potential across the intact human skin, outside negative and inside positive.[7] Most acupoints are measured at 5 mV higher than in nonacupoint areas.[5] This higher voltage at acupoint loci can be explained histologically and pathologically. The configuration of most acupoints is rich in nerve fibers and/or vasculolymphatic structures, and

once sensitized, inflammation may accumulate more fluids in the tissues of an acupoint. All these conditions may increase conductance and compensate the loss of resistance at acupoint loci according to Ohm's formula: $V = IR$.

Insertion of a metal needle makes a short circuit from the skin battery and thus creates a microcurrent, called a *current of injury,* moving from inside to outside. The tiny lesion created by an acupuncture needle causes negativity at the needling site and produces 10 mA of current of injury, which benefits tissue growth and regeneration.[8]

These microcurrents induced by the needling are not sufficient to initiate nerve pulses to the spinal cord; thus the microcurrents will not generate effects of "needling tolerance" like "morphine tolerance," meaning that repetitive needling will not reduce its therapeutic effect. In case of electroacupuncture stimulation of more than 3 hours' duration, the analgesic effect will gradually decline. Professor J.S. Han of the Beijing Medical University explained that possibly long-lasting electrical stimulation, especially with high frequencies such as 100 Hz, increases the release of cholecystokinin octapeptide (CCK-8), which is an endogenous antiopioid substance.[9]

NEEDLE MANIPULATION: MECHANICAL SIGNAL TRANSDUCTION THROUGH CONNECTIVE TISSUE

During acupuncture treatments, more than 90% of the needling elicits *de qi* sensation. *De qi* elicited by manipulation of the needles increases the effectiveness of muscle relaxation and helps relieve pain. (Warning: Caution should be taken in treating weak or older patients because they may not be able to tolerate even weak manipulation and may suffer from flare-up pain after treatment. For these patients, simple insertion of the needle to the proper depth is sufficient. Flare-up pain can be alleviated easily by inserting one or two needles at the painful site. No manipulation is suggested for some facial points because of the dense capillary bed in such areas, which could cause bleeding or bruising on the face.)

The research team of the University of Vermont College of Medicine demonstrated that manipulation promotes tissue healing by producing biomechanical, vasomotor, and neuromodulatory effects on interstitial connective tissue.[3]

When a needle is inserted into the body tissue, there is an initial coupling between the metal needle shaft and elastic/collagen fibers. This initial affinity is caused by both surface tension and electrical attraction between the metal needle and connective tissue charges. Once this wrapping has occurred, frictional force takes over. Then rotation of the needle increases the tension of the fibers by winding them around the needle, which pulls and realigns the connective fiber network

The experienced practitioner detects the needle resistance to rotation (needle grasp) while the patient feels *de qi* sensation. This needle grasp process deforms the extracellular matrix, fibroblasts attached to collagen fibers, and possibly capillary endothelial cells.

In response to this mechanistic deformation, cells generate cascades of cellular and molecular events, including intracellular cytoskeletal reorganization, cell contraction and migration, autocrine release of growth factors, and activation of intracellular signaling pathways and of nuclear binding proteins that promote the transcription of specific genes. These effects lead to the synthesis and local release of growth factors, cytokines, vasoactive substances, degradative enzymes, and structural matrix elements. Release of these substances changes the extracellular milieu surrounding needled tissues and finally promotes local healing. These effects may expand to distant connective tissues to spread the healing process with long-term effects. Thus mechanical signals produced by simple needle manipulations generate cascades of downstream physiologic healing effects.[10]

Clinical evidence shows that this mechanical signal transduction resulting from proper needle manipulation (rotation or "pistoning") may help desensitize sensory receptors and restore normal pain threshold. It is common, especially in treating acute injuries, for pain, tenderness, and swelling to subside during or shortly after needling.

LOCAL RELIEF OF CONCURRENT MUSCLE SHORTENING AND CONTRACTURE

Acupuncture effectively provides local relief of concurrent muscle shortening and contracture. All the local muscle pain stimulates the muscle to generate tender points, persistent involuntary contracture, and shortening of the muscles fibers, resulting in tense and stiff muscles. Four types of local muscle pain are most common: (1) mechanical, chemical, or physical (such as burning) injuries; (2) repetitive strain, overstretching, or a

long time of shortening beyond the muscle's tolerance when maintaining the same posture for a long time; (3) diseased viscera projecting pain to the body surface partially via mechanism of segmental neuronal reflex; and (4) referred pain associated with a diseased joint and its accessory structures.

Local muscle pain involves afferent sensory fibers (nociceptors), muscle fibers, and blood vessels. The nerve endings of sensory fibers contain neuropeptides substance P (SP), calcitonin gene-related peptide (CGRP), and somatostatin (SOM). Under pathologic conditions the neuropeptides can be released from the sensory nerve endings and influence basic tissue functions such as neuronal excitability, local microcirculation, and metabolism. When tissue-threatening (noxious) stimuli (mechanical, physical, or chemical) occur, the neuropeptides are released from the sensory nerve endings, which triggers a cascade of events leading to neurogenic inflammation. SP and CGRP cause vasodilatation and increase the permeability of the microvasculature. Histamine is liberated from mast cells when exposed to SP. All these substances diffuse to neighboring tissue, resulting in an expansion of the inflammation.

Once this neurogenic inflammation diffuses, fluids and proteins shift from the blood vessels into surrounding interstitial spaces. This process releases vasoneuroactive substances: bradykinin from protein (kalidin) in the blood plasma, and serotonin (5-hydroxytryptamine, 5-HT) from platelets. Leukotrienes and prostaglandins are released from the surrounding tissue cells at the injured site. All these substances increase the sensitivity of affected nerve endings. Thus the noxious stimuli result in tenderness (sensitized nociceptors) and then spontaneous pain (nociceptor excitation) in the localized region of muscle.

When nociceptors are sensitized, their firing threshold decreases. Under such physiologic alteration, any slight stimulus such as light pressure may cause the nerve ending to fire impulses to the CNS. This light pressure does not elicit any response from the normal unsensitized nerve ending. If the sensitization continues, it may further decrease the firing threshold of the nociceptors and the excited nociceptors may spontaneously discharge impulses to the CNS, which causes sensation of pain.

Repetitive strain or overuse injuries are common muscle activities that result in local muscle pain. If muscles are used for repetitive movement without adequate recovery time between movements or are held under a load in a relatively fixed position for prolonged periods, discomfort, soreness, or pain will develop following those activities, with peak discomfort during the first day or two. Pain makes muscles tender to palpation, restricted in range of motion, and sometimes slightly swollen. With this type of injury, some disorganization of striation of muscle fibers can occur, and a lack of myofibrillar regeneration could persist for up to 10 days.[11] Changes in blood chemistry have been noticed, including increases in plasma interleukin-1, acid-reactive substances, lactic dehydrogenase, serum creatine, phosphokinase, aspartate aminotransferase, and serum glutamic-oxaloacetic transaminase. Most of these enzymes are involved in muscle metabolism.

The literature on Chinese traditional acupuncture indicates that the diseased viscera project pain to predictable points or areas of the body surface. In general this is the manifestation of the segmental mechanism of viscerosomatic neuronal reflex. For example, inflammation of a kidney may cause tender points or painful spasm in the lumbar area, resulting in lower back pain with tender points palpable at the T10 to L2 level on the back muscle (erector spinae). For some patients additional tender points also appear in the neck region. This segmental mechanism plays an important role in treatment of the pain symptoms and is discussed in detail later. Needling these tender points associated with diseased organs relieves pain and other symptoms, such as cramping, inflammation, and ulcer.

Joint diseases and dysfunction can cause muscle pain. Because of the segmental reflex, the activity of sensory nerves influences the activity of efferent nerves from motor neurons of the same muscle; however, the sensory nerves of neighboring muscles and joints also affect this muscle. Stimulation of knee joint nociceptors excites afferent motor neurons of both flexor and extensor muscles.[12] It is possible that sensory input from a joint will lead to a contraction in neighboring muscles. Then the contracted muscles may put physical stress on the joint and its accessory structures, such as capsules, ligaments, and disks. All these structures will produce pain because they are richly innervated by sensory nerves.

All types of muscle pain of different pathophysiologies converge to produce similar phenomena: they produce tense, stiff, and shortened muscles and provoke the formation of tender points and enlarged contraction knots within the muscle. Some of the contraction knots, if not released immediately, become persistent muscle contracture, resulting in a chronic condition.

Those sensitized spots are also found in other soft tissues that are richly innervated by sensory nerves, such as tendons, ligaments, possibly periosteum, and superficial and deep fascia. Modern clinicians call these tender spots and contracture trigger points, *dermopoints, motopoints* (neuromuscular attachment points), *nodes,* and other terms, all of which represent some of the different aspects of the acupoints in traditional Chinese acupuncture.

Acupoints have different histologic composition and pathophysiologic phases (Chapters 1 and 2). Some acupoints consist mostly of sensitized nerve fibers; others, in addition to the sensitized nerve receptors, contain muscle contraction knots. Internal factors, such as diseased organs and arthritis, will sensitize acupoints all over the body. Remarkably their locations are highly predictable, partly because of a segmental mechanism or special tissue features associated with sensory nerve fibers. During acute injuries sensitized spots are provocatively formed according to the type of injury and body anatomy involved. For example, the mild ankle sprain (inversion injury) causes only elongation of ligaments on the lateral ankle, whereas a severe ankle injury may tear the ligaments between the fibula and tibia in addition to the lateral ligaments. Knowing anatomy helps in locating the most effective tender points for treatment. (To help locate the effective acupoints, the clinical chapters of this book describe some of the neuromusculoskeletal anatomy in relation to body mechanics.)

The muscle, tendon, or fascia that harbors tender or painful points may resist stretch and become tense, stiff, shortened, and painful. Most acupoints used for pain treatments are of muscular nature as discussed in Chapter 1.

Before we examine pathologic contracture, we review the membrane depolarization and five steps involved in healthy muscle contraction.

Depolarization can be described as follows. When a cell is not agitated, the outside of the cell membrane is electrically positive, the inside negative. When electric impulses or bioactive molecules stimulate the cell, positive Na^+ ions flow into the cell through the membrane so that the outside becomes less positive; this means the electricity flows into the cell. Then positive K^+ ions flow out from inside to restore positive polarity of the outside, which means that positive electricity flows out from the inside. Finally Na^+ ions are pumped out and K^+ ions are pumped in by molecular channels; so the concentration of Na^+ ions outside and K^+ inside is restored. This represents one cycle, and the process is called *depolarization* (Figure 3-1). The depolarization consumes metabolic energy.

All five steps of muscle contraction are related to depolarization and consumption of energy:

1. The electrical impulses from the CNS travel along the motor neuron fiber and reach the nerve terminal to depolarize the terminal membrane of the fiber (axon), which causes the terminal to release acetylcholine into the space of the neuromuscular junction.
2. The acetylcholine in the junction space depolarizes the membrane of the muscle cell (the postjunctional membrane).
3. In muscle cells, a membranous organelle called the sarcoplasmic reticulum (SR) is attached to the cell membrane and stores calcium. Depolarization of the cell membrane causes depolarization of the SR, which results in the release of calcium into the cell plasma.
4. The high concentration, of cytoplasmic calcium stimulates the coupling of two long, linear molecules, actin and myosin, and the two molecules move oppositely against each other so that the long, spindle-like muscle cells become shortened.
5. After this contraction, calcium ions are pumped back into the SR through molecular pumping mechanisms; so the concentration of cytoplasmic calcium declines, which

leads to decoupling of actin and myosin. Thus the muscle is relaxed to its original length. To maintain a posture, we voluntarily send impulses continuously to a group of muscles to maintain the coupling of actin and myosin so that muscles maintain contraction until we stop sending more impulses. Those processes represent normal physiologic contraction.

Now we compare the same steps of pathologic contraction with physiologic contraction. This process was discussed in Chapter 2, but is briefly reviewed here because it is an important mechanism in clinical acupuncture practice. Dr. D.G. Simons explained this process and called it the *energy crisis hypothesis.*"[13] We modify his hypothesis as follows (also see Figure 2-2, p. 22).

1. If afferent sensory nerves are sensitized (tender) or excited (pain), efferent motor nerves are activated to release excess acetylcholine into the neuromuscular junction space.
2. Excess acetylcholine causes longer depolarization of postjunctional membranes.
3. This results in longer depolarization of the SR membrane and leads to a longer period of high concentration of cytoplasmic calcium.
4. A high concentration of cytoplasmic calcium prolongs actin-myosin coupling. The sustained shortened muscle cell creates compression of the blood vessel. The compressed microcirculation (ischemia) provides less energy and oxygen supply, the results of local ischemia.
5. The actin-myosin coupling continues as the concentration of cytoplasmic calcium remains high and molecular pumps cannot return the calcium back to the SR because of low or no energy supply.

Thus the ischemia, hypoxia, low energy supply, and muscle shortening will continue and become a vicious circle (see Figure 2-2, p. 22) until appropriate treatment interrupts the vicious circle of energy crisis. The muscle contracture during such an energy crisis has a higher temperature than normal muscle tissue does. This pathologic contraction is an endogenous, not voluntary, impulse initiated and may persist indefinitely. Clinical experience shows that any method that interrupts the energy crisis will help relax the muscle and reduce muscle pain. Needling, electrical stimulation, physical stretch,

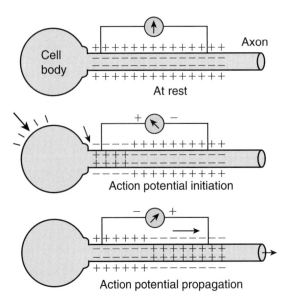

Figure 3-1   Diagram of depolarization of a nerve cell.

proper exercise, and drug injection are effective procedures used to break the energy-consuming vicious circle and to separate actin from myosin to relax the shortened muscle.

Manipulation of the needle has been suggested to deform connective fibers, and this mechanical signaling induces tissue healing. Clinical evidence shows that manipulation also helps to stretch muscles and breaks the energy crisis of some acupoints. Needling can precisely target and release endogenous contracture deep inside the muscles. These findings demonstrate the effectiveness of acupuncture procedures for muscle relaxation, restoration of local blood circulation, and promotion of tissue healing without any side effects. If local sensitization or endogenous contracture is acute and localized, muscle relaxation can be achieved immediately. Otherwise more treatments are needed to first destroy the endogenous contracture histologically and then promote tissue regeneration to replace the destroyed muscle fibers.

NEUROCHEMICAL MECHANISMS OF ACUPUNCTURE ANALGESIA

Neurochemical mechanisms of acupuncture analgesia (AA) have been intensively investigated in many Chinese, Japanese, South Korean, and North American universities. Professor Ji-shen Han's laboratory at Beijing Medical University, Professor Cao Xiao-ding's laboratory at the Shanghai Medical College of Fudan University, and Professor Bruce Pomeranz's laboratory at the University of Toronto have contributed solid scientific data explaining the neurochemical process of AA.

Recently Professor Zang Hee Cho and his research team at the University of California, Irvine, cooperated with Tian Tan Hospital in Beijing and have obtained new evidence by using functional magnetic resonance imaging (fMRI) techniques (Chapter 4). Our explanation of AA mechanisms is oversimplified for the purpose of this textbook. For example, after pain impulses reach the spinal cord, at least six neural pathways transmit those impulses from the spinal cord to the cerebral cortex, and numerous neurochemicals are released at different sites to modulate pain signals, such as three different endorphins (enkephalin, beta-endorphin, and dynorphin), cholecystokinin (CCK), serotonin, adrenocorticotrophic hormone (ACTH), SOM, substance P, vasoactive intestinal peptide (VIP), neurotensin, CGRP, gamma-aminobutyric acid (GABA), and more. Detailed

description of these interactions among the neurochemicals is beyond the scope of this clinical textbook. More detailed discussions are provided in Chapter 4.

The neurochemical mechanisms not only provide analgesia (pain relief) but also promote homeostasis and tissue healing and improve the immune system, the endocrine system, the cardiovascular system, other systems like the digestive system, and psychologic adjustment. These mechanisms explain why different problems, such as asthma, tinnitus, irritable bowel, gastric ulcers, and others, improve in the same course of pain treatment by acupuncture needling. Acupuncture restores the control system of the body and promotes self-healing, which are suppressed during the process of the disease or injury.

Mechanisms of pain perception and therefore its treatment involve the following parts of the nervous system:

1. The peripheral sensory nerve fibers, which are major components of acupoints
2. The spinal cord
3. The brain, particularly the brainstem, midbrain, thalamus, hypothalamus, pituitary gland, and cortex. They are all activated synergetically to modulate pain when needle lesions are induced by acupuncture treatment.

The quantitative nature of acupoint physiology discussed in previous chapters is the basis for our evaluation method and treatment protocol. Clinically we first select two types of acupoints (Chapter 5), local and distant, or symptomatic and homeostatic points. Local points are located in painful tissues and are more sensitive or are painful. In chronic cases these sensitized local points may stimulate neurons inside the spinal cord; they synapse with and finally sensitize those spinal neurons.[14]

Thus, when we stimulate the symptomatic acupoints, we also stimulate the sensitized neurons in the same segment of the spinal cord. This means we stimulate segmental circuits when we select local points. Distant points are located far from those local points, and their tenderness represents a homeostatic imbalance (Chapter 2).

Close attention should be directed to the phenomenon that homeostatic acupoints (HAs) become tender in a predictable sequence all over the body when homeostasis declines.[2] Everyone, including healthy persons, has a certain number of tender HAs all over the body. The difference between the healthy and the less healthy bodies is that the healthy ones have fewer tender HAs and the less healthy ones have more tender HAs. Those points, representing homeostatic changes, appear in predictable locations. In chronic cases more tender points are distributed all over the body. In a healthy person with an acute injury, tender points appear locally around the injured area. Clinically segmental (local) treatment may suffice for acute injuries, but both segmental (local or symptomatic) and nonsegmental (distal or homeostatic) points should be used for chronic symptoms to achieve optimal self-healing. Now it is clear that when we place needles into local painful points, AA is produced through segmental mechanism. If we use distal points, AA works through a nonsegmental mechanism. These mechanisms enhance one another.

Neural mechanisms in AA can be explained step by step as shown in Figure 3-2. Pain (cell 1) sends messages to the spinal cord, where they are relayed up through pathways (cell 2) to the brain centers, thalamus, and cortex; these messages are perceived as pain (see Chapter 4). When we use acupuncture to treat this pain, we select both local (segmental circuit) and distal (nonsegmental circuit) acupoints. Wherever we insert a needle into a patient's body, the needling stimulates afferent sensory receptors of small-diameter nerves in the skin and muscles, as discussed previously (cutaneous A-delta and C fibers, muscular type III and IV fibers, sometimes type II fibers).

Let us start with the examination of segmental mechanism. During the needling of a local point in the painful area, the impulses travel from the acupoint (cell 5) to the spinal cord (cell 6) to activate spinal neurons (cell 7) and secrete enkephalin and dynorphin to inhibit the pain messages. Next the needle impulses are relayed through cell 6 to the midbrain (cells 8 and 9) and the pituitary. The midbrain uses enkephalin to activate the raphe descending pain-inhibition system (cell 11).

The pain-inhibition system (cell 11) secretes monoamines, serotonin, and norepinephrine to inhibit pain transmission through dual functions:

1. Inhibition of ascending pain messages
2. Activation of spinal cord neurons (cell 7) synergetically with cell 6 to inhibit any incoming pain message from cell 1. The hypothalamus/pituitary, activated by the needling signals from the spinal cord (cell 6), releases beta-endorphin into the blood and cerebral spinal fluid, promoting physiologic analgesia and homeostasis of

numerous systems, including the immune system, cardiovascular system, respiratory system, and tissue healing. The hypothalamus/pituitary also secretes ACTH to activate the adrenaline gland to modify pain sensation and immune reaction. This HPA-axis is part of the central mechanism of acupuncture and will be discussed in Chapter 4.

Finally the needling signals generate neuronal activities in the highest brain level, the neocortical area. Professor Zang-Hee Cho and his research team provided the first scientific evidence for this central processing.[15] This cortical processing is responsible for the modulation of pain perception.

It is clear that when distal points (nonsegmental circuit) are selected, the needle impulses bypass spinal cord neuron 7 and travel directly to the supraspinal level: the midbrain and pituitary/hypothalamus. Segmental circuits (local points) activate the spinal cord, in addition to the midbrain and pituitary/hypothalamus. To achieve maximal results, both segmental (symptomatic acupoints) and nonsegmental (homeostatic acupoints) circuits should be used.

To summarize, local points (also called Ashi, segmental, or symptomatic acupoints) directly inhibit pain messages, and distal (homeostatic) points promote systemic homeostasis. They synergistically enhance pain relief and healing.

Using this scientific rationale, the physiology of the acupoint system, and our clinical evidence, we designed an Integrative Neuromuscular Acupoint System (INMAS) protocol using both segmental and nonsegmental mechanisms for practically every kind of peripheral pain symptom. In general, symptomatic acupoints (SAs) are selected for specific symptoms, and HAs are selected for nonspecific effect to restore systemic homeostasis. Thus our INMAS protocol, which combines SAs, HAs, and paravertebral acupoints (PAs), can be applied to a variety of symptoms recorded in the classic acupuncture literature. Please note that PAs and SAs are on the peripheral nerves of the same segments.

BLOOD COAGULATION SYSTEM AND IMMUNE COMPLEMENT SYSTEM

A needle-induced lesion is a minute trauma to the tissue cells and mostly causes invisible tiny internal bleeding. This lesion activates the restorative con-

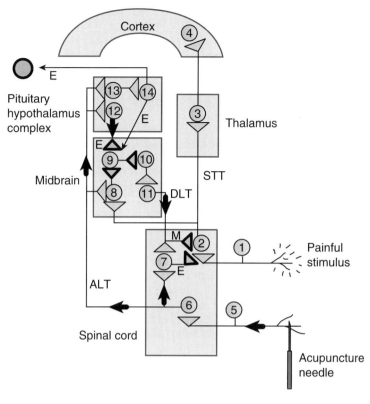

Figure 3-2 Neural mechanism of acupuncture analgesia. *E,* Endorphins; *M,* monoamines; *ALT,* anterolateral tract; *DLT,* dorsolateral tract; *STT,* spinothalamic tract. (Redrawn from Stux *G,* Hammerschlag *R,* editors: *Clinical acupuncture scientific basis,* Berlin, 2001, Springer.)

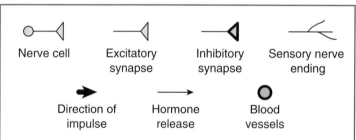

trol mechanisms involving the neuroendocrine-cardiovascular–mediated immune response, and thus promotes tissue healing and homeostatic restoration, resulting in systemic healing of the whole body in addition to local healing of the pathological symptoms.

Needling-induced chemicals from lesioned connective tissue such as collagen fibers and mast cells activate blood coagulation factor XII (the Hageman factor). In addition to causing blood coagulation, factor XII activates other factors to attract immune cells to the site of needling. The lesioned tissue cells stimulate mast cells and produce peptides such as bradykinin and histamine, whose peripheral function includes vasodilatation

and increased vascular permeability and immune-related cytokines.

The enhanced vasodilatation of capillaries improves blood flow to the site and enables immune cells to move from the blood circulation to trigger the defensive immune reaction around the needling lesion. Chemicals are released to activate immune cells and excite nociceptive sensory fibers.

When the needle is removed, tissue repair processes are stimulated, lesioned cells are digested, and protein synthesis is mobilized. The lesion-induced healing is directed by systemic neurohormonal mechanisms. The pituitary starts to increase the blood volume of ACTH, which triggers synthesis and the secretion of physiologic corticosteroids and other hormones . This process protects the body from stress, including reduction of the inflammatory reaction (see Chapter 4). Descending neural control systems from the brain inhibit and desensitize the nociceptive neurons in the spinal cord and peripheral nerve endings, and balance the ANS, which normalizes blood flow and energy metabolism. Finally the body's homeostasis is improved or restored and local tissue healing and pain relief are accelerated.

SUMMARY

Acupuncture needling therapy is a drugless inoculation of minute "traumas" or lesions into the body to restore the mechanisms of self-healing, including autonomic homeostasis, tissue healing, and pain relief. At the needling site, a cutaneous microcurrent circuit is built to produce a current of injury (about 10 mA), which stimulates tissue growth. Mechanical stimulation from the needle, especially from needle manipulation, deforms the connective collagen and elastic fibers, which transduces signals for tissue healing and gene transcriptions.

The needling and its lesion also induce a local antiinflammatory reaction against the intrusive lesion. Endogenous muscle contracture (nonvoluntary muscle contraction), which creates an energy crisis in shortened muscles, can be relaxed by needling the corresponding acupoints to restore normal muscle physiology. Neurophysiologically there are segmental and nonsegmental neural mechanisms. Needling signals from symptomatic (segmental) points are processed at both the spinal cord and supraspinal cord centers (midbrain, thalamus, pituitary, and cortex); stimulation signals from distant homeostatic (nonsegmental) points may be directly relayed to supraspinal cord centers. Both mechanisms enhance one another to activate descending control systems, which includes the secretion of chemicals and hormones into the blood and cerebrospinal fluid to restore homeostasis and neural modulation of pain relief.

Patients respond differently to acupuncture treatments because of their physiological differences. About 28% of the clinic population are excellent responders, 64% good and average responders, and 8% weak or nonresponders.[2]

Differentiation of patients and prediction of prognosis are important parts of the treatment procedure in acupuncture therapy. Understanding the needling mechanisms facilitates development of a practical protocol for all pain symptoms. Our INMAS protocol (see Chapter 5) simplifies the process of point selection. INMAS provides a standardized protocol required by Western medicine and ensures the personalized treatment practiced in TCM. Our 16-point quantitative evaluation method provides a generally predictable prognosis of pain management.

This chapter discusses the peripheral effects of acupuncture stimulation. Chapter 4 presents a discussion of the central effects of acupuncture stimulation. To help understand both peripheral and central mechanisms, a brief outline of both mechanisms is provided here.

It is clear that acupuncture stimulation, with both peripheral and central effects, activates the physiologic processes of built-in complex survival mechanisms to restore and maintain homeostasis. The peripheral effects involve the creation of needle-induced lesions, cutaneous microcurrent, mechanical signal transduction through connective tissues, local relief of muscle shortening and contracture, and other local neuroendocrine-immune reactions. The central effects are a form of CNS response resulting from peripheral sensory stimulation. This response includes the neural immune interaction, the humoral and ANS, especially vagus nerve pathways, and the neural efferents based on other hypothalamic neural circuits. It should be emphasized that the peripheral and central effects of acupuncture stimulation are physiologically inseparable.

Newly available molecular imaging tools such as high-resolution and high-sensitivity molecular-imaging positron emission tomography (PET) and high-field fMRI enable us to investigate the mechanisms of the human brain, especially the higher brain (the cortex), such as neurochemical and hemodynamic responses in vivo to acupuncture stimulation. The information gained from these tools will promote better understanding of the mechanisms of acupuncture and help to select more effective clinical procedures.

The central effects of acupuncture stimulation activate the four front lines of homeostasis: (1) the nervous system, (2) the immune system, (3) the endocrine system, and (4) the cardiovascular system controlled by neural pathways such as the ANS, especially the vagus nerve pathway. These built-in homeostatic survival mechanisms are discussed briefly in Chapter 4.

All the available scientific data definitely support and justify the INMAS (see Chapter 5) and its clinical application. Both laboratory and clinical data match and agree with each other. The following points explain how the fMRI data support clinical procedures.

1. Some acupoints produce more analgesic effects than others.

   Acupoints are neurogenic. Stimulation of any sensory and postganglionic nerve endings in the body produces analgesic effects both locally and systemically. Nevertheless, certain acupoints associated with certain nerve structures such as major nerve trunks or other particular anatomic configurations (see Chapters 1 and 2) produce more effective analgesia or therapeutic results. The 24 HAs listed in Chapter 5 (also see the inside cover) are such acupoints. These 24 HAs represent the most important acupoints in the classic meridian system and contain the major features of neuromuscular configurations. In plain language, as Professor Cho said in a *Newsweek* interview, "We may find that one well-placed needle can do what we now do with 20."[16] In Chapter 4, readers will find that in fMRI experiments, stimulation of both homeostatic acupoint H5 deep peroneal (Liv 3, Taichong) and a "sham" acupoint produce analgesic effects, but H5 reduces more pain signals in the cerebral cortex.

2. Twenty-four homeostatic acupoints are standardized for every patient and used for AA, regardless of the specific cause of the pain symptoms.

   Clinically we should select the acupoints that are able to produce more AA effects. fMRI data (see Chapter 4) and electrophysiologic data (Ma, Y.-T. , unpublished) indicate that, at least in AA, stimulation of any acupoint activates similar analgesic effects at supraspinal levels, such as in the midbrain and cortices. This means that any randomly selected acupoint may produce pain relief. However, symptomatic acupoints activate both peripheral and central analgesic mechanisms, whereas distal points such as distal homeostatic acupoints activate mostly central analgesic mechanisms. Thus it is very important to select more effective SAs. To achieve this, a clinician should have a practical knowledge of pathophysiology, anatomy, and body mechanics. We have provided this basic knowledge in the clinical chapters.

   Clinical data also suggest that 24 HAs produce AA in more than 92% of all patients (see Chapter 6) with different pain symptoms. Application of these 24 HAs simplifies clinical procedure while providing sufficient AA effects.

3. More about acupoint specificity: the segmental principle.

   Both fMRI and clinical data agree in that stimulation of any sensory nerve endings produces AA effects in the spinal cord and brain. The difference among the stimuli to different acupoints is that some points produce more AA effects than others. In clinical practice, however, practitioners need to consider the segmental nature when selecting some acupoints (see Chapter 5). For example, when treating elbow problems, PAs along C4-T1 are selected because SAs in the elbow and PAs along C4-T1 belong to the same spinal segments. In the same way, paravertebral acupoints along L2-L5 are selected for treating knee pain. These combinations of SAs (such as in the elbow or the knee) with PAs are based simply on the segmental innervation of the spinal nerves.

References

1. Pomeranz B: Acupuncture analgesia—basic research. In Stux G, Hammerschlag R, editors: *Clinical acupuncture scientific basis,* Berlin, 2001, Springer.
2. Dung HC: Physiology in acupuncture. In *Anatomical acupuncture,* San Antonio, Texas, 1997, Antarctic Press.
3. Langevin HM, Yandow JA: Relationship of acupuncture points and meridians to connective tissue planes, *Anat Rec* 269(6),257-265, 2002.
4. Levine JD, Fields HL, Basbaum AI: Peptides and the primary afferent nociceptor, *J Neurosci.*13:2273-2286, 1993.
5. Becker O, et al: Electrophysiological correlates of acupuncture points and meridians, *Psychoenergetic Systems* 1:195-212, 1976.
6. Melzack R, Katz J: Auriculotherapy fails to relieve chronic pain, *JAMA* 251:1041 1043, 1984.
7. Jaffe L, et al: The glabrous epidermis of cavies contains a powerful battery, *Am J Physiol* 242:R358-R366, 1982.
8. Pomeranz B: Effects of applied DC fields on sensory nerve sprouting and motor nerve regeneration in adult rats. In Nuccitelli R, editor: *Ionic currents in development,* New York, 1986, Alan R Liss.
9. Han JS, Tang J, Huang BS: Acupuncture tolerance in rats: antiopiate substrates implicated, *Chin Med J* 92:625-627, 1979.
10. Langevin HM, Churchill DL, Cipolla M: Mechanical signaling through connective tissue: a mechanism of the therapeutic effect of acupuncture, *FASEB J* 15:2275-2282, 2001.
11. O'Reilly KP, Warhol MJ, Fielding RA, et al: Eccentric exercise-induced muscle damage impairs muscle glycogen repletion, *J Appl Physiol* 63:252-256, 1987.
12. He X, Proske U, Shcaible H-G, et al: Acute inflammation of the knee joint in the cat alters responses of flexor

motoneurons to leg movements, *J Neurophysiol* 59:326-340, 1988.

13. Simons DG: Referred phenomena of myofascial trigger points. In Vecchiet L, et al, editors: *Pain research and clinical management: New trends in referred pain and hyperalgesia, vol 27,* Amsterdam, 1993, Elsevier.

14. Dubner R, Ruda MA: Activity dependent neuronal plasticity following tissue injury and inflammation, *Trends Neurosci* 15:96-103, 1992.

15. Cho Z-H, et al: Functional magnetic resonance imaging of the brain in the investigation of acupuncture. In Stux G, Hammerschlag R, editors: *Clinical acupuncture,* Berlin, 2001, Springer.

16. Cowley G: Now, 'integrative' care, *Newsweek* December 2, 2002, p. 50

CHAPTER 4

The Neural Bases of Acupuncture: Central Mechanisms

BASIC CONCEPTS: BRAIN, ORGANS, AND ACUPUNCTURE

New Imaging Techniques and Understanding the Brain

Based on recent developments in neuroscience, it is possible to recognize many classes of diseases that are directly or indirectly related to our brain and spinal cord, collectively known as the central nervous system (CNS). Early work on the β-endorphin theory suggests that cortical involvement follows acupuncture stimulation. Indeed numerous hypotheses on acupuncture analgesia (AA) can be successfully explained by neuronal mechanisms that correlate with the brain, such as the humoral and autonomic nervous functions of the hypothalamus and the brainstem. It is increasingly clear that acupuncture stimulation leads to activation and deactivation of the upper parts of the brain or upper cortical areas via various spinal tracts. In return its reflexes project back to the lower parts of the brain, from the upper brain via the brainstem, where it is believed that many survival-related autonomic functions are regulated.

A vast amount of clinical experience with traditional acupuncture has been gained over thousands of years.[1-6] On the other hand, over the last several decades, Western medicine has progressed rapidly in both techniques and physiologic understanding of disease. The mechanisms of treatment have benefited from numerous newly developed medical techniques, such as X-ray computed tomography (XCT) and magnetic resonance imaging (MRI). With these developments it is now possible to visualize the inner organs of our living human body as well as the brain in vivo. More recently the development of functional imaging devices such as positron emission tomography (PET)[7-9] and functional MRI (fMRI)[10-12] has brought about a revolution in our understanding of the brain. PET and fMRI now allow us to image minute changes in glucose utilization as well as

oxygen consumption in different parts of the brain. These techniques allow us to observe the brain's energy metabolism and oxygenation status with a spatial and temporal resolution never before possible.[9] Most importantly these technical advances allow us to investigate cortical responses of the brain as a function of acupuncture stimulation, such as the correlation of a specific stimulation with a specific cortical response.[13-15] Direct observation of the human brain in vivo while the body is receiving acupuncture stimulation opens a new era in acupuncture research. In addition this information on cortical activation provides clues about how acupuncture works, that is, the nature of the mechanisms involved in acupuncture treatment. These remarkable developments have the potential to finally unravel the millennia-old enigma of acupuncture.

Neural Substrates of Pain Signal Processing

Let us examine the analgesic effect of acupuncture, one of the commonest modalities in acupuncture treatment. First it is necessary to study the basic pain mechanism, from which will follow an explanation of how AA works. In an experiment, pain stimulation was induced by immersion of the index finger into a bath of hot water (about 52° C) for a period of 30 seconds.[16] The activation of cortical areas caused by pain stimulation was obtained by fMRI and is shown in Figure 4-1. Three areas are notably involved with pain signal processing and these are indicated by three rectangles (the dorsal anterior cingulate cortex [dACC], the caudal anterior cingulate cortex [cACC], and the rostral anterior cingulate cortex [rACC]) to illustrate more completely the details of the activation pattern. These three areas were chosen because they are believed to be the most significant cortical areas concerned with pain processing, that is, dACC for pain signal "riveting or attention-focusing," cACC for "perception" of the emotional component of

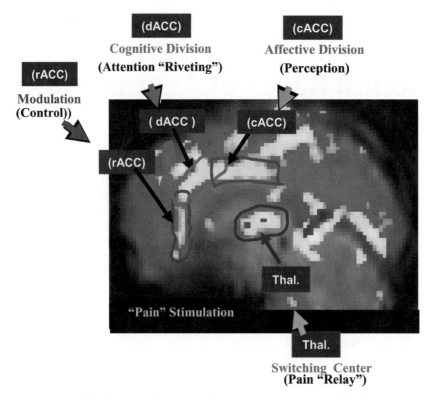

Figure 4-1   Neural substrates of pain signal processing. Activation of the key pain processing cortical areas. Three areas are noted that are believed to be the major cortical areas involved in pain processing: the dorsal anterior cingulate cortex (dACC) for pain signal riveting or attention focusing, the caudal anterior cingulate cortex (cACC) for perception of the emotional component of pain, and the rostral anterior cingulate cortex (rACC) for modulation or control of pain. In addition, the thalamus, the main relay station, is also shown.

pain, and rACC for "modulation or control" of pain.

The thalamic areas, believed to be the major components of pain signal relay and attention selection centers, are also activated. A most intriguing aspect of this study is that the time-differential activation pattern provides important clues about how various parts of the cingulate cortex are involved in the perception and modulation of pain and in pain processing.[16] For instance the rACC is activated during the last minutes of observation, suggesting that some form of the pain modulation process (e.g., the release of endogenous opioids, which initiate the inhibitory process by a stress effect resulting from sustained pain) is taking place at this late period because of sustained pain, as discussed by Zubieta et al.[17] Considering the fact that all the cingulate cortices, dACC, cACC, and rACC, together with the thalamus, are activated as a result of pain stimulation, one can hypothesize that the

main part of the pain signal processing is a central process rather than a peripheral process. Pain signal relay, attention focusing, pain perception, and modulation or control are all processed in the brain's center, the cortical and subcortical centers of the brain, including the ACC and the thalamus. This dynamic pain processing pathway appears to provide key information for understanding pain relief mechanisms, such as AA.

ACUPUNCTURE ANALGESIA AND ITS NEURAL SUBSTRATES

Observation of Acupuncture Analgesia by Functional Magnetic Resonance Imaging

Meridian (Homeostatic) Acupoint   The pain and pain-relief mechanisms involved in AA are complex, and science has yet to provide a convincing physiological explanation of them. Although acupuncture has been used for many centuries,[1-6] scientific evidence for the physiology and efficacy of pain treatment has not been established. Possible mechanisms for pain relief in AA have been studied in the West since 1965, beginning with the pioneering work of Melzack and Wall.[3] Although rigorous scientific explanations are rare and other evidence is mostly anecdotal, acupuncture has been reported to successfully treat many classes of disease, and be especially effective for the control of pain.[1-6,18] As discussed in the previous section, brain imaging tools such as PET and fMRI have made it possible to visualize directly brain function in vivo. fMRI experiments using the new data-processing technique known as dynamic regression analysis are providing the opportunity to study physiologically modulated cortical activation due to "pain stimulation" as well as "pain stimulation after the administration of acupuncture."[16] For the AA study, thermal stimulation was applied in the same way as in the pain study (i.e., immersing the index finger into a bath of hot water with a temperature of 52° C for a duration of 30 seconds). This stimulation resulted in a sequence of different sensations: feelings of heat, unpleasantness, extreme pain, and unbearable pain. Acupuncture stimulus was applied (or administered) to the meridian (homeostatic) acupoints H5 deep fibular (peroneal, Taichong) with manual twirling or rotating of the needle for 30 seconds (approximately one rotation per second), resting for 30 seconds without twirling the needle, and then repeating five

times without removing the needle, after which the needle was removed for the remainder of the data acquisition period.[19,20] Application of the pain stimulation was continued for 4 minutes after completing the acupuncture stimulation. From this experiment some new observations were made about the relationship between cortical activation and pain as well as the pain-relief mechanism of acupuncture. The experimental data suggest that the cortical areas related to pain signal relaying, attention-focusing or riveting, and perception are the anterior cingulate gyrus and the thalamic areas, as mentioned earlier.[16] The experimental results obtained from "pain" and "acupuncture + pain" stimulation are illustrated in Figure 4-2. The activation pattern resulting from pain stimulation alone showed activation of various cortical areas, including the cingulate cortex, the thalamus, and the motor areas (see Figure 4-1). On the other hand, the "acupuncture + pain" experiment revealed a significant decrease in activation of the ACC and the thalamic areas as well as the motor areas. Most of the activations seen in the cingulate cortex and the thalamic nuclei with pain alone become diminished after acupuncture, suggesting that the administration of acupuncture indeed desensitizes or blocks pain perception.[20]

"Sham" Acupoints: Comparison of Meridian (Homeostatic) and "Sham" Acupoint Stimulation As shown in the previous study on "pain" and "pain with administration of acupuncture,"

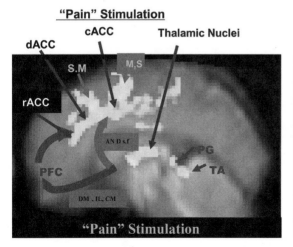
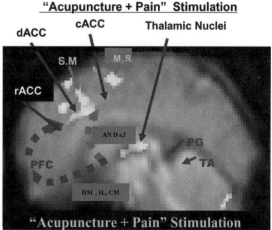

Figure 4-2 Cortical activation maps resulting from "pain" stimulation and "acupuncture + pain" stimulation, respectively. A significant decrease in activation is seen in most of the pain signal processing areas, which include the cingulate cortex and the thalamus.

there appears to be substantial deactivation of the cortical areas when acupuncture is administered compared to when it is not, especially in areas involved with pain signal processing. One of the most interesting aspects of acupuncture, however, is the point specificity, that is, how accurately the acupoint must be localized and how the outcome of the acupuncture treatment is affected by uncertainty in localization. This question of point specificity was studied by comparing the result of traditional "meridian" acupoint stimulation with the result of stimulating "sham" points.[19,20] Please note that the "meridian" acupoint Liv 3 Taichong used in these experiments is one of the 24 homeostatic acupoints (HAs) H5 deep fibular (peroneal) described in Chapter 5. All 24 of these HAs are in fact major meridian acupoints in the traditional acupuncture system (see Appendix II). "Sham" points are deliberately chosen as much as a few centimeters away from the traditional meridian acupoints. This study was a comparison of two sets of experiments, namely, one with "pain" versus "meridian acupuncture + pain" and the other with "pain" versus "sham acupuncture + pain." Figure 4-3 shows the results.[19,20]

When the results of "pain" versus "sham acupuncture + pain" (see Figure 4-3, C and D) are compared with the traditional "pain" versus "meridian acupuncture + pain" results (see Figure 4-3, A and B), there appears to be very little difference, which suggests that sham and meridian acupuncture might share a common mechanism.

This finding also brings into question the point specificity of acupuncture, at least in the case of AA.[20]

The similarity of the activation patterns in the two cases of meridian and sham acupuncture supports the hypothesis that the effect of acupuncture, at least for AA, is simply the effect of the stress-induced hypothalamic-pituitary-adrenal (HPA) axis response (the pathways are discussed more specifically below). That is, decreased activation may be due to "sustained pain stress" rather than to stimulation of a specific point as is taught in traditional acupuncture.[17,21] Acupuncture or acupuncture-like sensory stimulation induces activation of the HPA axis and therefore activation of the endogenous central opiate circuitry, thereby reducing or inhibiting the ascending pain signals.

HYPOTHESIS OF ACUPUNCTURE MECHANISMS

Hypothesis of Acupuncture Mechanisms and Neural Substrates

Humoral, Neural, and Immune Responses Related to Acupuncture   As already described, acupuncture therapy has demonstrated efficacy in several clinical areas; among these is pain. Although the understanding of pain has progressed immensely in the last two decades,[1-6,18] the underlying mechanisms of acupuncture in general and its analgesic effect in particular are still not clearly delineated.

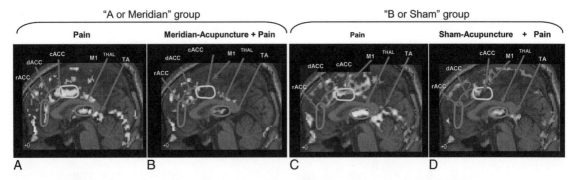

Figure 4-3   Comparison of the functional magnetic resonance imaging (fMRI) results of "pain" versus "meridian acupuncture + pain" and "pain" versus "sham acupuncture + pain" experiments. **A,** The activation pattern resulting from pain stimulation of the A group. **B,** Pain after the administration of "meridian" acupuncture stimulation of the A group. **C,** Pain stimulation of the B group. **D,** Pain after the administration of "sham" acupuncture of the B group. Both meridian or A group and sham or B group acupuncture show substantially decreased activity in most of the areas compared with pain stimulation alone, namely, the dorsal anterior cingulate cortex (dACC), the caudal ACC (cACC), and the rostral ACC (rACC) as well as the thalamus.

The leading hypotheses include the effects of local stimulation, neuronal gating, the release of endogenous opiates, and the placebo effect. Accumulating evidence suggests that the CNS is essential for the processing of these effects via its modulation of the autonomic nervous system (ANS), the neuroimmune system, and hormonal regulation. Because these processes are programmed into basic survival mechanisms, it appears vital to seek an understanding of the effects of acupuncture within a framework of neuroscience.

In view of the preceding results, we propose a model that incorporates the stress-induced HPA axis model of Maier et al[22] and Akil et al,[23] the cholinergic antiinflammatory action model of Tracey et al,[24-26] and the recently observed neuroimaging results of Cho et al,[19,20] Zubieta et al,[17] and Petrovic et al.[21] As already mentioned, over the last two decades there have been numerous developments in neuroscience concerning pain, the ANS, the immune system, and functional brain imaging.[27-33] The underlying mechanisms of acupuncture, however, have appeared too diverse to be understood in a quantitative and rational manner and require further study. Because acupuncture therapy is claimed to be effective in many conditions, including acute pain, investigators have attempted to explain the underlying mechanism of acupuncture in many different ways: as an effect of local stimuli, a neural reflexive response, a humoral outflow response, and a placebo effect.[1-6,34] In addition, physiologic studies using animal models and human subjects have also been developed to explain AA and these have generated increasing scientific support and enhanced the credibility of acupuncture as a treatment option.[1-6]

One clear fact is that the CNS controls the autonomic processes related to visceral reactivity; cognitive processes related to pain perception, learning, and memory; and other physiologic processes related to pain. Regardless of which pathways are being contemplated, whether it is supposed to work by neural, humoral, or neuroimmunologic interactions, it appears inevitable that the brain is involved in the behavioral effects of acupuncture. The CNS is precisely the network that is essential for information processing between afferent stimuli (inputs) and efferent responses (outputs), as well as control of stress hormones, the ANS, and even the immune system, all of which are essential for survival. On the other hand, recently developed brain imaging techniques, such as PET and fMRI, are beginning to shed light on the workings of the human brain, including acupuncture-related cortical responses.[7-15] Because

these techniques provide the opportunity to observe neuronal activities directly, both spatially (anatomically) and temporally (in a time-dependent manner), they allow quantitative analysis of the living brain while it is engaged in deliberate actions (e.g., acupuncture or acupuncture-like stimulation). As a result recent acupuncture research has been directed increasingly toward neuroimaging, with molecular science and pharmacokinetics as its bases.[16-20]

In this section, we briefly review how the scientific understanding of acupuncture has recently evolved based on neuroimmunophysiologic and molecular aspects, and evidence obtained by functional brain imaging.[13-21,27-34] In addition, we propose a hypothesis, as well as a model, of the acupuncture mechanism that includes the stress-induced HPA-axis hypothesis,[22,23] the neural-immune interaction of the cholinergic antiinflammatory activity hypothesis,[24-26] and the recently obtained neuroimaging evidence.[17,19-21]

Immune Neural Interaction and the Hypothalamic-Pituitary-Adrenal Axis Hypothesis

Let us first look at the recent series of studies conducted by Maier et al and Tracey and colleagues,[22-26] which describe the interactions between the immune system and the brain as well as the effects of the ANS on immune functions; they also begin to show how the brain controls certain types of inflammation and therefore pain. In particular, Tracey's review provides interesting and important clues for the formulation and understanding of acupuncture mechanisms. For example, it explains that inflammatory information is transmitted through sensory nerves to the hypothalamus, where input signals are processed, resulting in an antiinflammatory output via the humoral system and the ANS via the well-known HPA axis, as briefly described earlier. The similar idea that acupuncture is involved in the immune system has recently been supported by observations under various clinical conditions, and it has been suspected that acupuncture might affect immune modulation.[27,28] Although actual scientific evidence has yet to be confirmed, the work on neuroimmune and autonomic reflexes by Maier et al (see also Besedovsky et al[29]) and Tracy and colleagues could form an important basis for understanding the acupuncture mechanism as a neural-immune reflex.[24-26] More specifically they have discovered that tumor necrosis factor alpha (TNF-α) and other cytokines (e.g., interleukin-1β) exist in the brain and directly interact with the inflammatory immune system in the periphery or vice versa (i.e., from periphery to brain). By communicating with the brain it produces neural outflows via humoral and ANS pathways.[23-26] For example, parasympathetic nerve endings release acetylcholine (ACh), which has a resulting antiinflammatory effect; that is, the immune system interaction appears to suppress the synthesis of inflammatory cytokines, such as TNF-α and interleukin-1β (IL-1β). This observation of the cholinergic suppression of inflammatory cytokines is a new factor that could play an important role in understanding the mechanisms of acupuncture.[24]

In addition, the blood-borne pathway contributes via the circumventricular (CV) area, including the postrema and subfornical organs.[23] The dorsal vagal complex and the dorsal motor nucleus of the vagus nerve are also known to respond to circulating TNF concentrations and activate the HPA axis, thereby inducing the release of glucocorticoids and other hormonal substances (e.g., melanocyte-stimulating hormone [MSH], spermine), which subsequently further suppress inflammatory cytokine synthesis such as IL-1b and TNF-α.[24,25]

Different Modes of Acupuncture or Acupuncture-like Stimuli

Based on Tracey's concept of vagus nerve stimulation, and including possible reflexive factors that have an antiinflammatory effect on the inflamed area,[24,25,29] the hypothesis of afferent vagus nerve stimulation can be extended to incorporate somatic stimulation. In other words, the afferent visceral and somatic acupuncture signals that can be transmitted to the supraspinal level for the induction of the reflexive antiinflammatory signals, through both humoral and neural mechanisms, could be important components of acupuncture. These are summarized in Figure 4-4. In other words, several different modes of acupuncture or acupuncture-like sensory stimuli can be noted as follows:

1. Efferent vagus nerve acupuncture (EVA) or efferent vagus nerve stimulation
2. Afferent vagus nerve acupuncture (AVA) or afferent vagus nerve stimulation
3. Afferent somatic nerve acupuncture (ASA) or afferent somatic nerve stimulation

Through each different afferent and efferent stimulus, a number of distinctive descending antiinflammatory signals, both direct and reflexive, will be induced (see antiinflammatory efferent shown in the inset of Figure 4-4) as a result of the afferent

cytokine signaling of TNF-α, IL-1β, and high-mobility group B-1:

1. A direct antiinflammatory efferent (signal I) resulting from EVA via the dorsal motor nucleus of the vagus (DMV)
2. An antiinflammatory efferent (signal II) resulting from AVA via the nucleus of solitary tracts (NST) and the resulting humoral and ANS reflexives by the hypothalamus or via the HPA axis
3. An antiinflammatory efferent (signal III) resulting from the ASA via brainstem nuclei other than NST and the resulting humoral and ANS reflexives (especially the sympathetic outflows) by the hypothalamus or via the HPA axis

As Tracey and colleagues demonstrated, efferent vagus nerve stimulation (e.g., EV acupuncture) resulted in an increase of efferent vagus nerve cholinergic activity, which had an antiinflammatory effect as a result of suppressing inflammatory cytokines, such as TNF-α, IL-1β, and HMGB-1. These facts suggest that afferent vagus nerve stimulation, or AVA, would work in a similar way, possibly via the supraspinal reflex (the HPA axis), and would have a more global and nonspecific reflexive effect confined mostly to the visceral organs. The most widely used acupuncture stimulation, however, appears to be ASA by the insertion of acupuncture needles into the cutaneous tissues or skin and muscle. One could expect that it might also have a similar effect, possibly with even broader and more diffuse efferent nerve activities, covering both generalized sympathetic and vagus or parasympathetic nerve activities, as shown in the efferent nerve signals, such as signal III (see Figure 4-4). The latter may also work via the HPA axis (see discussion of neural substrates and afferents below, and shown in Figure 4-5).

Afferents to the Paraventricular Nucleus of the Hypothalamus and the Neural Substrates

To substantiate the preceding discussions, it is worthwhile to look at the stress-related circuit, which could provide important clues. The most promising model so far is that of the stress-induced HPA cortical or adrenal medullary (HPA) axis.[22,23] We propose to extend this model to a broad-sense HPA (BS-HPA) axis, which includes the neuroimmune interactions, ANS outflows, and other neural projections, such as the projection to the

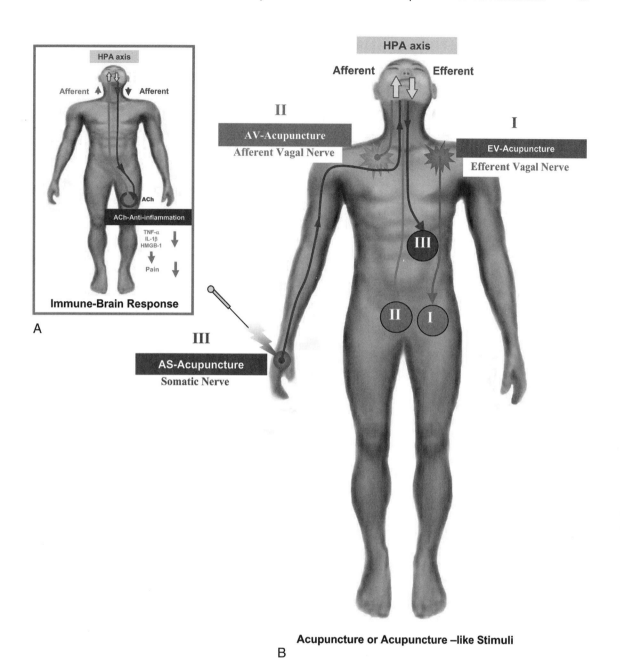

Figure 4-4   Three modes of efferent or outflows as a result of acupuncture or acupuncture-like stimuli. **I,** Efferent pathways due to efferent vagus (EV) nerve acupuncture or stimulation. **II,** Efferent pathways due to afferent vagus (AV) nerve acupuncture or stimulation. **III,** Efferent pathways due to afferent somatic (AS) nerve acupuncture or stimulation. *HPA axis,* Hypothalamus-pituitary-adrenal axis; *TNF-α,* tumor necrosis factor-α; *IL-1β,* interleukin-1β; *HMGB-1,* high mobility group B-1.

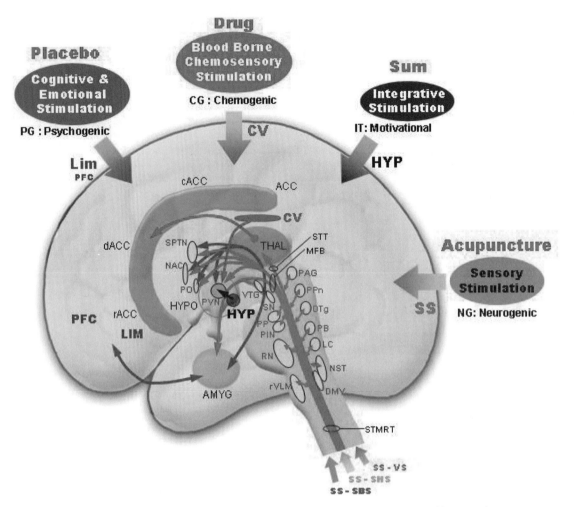

Figure 4-5 Possible outflows resulting from acupuncture or acupuncture-like stimulus. Four major input signals are possibly involved in stress-induced hypothalamic-pituitary-adrenal (HPA) axis: sensory (via the somatic and vagus nerve) stimulus, cognitive and emotional (via the prefrontal area and limbic system) stimulus, blood-borne chemosensory (via the circumventricular area), and the final integrative component (via the hypothalamus). These inputs are believed to be projected to the paraventricular nucleus (PVN; the medial parvocellular part) of the hypothalamus, which would then generate the outflows. *HYPO,* Hypothalamus; *THAL,* thalamus; *AMYG,* amygdala; *PFC,* prefrontal cortex; *ACC,* anterior cingulate cortex; *RN,* raphe nuclei; *PAG,* periaqueductal gray; *PIN,* posterior-interpeduncular nucleus; *DMV,* dorsal motor nucleus of vagus; *PP,* peripeduncular nucleus; *rVLM,* rostral ventrolateral medulla; *SPTN,* septal nucleus; *NAC,* nucleus accumbens; *PO,* preoptic nucleus; *PVN,* paraventricular nucleus; *VTG,* ventral tegmental area: dopaminergic; *SN,* substantia nigra: dopaminergic; *LC,* locus caeruleus: noradrenergic; *PB,* parabrachial nucleus: noradrenergic; *DTg,* dorsal tegmental area: cholinergic; *rACC, dACC, cACC,* rostral, dorsal, caudal ACC; *PPn,* pontine peduncular nuclei: cholinergic; *MFB,* medial forebrain bundle; *STT,* spinothalamic tract; *CV,* circumventricular organs; *LIM,* limbic system; *HYP,* hypothalamic integration; *SS,* sensory stimulation; *SS-SBS,* SS-somatic body sensory; *SS-SHS,* SS-somatic head & special; *SS-VS,* SS-visceral sensory.

periaqueductal gray-raphe axis. This model appears appropriate because the hypothalamus is also the origin of the ANS as well as other neural outputs.[35]

It is well known that vagus nerve stimulation may have a reflexive antiinflammatory effect on an inflamed area. This discussion extends the afferent vagus nerve stimulation hypothesis to the somatic stimulation, including the ASA, which will be projected to the supraspinal level for the induction of the reflexive antiinflammatory signals through the BS-HPA axis, that is, via the neuroimmune interactions, humoral system, ANS, and other neural systems.[22-26]

In summary, four major input signals are possibly involved in the stress-induced HPA axis: the sensory stimulus (via the somatic and vagus nerves), the cognitive and emotional stimulus (via the prefrontal area and limbic system), the blood-borne chemosensory stimulus (via the circumventricular area), and the final integrative component (via the hypothalamus). These inputs are believed to be projected to the paraventricular nucleus (PVN; the medial parvocellular part) of the hypothalamus, which would then generate the outflows.[23] The cognitive and emotional stimulus might have a relationship to a psychogenic stimulus, such as a placebo,[21] whereas the blood-borne chemosensory stimulus is related to drug administration. The somatic and vagus nerve stimulation can be considered neurogenic stimulation, which possibly can be related to acupuncture or acupuncture-like sensory stimuli. The internal hypothalamic inputs to the PVN, such as the daily rhythmic variation of glucocorticoids and the condition of hunger (motivational) or satiety, could be important adjuncts to the modulation of the various effects of input stimuli, including acupuncture.

These four inputs then converge onto the PVN, that is, from the group that consists of the limbic system and the prefrontal cortex, the circumventricular (CV) area, the sensory stimuli pathways (SS), and the hypothalamus itself (HYP) (see Figure 4-5). These four inputs are shown together with various nuclei possibly involved with activation of the stress-induced HPA axis. Because our discussion here is limited to acupuncture, we will also limit it to sensory stimulation. Among the four afferents, the major afferents related to acupuncture needling are the SS pathways. Sensory stimulation consists of three major inputs or afferents, which will be projected to the PVN, possibly via activation of various neurons in the brainstem area. These pathways include one from the body (somatic-body sensory, SS-SBS); one from the head and facial regions (somatic head and special-

sensory afferents, SS-SHS, such as the visual and auditory pathways); and the visceral afferent (visceral sensory, SS-VS). These are probably the sensory stimuli that are acupuncture-related, and we call them *neurogenic components,* except for some parts of the visual and auditory aspects of SS-SHS. Most of the bodily somatic sensory stimuli excite the midbrain periaqueductal gray (PAG), the peduncular pontine (PPn), the dorsal tegmental nucleus (DTg), and the parabrachial nucleus (PB), among others. Some of the nociceptive inputs are believed to activate the PAG from where a projection is made to the PVN. Both the PPn and the DTg neurons are cholinergic and are believed to be projected to the PVN. The facial somatic inputs are also believed to terminate on the same areas (PAG, PPn, DTg). Some of the special sensory stimuli are believed to terminate at the peripeduncular nucleus (PP) and the posterior interpeduncular nucleus (PIN) as well as the PPn and the DTg. Because of the geometric proximity, visceral inputs are believed to terminate in and excite the dorsal and ventral medullary areas, including the nucleus of the solitary tracts (NST, areas A2 and C2) and rostral ventrolateral medulla (rVLM, areas A1, C1, C3). In the dorsolateral medulla, the NST and the LC (locus caeruleus) are the two major noradrenergic neuronal sites, and their outputs are believed to project to the PVN via the parabrachial nucleus following the medial forebrain bundle (MFB). Neurons at the lower and rostral ventrolateral medullary (rVLM) areas are adrenergic (C1, C3) and project to the PVN, again via the MFB. Serotonergic neurons in the dorsal raphe are also believed to be projected to the PVN as well as to the ventral raphe nuclei (B6, B7, B8), although direct involvement of these nuclei with the PVN is not known. In addition, the somatic sensory information conveyed to the thalamus, especially to the ventroposterolateral (VPL) or ventroposteromedial (VPM) nucleus of the thalamus, projects to the corresponding somatosensory cortex and then possibly to the secondary somatosensory cortex.

Parts of the neuronal projections from the PAG and other cholinergic neurons also project to the midline thalamic areas, such as the dorsomedial and intralaminar nucleus as well as the anterior nucleus of the thalamus, and then project to the ACC and also to the prefrontal cortex. The ACC is believed to be the signal processing center for incoming pain signals, including attention focusing, perception of the affective component of pain, and modulation.[19,20] Painful stimuli are believed to project to both the somatic and visceral afferents and also to the amygdala, the pain activating center, and finally to the PVN via the stria terminalis as shown in Figure 4-5. The hippocampus (not shown) is believed to play a key role in the negative feedback of glucocorticoids in the HPA axis.[29] These inputs, plus emotional and motivational information generated from the hypothalamus itself, are believed to be integrated by various nuclei within the hypothalamus. They project to the PVN, which then generates the outflow, as discussed in the following section.

Those four major inputs (SS, LIM, CV, and HYP) are shown in Figure 4-5. We can conceptualize these connections in common lay terms, such as *placebo, drug, motivational,* and *acupuncture.* For example, cognitive and emotional stimulation might have a relationship to more generally known psychogenic stimulation, such as the placebo effect, whereas the blood-borne chemosensory stimulation has a relationship to drug administration. Similarly the somatic and vagus nerve stimulation can be considered a form of related neurogenic stimulation, such as acupuncture needling.

Finally the internal hypothalamic inputs to the PVN, such as the daily rhythmic variation of glucocorticoids and the hunger (motivational) or satiety condition, could be an important adjunct to modulation of the various perceptual and healing effects of acupuncture. When the body has an insufficient level of glucocorticoids, it is most sensitive to input stimuli and also most vulnerable to the changes it encounters. The HPA axis is therefore most sensitive to the change of glucocorticoid level when the level is lowest, such as in the evening.[23]

Efferents (or Outflows) from the Hypothalamus

Major efferents or outflows from the PVN (and also perhaps from the PVN and the arcuate nucleus of the hypothalamus) that possibly result from acupuncture or acupuncture-like sensory stimuli may be conveyed via five distinctive pathways. The first group of pathways (group 1) is humoral, originating from the traditional HPA axis and projecting to the various organs in the body and the brain via the bloodstream. One is the pathway to the inflammatory area where immune-related leukocytes, such as macrophages, are induced, and the other is the pathway to the supraspinal CNS, as shown in Figure 4-6. The humoral pathway (no. 1) targets the macrophages in the inflammatory area and releases a number of antiinflammatory cytokines and hormones, including antiinflammatory cytokines such as IL-10, glucocorticoids, melanocyte stimulating hormone, spermine, and

oxytocin. These cytokines and hormones act on the macrophages as suppressors of inflammatory cytokine synthesis, such as synthesis of TNF-α, IL-1β, and HMGB-1 at macrophages, thereby reducing inflammation and pain. Another humoral outflow (outflow no. 1) is the β-endorphin-releasing humoral pathway. Because corticotrophin releasing hormone (CRH) from the PVN of the hypothalamus activates proopiomelanocortin (POMC) at the corticotrope in the anterior pituitary, which is the precursor of both adrenocorticotrophic hormone (ACTH) and β-endorphin, it is conceivable that the HPA axis induces the release of β-endorphins, thereby projecting to diffuse areas within the brain. That is, since β-endorphins are likely to be released as a result of activation of the HPA axis, therefore β-endorphins are released as a result of stimulation.

The second group of pathways (group 2) is neural as well as humoral. It is the hypothalamic autonomic-sympathetic nervous system, which drives the release of norepinephrine (NE) at the adrenal medulla. This is the neurohumoral pathway that releases NE through the systemic bloodstream.

The third group (group 3) is neural, that is, the noradrenergic sympathetic outflow, which probably originates from the hypothalamic autonomic nervous systems of the sympathetic (HAS) axis via the spinal cord (intermediolateral zone). Here again NE is released and expected to produce IL-10 by activation of the β-AR, similarly to pathway 2. NE is usually considered an excitatory neurotransmitter working opposite to ACh in the ANS; this pathway is traditionally known to have numerous adverse effects, such as an increase in heart rate and vasoconstriction. Recent findings suggest, however, that there is also a beneficial effect, such as production of antiinflammatory cytokine, IL-10, as mentioned previously; therefore, NE is also an antiinflammatory agent working in synergy with Ach, which suppresses inflammatory cytokines.[24-26]

The fourth group (group 4) is the HAP vagus nerve outflow, which is cholinergic. It is directed to macrophages and interacts with nicotinic acetylcholine receptor nAChR-α7, thereby suppressing the synthesis of TNF-α and IL-1β.[24] The antiinflammatory effect of this cholinergic pathway is recently discovered and strongly suggests that the vagal nerve outflow activity resulting from the afferent vagus nerve stimulation or other sensory stimuli would be an important antiinflammatory activity and could be related to one of the beneficial effects of acupuncture or acupuncture-like stimuli.[24,28]

The last group (group 5) is neural. It is neither sympathetic nor parasympathetic and is coupled

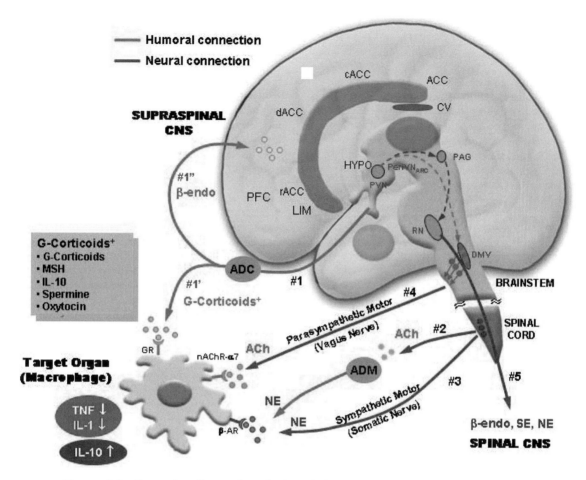

Figure 4-6   Five major efferents from the hypothalamic paraventricular nucleus (PVN) related to the broad-sense hypothalamic-pituitary-adrenal (BS-HPA) axis, which would have an effect on the suppression of cytokines and pain at the inflamed areas as well as other central nervous system (CNS) regions. This BS-HPA axis appears to play a key role in acupuncture. The humoral pathways (1′, 1″, and 2) target macrophages in the inflammatory area and other diffuse areas of the higher brain and release numerous antiinflammatory cytokines and hormones, which act on the macrophages as suppressors of the inflammatory cytokines and also act as a beneficial factor to other areas of the brain (for example β-endorphins). The neural pathways (3 and 4) include both sympathetic and parasympathetic outflows that release norepinephrine (NE) and acetylcholine (ACh). A recent study found that NE is also an antiinflammatory agent working in synergy with ACh, which suppress the inflammatory cytokines. The last group of pathways (no. 5) is neural and appears coupled directly from the periventricular nucleus and possibly the arcuate nucleus of the hypothalamus-PAG-raphe axis to the dorsal horn of the spinal cord, where inhibitory action takes place. The latter is the well-known central descending pain inhibitory pathway that inhibits the ascending pain signal from the periphery. *ACC*, Anterior cingulate cortex; *rACC, cACC, dACC,* rostral, caudal, dorsal ACC; *LIM,* limbic system; *CV,* circumventricular organs; *PFC,* prefrontal cortex; *ADM,* adrenal medulla; *ADC,* adrenal cortex; *HYPO,* hypothalamus; *PeriVN$_{ARC}$,* periventricular & arcuate nucleus; *PAG,* periaqueductal gray; *RN,* raphe nucleus; *DMV,* dorsal motor nucleus of vagus; *GR,* glucocorticoid receptor; *nAChR-α7,* nicotinic ACh receptor α7; *β-AR,* β-adrenergic receptor; *TNF,* tumor necrosis factor; *G-Corticoids,* glucocorticoids; *IL-1,* interleukin-1; *IL-10,* interleukin-10; *β-endo,* β-endorphin; *SE,* serotonin.

directly from the PVN, then to the arcuate nucleus of the hypothalamus to the PAG, and then to the ventral raphe nucleus (raphe magnus) and dorsal horn of the spinal cord. This neural pathway is the well-known central descending pain-inhibitory pathway in the spinal cord acting on the ascending pain signal pathway from the periphery.[2-6,18,34] This fifth pathway is interesting because its effect can be observed by neuroimaging in conjunction with acupuncture or acupuncture-like stimuli and pain, which was discussed earlier and will be reiterated in the following section.

EVIDENCE SUPPORTING THE BROAD-SENSE HYPOTHALAMIC-PITUITARY-ADRENAL AXIS HYPOTHESIS

As discussed in the study involving the use of sham acupoints, the fMRI observations of "pain" and "pain with administration of acupuncture" revealed several interesting results and provide clues to an explanation of basic acupuncture mechanisms. The results of another set of experiments similar to the previously discussed fMRI study, which consists of "pain," "meridian acupuncture + pain," and "sham acupuncture + pain," are shown in Figure 4-7.[19,20]

Comparison of the results from the preceding three experimental paradigms provides the following conclusions. First, as shown in Figure 4-7, *A,* cortical activation by pain alone clearly demonstrates that pain activates most of the known pain processing centers, such as the dACC, the cACC, and the rACC together with the supplementary and premotor as well as the primary motor areas.[16] Also, the thalamic areas are activated as expected; the thalamus is the main relay station of the pain sensory signal to the upper cortical areas, including the cingulate cortex. Although other cortical areas are involved and are activated, this midline view shows clearly the most distinct cortical areas that are activated robustly, including not only the ACC and the thalamus but also the supplementary and the motor areas (SMA and M1), which are also consistently activated.[16]

Second, Figure 4-7, *B,* shows an activation pattern resulting from pain stimulation after the administration of acupuncture needling in which activity decreased substantially in most of the areas once activated by pain stimulation alone, namely, the dACC, the cACC, and the rACC, the three most often activated areas together with motor areas (SMA, M1). Again activation of the thalamic area also decreases. These changes in activation on

administration of acupuncture based on the traditionally described acupoints (known as the *meridian* acupuncture points) clearly demonstrate that the pain processing areas are desensitized as a result of acupuncture administration or stimulation. This part of the study is based on traditional acupuncture theory, which designates the acupoints and claims specificity for each acupuncture point. However, the "point specificity" of acupuncture (the idea that the acupoints are specific according to the meridian theory) has been challenged by many Western medical researchers and has also been the subject of great controversy.[2,17,21]

Third, to test this "point specificity" question, a "sham acupuncture" study was carried out in which the site of needle stimulation was deliberately chosen to be different from the traditional meridian acupuncture points. The result of this study is shown in Figure 4-7, *C,* and is strikingly similar to that obtained by using the meridian acupoints. This suggests that the point specificity of acupuncture is in question, at least in the case of acupuncture analgesia.[20]

The implication of these findings is that acupuncture or acupuncture-like sensory stimulation induces the activation of the HPA axis and therefore activation of the endogenous central opiate circuitry, as discussed earlier (e.g., no. 5, shown in Figure 4-6), thereby reducing or inhibiting the ascending pain signals. This descending pain inhibitory theory supports the decreased activation observed in this acupuncture experiment (see and compare Figures 4-7, *A* to *C*),[19,20] and is consistent with data obtained by Zubieta et al[17] and also with the results of Petrovic et al.[21] These data again confirm that the effect of acupuncture, especially that of analgesia, is mediated by the BS-HPA axis response to the sensory stimulus; that is, acupuncture's sustained pain stimulation enhances stress-induced analgesia.

SUMMARY

New molecular and neurophysiological research is increasingly producing the results of stress effect studies,[22,23] antiinflammatory immune response studies,[24-26] neuroimmune-based acupuncture research,[27,28] and more recently neuroimaging-based acupuncture research.[16-21]

These researches strongly support the view that acupuncture mechanisms can be explained on molecular and neurophysiologic bases, including neuroimmune interactions, specifically via the BS-HPA axis mechanism. The BS-HPA axis hypothesis not only shares the well-known central descending

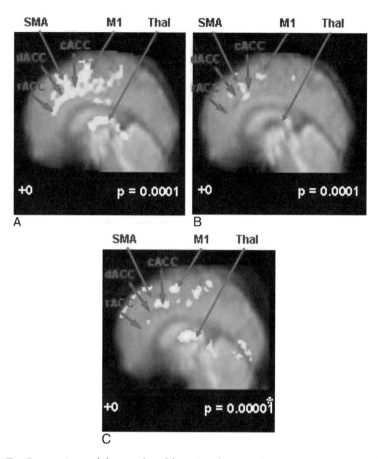

Figure 4-7 Comparison of the results of functional magnetic resonance imaging (fMRI) of "pain," "meridian acupuncture + pain," and "sham acupuncture + pain" experiments. **A,** Cortical activation by pain alone clearly demonstrates that the pain indeed activates most of the known pain processing centers such as the dorsal anterior cingulate cortex (dACC), caudal anterior cingulate cortex (cACC), and rostral anterior cingulate cortex (rACC) together with the supplementary and primary motor areas. **B,** Activation pattern resulting from pain stimulation after the administration of "meridian" acupuncture shows substantially decreased activity in most of the areas that were once activated by pain stimulation alone, namely, the dACC, the cACC, and the rACC. **C,** Same as **B** with "sham" acupuncture. These data strongly suggest that the point specificity claimed by classic acupuncture literature is not entirely true. *rACC, dACC, cACC,* Rostral, dorsal, caudal ACC; *SMA,* supplementary motor area; *M1,* primary motor; *Thal,* thalamus.

pain-inhibitory theory involving endogenous opioids, but it also suggests that there is a possible antiinflammatory mechanism in conjunction with neuroimmune pathways and the cholinergic antiinflammatory mechanism.[23-26,29]

Based on the discussion presented here, acupuncture may be working through several different modes within the frame of the BS-HPA axis response, as shown in Figure 4-6. These modes include the following:

1. The ANS neural pathway—a fast and immediate response mode of the nervous system, including the hypothalamic autonomic nervous systems of sympathetic (HAS) and parasympathetic (HAP) pathways (see pathways 3 and 4 in Figure 4-6)
2. The humoral pathways (slower but more diffused) and the mixed mode, including the opioid system, the endocrine system, and the neurohumoral system in conjunction

with the hypothalamus (i.e., the classic stress-induced HPA axis), which includes neuroimmunologic action (see pathways 1′ and 1″ and 2 in Figure 4-6)[25,32]

3. The non-ANS neural pathway—The classic descending pain inhibitory pathways involving central endogenous opioids (see pathway 5 in Figure 4-6), that is, the hypothalamic-pituitary-PAG-raphe-spinal cord axis originating from the PVN and the arcuate nucleus of the hypothalamus. With these models and the experimental evidence presented herein, one may hypothesize that the mechanism behind acupuncture is a form of CNS response that results from sensory stimulation. This hypothesis may be based on the HPA axis in a broad sense (BS-HPA axis) involving both the neuroimmune interaction, the humoral and ANS pathways, and the neural efferents based on other hypothalamic neural circuits affected by acupuncture or acupuncture-like sensory stimuli.

What seems important at this time is to investigate the specifics of various acupuncture modalities, in respect of both input and outflow. The mechanisms behind acupuncture treatment, such as the details of the HPA axis–based treatment effect or AA, are on the verge of verification with the help of newly available molecular imaging tools such as high-resolution and high-sensitivity molecular imaging PET and high-field fMRI. These imaging techniques enable us to investigate changes in both the neurochemical and hemodynamic responses that result from external stimuli, such as acupuncture needling or acupuncture-like sensory stimuli. It is hoped that with these new tools we will soon be able to shed light on the mechanism of acupuncture, a millennia-old Oriental medical practice that is often surprisingly efficacious for certain illnesses, including acute pain and inflammatory diseases. With all these scientific developments, the challenge is to investigate further the specifics of each case in connection with the various input parameters, such as point selection and combination, stimulation intensity, frequency (in the case of electroacupuncture), duration of stimulation, and the repetition rate, among others, all of which can affect the outcome of acupuncture stimulation. In addition, various physiologic differences, such as body constitution, pathologic conditions, and the daily rhythm of humoral secretion (such as glucocorticoids), will certainly be important parameters to which attention must be paid.

References

1. National Institutes of Health: NIH Consensus Development Statement on Complementary Medicine, 1997. Question 1. Available at: http://odp.od.nih.gov/consensus/statements/cdc/107/107stmt.html.
2. Filshie J, White A, editors: *Medical acupuncture: a Western scientific approach,* Edinburgh and London, 1998, Churchill Livingstone.
3. Melzack R, Wall PD: Pain mechanisms: a new theory, *Science* 150:971-979, 1965.
4. Pomeranz B: The scientific basis of acupuncture. In Stux G, Pomeranz B, editors: *The basics of acupuncture,* Berlin, 1991, Springer-Verlag.
5. Takeshige C, et al: Descending pain inhibition involved in acupuncture analgesia. *Brain Res Bull* 29: 617-634, 1992.
6. Stux G, Hammerschlag R: *Clinical acupuncture*, Berlin and Heidelberg, 2000, Springer-Verlag.
7. Cho ZH, Chan JK, Ericksson L: Circular ring transverse axial positron emission camera for 3-D reconstruction of radionuclides distribution, *IEEE Trans Nucl Sci* 23: 613-622, 1976.
8. Phelps ME, Mazziotta JC: Positron emission tomography: human brain function and biochemistry, *Science* 228: 799-809, 1985.
9. Raichle ME: Behind the scenes of functional brain imaging: a historical and physiological perspective, *Proc Natl Acad Sci U S A* 95:765-772, 1998.
10. Ogawa S, et al: Intrinsic signal changes accompanying sensory stimulation: functional brain mapping with magnetic resonance imaging, *Proc Natl Acad Sci U S A* 89: 5951-5955, 1992.
11. Kwong KK, et al: Dynamic magnetic resonance imaging of human brain activity during primary sensory stimulation, *Proc Natl Acad Sci U S A* 89:5675-5679, 1992.
12. Cho ZH, Ro YM, Lim TH: NMR venography using the susceptibility effect produced by deoxyhemoglobin, *Magn Reson Med* 28:25-38, 1992.
13. Cho ZH, et al: New findings of the correlation between acupoints and corresponding brain cortices using functional MRI, *Proc Natl Acad Sci U S A* 95:2670-2673, 1998.
14. Wu MT, et al: Central nervous pathway for acupuncture stimulation: localization of processing with functional MR imaging of the brain—preliminary experience, *Radiology* 212:133-141, 1999.
15. Hui K, et al: Acupuncture modulates the limbic system and subcortical gray structures of the human brain: evidence from fMRI studies in normal subjects, *Hum Brain Mapp* 9:13-25, 2000.
16. Cho ZH, et al: Pain dynamics observed by fMRI using a differential regression analysis technique, *J Magn Reson Imag* 18:273-283, 2003.
17. Zubieta JK, et al: Regional mu-opioid receptor regulation of sensory and affective dimensions of pain, *Science* 293: 311-315, 2001.
18. Han JS: Acupuncture: neuropeptide release produced by electrical stimulation of different frequencies, *Trends Neurosci* 26:17-22, 2003.
19. Cho ZH, et al: fMRI neurophysiological evidence of acupuncture mechanisms, *Med Acupuncture* 14:16-22, 2002.
20. Cho ZH, et al: Acupuncture: the search for biologic evidence with functional magnetic resonance imaging and positron emission tomography techniques, *J Altern Complement Med* 8:399-401, 2002.
21. Petrovic P, et al: Placebo and opioid analgesic: imaging a shared neural network, *Science* 295:1737-1740, 2002.

22. Maier SF, et al: The role of the vagus nerve in cytokine-to-brain communication, *Ann N Y Acad Sci* 840:289-300, 1998.

23. Akil H, et al: Overview: thyroid and adrenal axes. In Zigmond MJ, et al, editors: *Fundamental neuroscience: neuroendocrine systems, vol I,* San Diego, 1999, Academic Press.

24. Tracey KJ: The inflammatory reflex, *Nature* 420:853-859, 2002.

25. Tracey KJ, et al: Anti-cachectin/TNF monoclonal antibodies prevent septic shock during lethal bacteraemia, *Nature* 330:662-664, 1987.

26. Wang H, et al: Nicotinic acetylcholine receptor alpha7 subunit is an essential regulator of inflammation, *Nature* 421:384-388, 2003.

27. Son YS, et al: Antipyretic effects of acupuncture on the lipopolysaccharide-induced fever and expression of interleukin-6 and interleukin-1beta mRNAs in the hypothalamus of rats, *Neurosci Lett* 319:45-48, 2002.

28. Mori H, et al: Unique immunomodulation by electroacupuncture in humans possibly via stimulation of the autonomic nervous system, *Neurosci Lett* 320:21-24, 2002.

29. Besedovsky H, et al: Immunoregulatory feedback between interleukin-1 and glucocorticoid hormones, *Science* 233:652-654, 1986.

30. Libert C: Inflammation: a nervous connection, *Nature* 421:328-329, 2003.

31. Derbyshire SWG: Measuring our natural painkiller, *Trends Neurosci* 25:67-68, 2002.

32. Giardino L, et al: Daily modifications of 3H-naloxone binding sites in the rat brain: a quantitative autoradiographic study, *Chronobiol Int* 6:203-216, 1989.

33. Jones AK, et al: In vivo distribution of opioid receptors in man in relation to the cortical projections of the medial and lateral systems measured with positron emission tomography, *Neurosci Lett* 126:25-28, 1991.

34. Han JS, et al: Enkephalin and beta-endorphin as mediators of electro-acupuncture analgesia in rabbits: an antiserum microinjection study, *Adv Biochem Psychopharmacol* 33: 369-377, 1982.

35. Cho ZH, Wong EK, Fallon J: *Neuro-acupuncture,* Los Angeles, 2001, Q-Puncture Inc.

CHAPTER 5

Integrative Neuromuscular Acupoint System

INTRODUCTION

The classic Chinese acupuncture system was first described in the *Yellow Emperor's Canon of Internal Medicine (Huangdi Neijing)*, which dates back to between 500 and 200 BC, and is still the "bible" of classic acupuncture. At the time when it appeared the "Canon" was a masterpiece extraordinarily ahead of its time.

The traditional Chinese acupuncture system used today is more elaborate than that of the "Canon." It comprises an intricate system of 14 meridians with 361 points. Each point is believed to have a fixed location and a specific quasipharmacologic function, which practitioners are expected to know by heart. Currently traditional acupuncture has grown to include approximately 2500 additional extra-channel meridian acupoints that are applied individually as necessary.

We believe that one reason acupuncture is only marginally accepted by the Western medical community is that the archaic and time-consuming intricacies of the classic acupuncture system make understanding, learning, and applying it excruciatingly difficult.

To overcome these problems, we developed and present here a unique acupoint system, the Integrative Neuromuscular Acupoint System (INMAS). INMAS is a user-friendly system that applies biomedical concepts to interpret the basic mechanisms of the acupoint system and its clinical procedures, while preserving the essential principle of classical acupuncture: Treat the whole person, not only the diseased organ; treat the root of the symptom, not only the symptom.

The INMAS protocol resonates with the Western practitioner, thus facilitating its incorporation into pain management. Mechanisms of acupuncture are clarified in terms of their peripheral and central effects (see Chapters 3 and 4) and are explained using basic neuroscientific terminology and concepts that are based on the scientific and clinical discoveries of the last 40 years.

INMAS provides a simple anatomic acupoint system, a reliable and reproducible quantitative method to evaluate patients and predict the outcome of the treatment, and a standardized treatment protocol. This protocol provides the standardization that Western medicine requires, while maintaining the individualized approach practiced in traditional Chinese medicine (TCM).

THREE TYPES OF ACUPOINTS

The INMAS consists of three types of acupoints: homeostatic acupoints (HAs), symptomatic acupoints (SAs), and paravertebral acupoints (PAs). Each type has distinct pathophysiologic features as explained below.

1. Twenty-four HAs.

   Healthy persons have fewer tender acupoints in their bodies. As homeostasis of the body declines, more tender acupoints gradually develop. These tender acupoints appear in predictable locations and in predictable sequential orders. These acupoints are the HAs.

   Because tender HAs appear in predictable locations, the name of each homeostatic acupoint can be clearly defined by its associated nerve or gross anatomic landmark and can be easily located by practitioners.

   A healthy person may have only a few tender HAs, whereas a sick person can have more than 100. Persons with fewer tender HAs need fewer acupuncture treatments to achieve pain relief. Thus, the number of tender HAs in the body represents the self-healing potential of the person. The appearance pattern of tender HAs in the body is almost the same in everyone.

   A chronic pathological condition can gradually result in more than 100 tender HAs in the body. Usually other tender HAs develop around what are known as the *24 primary HAs* that appear first in the body. For instance, the H1 deep radial acupoint (Figure 5-1) is tender in almost everyone. If homeostasis declines or if an elbow or arm is injured, more tender acupoints appear along the deep radial nerve from H1 distally toward the wrist. Thus, the practitioner need only remember the 24 primary HAs to know all other potential HAs.

Palpation of all primary 24 HAs also helps the practitioner to locate the origin of referred pain, which is often a challenging puzzle in pain management. Clinically pain is often referred from one HA to another HA.

The use of primary HAs is *standardized* in every case (see below). Needling HAs follows the concept of TCM, which emphasizes balance between *yin* and *yang* and treatment of *ben*, the root of the symptoms.

Note that an HA also can be an SA (see next section). For example, although the H8 infraspinatus acupoint (see later discussion) is an HA, this point becomes more tender in patients with shoulder pain and is then, in fact, an SA.

2. Symptomatic acupoints (SAs or *Ashi* points).

SAs display individualized patterns of pain symptoms; thus SAs vary in everyone. Many practitioners call SAs local points, or Ashi points according to traditional acupuncture practice. Some examples of SA formation include the following.

In patients with respiratory symptoms such as asthma, tender acupoints can be found on the neck, arms, upper back, and front chest. Some of the peripheral nerves from C2 to T12 may contribute to the formation of these tender acupoints.

Tender acupoints in patients with lower back pain often appear around lower back HAs: H15, H14, H16, H18, and H22.

Unlike HAs, whose formation is predictable in terms of their locations and sequence, SAs develop in relation to the injuries of each patient and their formation is unpredictable and individual.

When treating a patient with pain, the practitioner should carefully palpate the injured area to find the SAs.

3. Paravertebral *(Huatuo Jiaji)* acupoints (PAs).

Paravertebral acupoints are located along both sides of the spine on the back muscles, from the base of the skull down to the sacral area. In classic acupuncture, some of those points are called *Huatuo Jiaji* points, some back *shu* points. These points consist of nerve fibers from the posterior primary rami of the spinal nerves. PAs are closer to the root of spinal nerves and sympathetic trunk ganglia. Clinical evidence shows that these acupoints may be more effective than other acupoints in balancing the activity of the autonomic nervous system, even though every other acupoint in the body may also balance autonomic activity.

In addition, needling PAs relaxes back muscles, thereby easing pressure on the vertebral joints. This function improves most symptoms related to the back muscles and the spine, such as radiculopathy and osteoporosis.

Sometimes particular PAs may become tender, in which case they are also regarded as SAs. For example, a patient with stomach pain or an ulcer has tender points that are palpable around the xiphoid process in front, but on the back tender points may appear on one side or on both sides along T7-T12.

From a clinical perspective, unlike HAs and SAs, PAs do not have exact locations because the cutaneous branches from neighboring spinal nerves overlap each other. To achieve the best efficacy from the needling stimuli, it is better to needle all the neighboring spinal nerves. For example, if postherpetic pain is related to T5-6 spinal nerves, it is better to needle the area from T4 to T7.

Clinically PAs are selected according to their neurosegmental or dermatomal relation to SAs. PAs are used to enhance the desensitization of SAs and balance the autonomic nervous system. For example, if SAs appear on the upper extremities, PAs along C4-T1 are selected. If SAs appear on the lower extremities, PAs along L2-S4 are selected.

The combination of the three types of acupoints forms a universally standardized protocol for all pain symptoms; at the same time this protocol ensures an individualized approach, as is practiced in TCM, by identifying and treating the specific SAs of each patient. In other words, when treating patients, primary HAs are the same for every patient, whereas SAs are individualized symptomatic

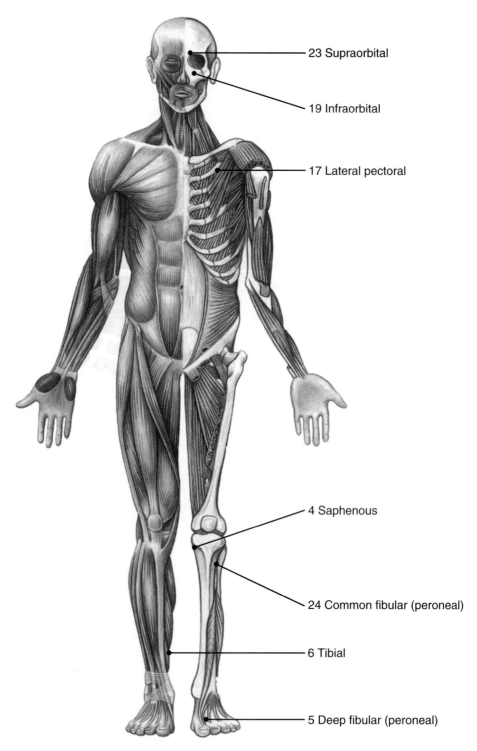

Figure 5-1   Twenty-four homeostatic acupoints (HAs). The number of each acupoint indicates the sequence of phase transition from latent to passive phase. For example, H2 becomes tender after H1 does. (Modified from Abrahams P, Hutchings R, Marks S: *McMinn's color atlas of human anatomy*, ed 4, London, 1997, Mosby.)

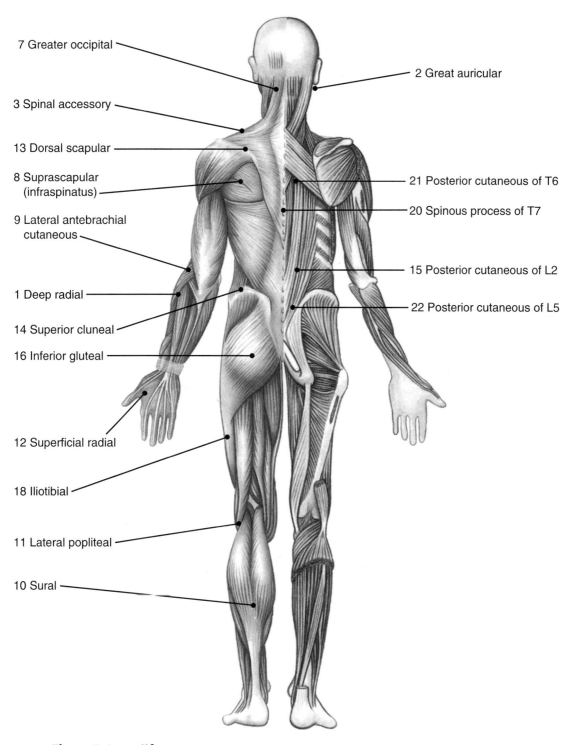

7 Greater occipital

2 Great auricular

3 Spinal accessory

13 Dorsal scapular

8 Suprascapular (infraspinatus)

21 Posterior cutaneous of T6

20 Spinous process of T7

9 Lateral antebrachial cutaneous

15 Posterior cutaneous of L2

1 Deep radial

22 Posterior cutaneous of L5

14 Superior cluneal

16 Inferior gluteal

12 Superficial radial

18 Iliotibial

11 Lateral popliteal

10 Sural

Figure 5-1, cont'd

points. Different SAs require different PAs according to their neurosegmental connection. Thus this protocol contains both standardization and individualization.

The following example explains how we can use one principal protocol to treat two different pain symptoms, elbow pain and knee pain. More detailed instruction is provided in Chapter 6.

Patient A (with elbow pain)	Patient B (with knee pain)
HAs Primary HAs	Primary HAs (same as patient A)
SAs Locate SAs in elbow and arm	Locate SAs in the knee, thigh, and leg
PAs Use PAs along C4-T1	Use PAs along L2-5

THE RANDOM AND PREDICTABLE PATTERNS OF TENDER ACUPOINT FORMATION

All acupoints consist of peripheral nerve fibers, including the sensory and postganglionic nerve fibers and other soft tissues (see Chapter 1). Acupoints become tender in two distinguishing patterns: the *random* pattern of SAs and the *predictable* pattern of HAs.

As previously explained, when homeostasis declines, homeostatic acupoints are gradually transformed from a latent phase (nonsensitive) to passive or active phases. In general, HAs appear symmetrically in predictable locations and predictable sequential order in the human body, and this is referred to as the predictable pattern of tender HA formation. There can be more than 100 HAs in some patients; the first 24 HAs are shown in Figure 5-1. All other HAs appear around these 24 primary HAs, as discussed previously.

Acute injury or acute disease always sensitizes some localized sensory nerves (tender acupoints). These tender acupoints can appear anywhere in the area affected by the injury or disease. This is the random pattern of SA formation.

The SA random pattern and HA predictable pattern of tender acupoint formation often coexist. For instance, primary acupoint H1 (deep radial; see later discussion) is tender in all healthy and unhealthy people alike. Patients with neck, shoulder, elbow, wrist, and hand pain have a common tender primary acupoint H1 deep radial as well as different, random additional tender acupoints around the H1 deep radial.

The three pathophysiologic phases of acupoints reveal the quantitative and qualitative dynamics of an acupoint: when pathologic factors persist, the number, size, and sensitivity of tender HAs and SAs increase. With proper treatment, the number of tender acupoints decreases and the sensitivity of each acupoint subsides (see Chapters 2 and 3). In the absence of proper treatment or when the self-healing potential is impaired, the size of an acupoint will increase and it will finally become a permanent pathologic structure such as a palpable nodule in the muscle.

There are no "sham" acupoints (see Chapter 4). Stimulated by acupuncture needling, any sensory nerve fiber, sensitized or not sensitized, will produce and send electrical signals to the spinal cord and the brain. Important acupoints, such as the 24 primary acupoints, provide stronger signals, and "sham" acupoints provide weaker signals.

Electrophysiologic experiments show that certain nerve fibers, when sensitized, will generate stronger signals by normal mechanical or thermal stimulation (unpublished data, Dr. Yun-tao Ma). Clinically important acupoints often produce more needle sensation *(de qi),* such as aching, soreness, numbness, heaviness, pressure, or electric shock. Therapeutically these acupoints produce strong signals and are more effective than acupoints with weaker signals.

All three types of acupoints must be combined to achieve the best therapeutic results when treating any symptom. The following is one example of how to combine three types of acupoints to treat a patient with knee pain. First, have the patient assume a supine position and palpate the area around the knee to find and then needle these local SAs. Then palpate and needle the HAs accessible in the supine position. Finally, turn the patient over to a prone position and needle tender points in a popliteal area and the PAs around L2-S2, plus HAs accessible to this position in the shoulder and neck areas. This combination, including both local (SAs) and distal points (HAs), provides the best efficacy. The number of acupoints needled for each treatment depends on the severity of the injury, the homeostatic status of the patient, and his or her needling tolerance. We discuss this in greater detail in later chapters.

NEUROANATOMY OF 24 PRIMARY HOMEOSTATIC ACUPOINTS

For 30 years Dr. H.C. Dung studied the pathophysiology of HAs in both clinical practice and laboratory research. He found that as many as 110 HAs may develop when homeostasis declines. Of these, 24 acupoints are the most important, as discussed previously.[2]

This discovery of HAs and their quantitative relation to homeostasis makes it possible to evaluate the pathophysiological condition (the self-healing potential) of a patient and predict the duration and prognosis of the acupuncture treatment (Chapter 6).

The 24 primary acupoints are named with their homeostatic sequence number, followed by the name of the related peripheral nerves or anatomic landmarks (see Figure 5-1). Consider, for example, the H1 deep radial acupoint. H1 means that this acupoint is the first of all the HAs to become tender on the body, and *deep radial* indicates that this acupoint is located on the deep radial nerve. Acupoint H19 infraorbital is located on the infraorbital foramen where the infraorbital nerve emerges and usually becomes tender after the H18 iliotibial point.

Needling safety and efficacy should be the primary concern of a practitioner. For example, when working in the region of the upper and lower extremities, the risk of an accident is low. In other body regions, a practitioner should be careful to avoid causing injury to the vital organs, such as the lung or the heart. With experience each practitioner can create his or her own needling method in treating each patient, keeping in mind that no two patients are identical.

All the acupuncture needling methods described in the following section apply to prone or supine positions. The actual location of an acupoint varies in different patients. To achieve the best results, a practitioner should *always* palpate the body to locate the actual acupoints before needling them. The 24 primary homeostatic acupoints (see Figure 5-1) are described below according to body region.

Homeostatic Acupoints on the Head and Neck

The five primary homeostatic acupoints are two on the face; two on the neck; and the fifth acupoint, H3 spinal accessory, on the shoulder bridge region. The H3 spinal accessory acupoint is included in this section because it is innervated by the spinal accessory nerve, which contains both cranial and cervical nerve roots.

H19 Infraorbital This acupoint is located exactly on the infraorbital foramen (Figure 5-2).

The infraorbital nerve, a cutaneous nerve from the maxillary branch (V2) of the trigeminal nerve, passes the foramen and innervates the facial skin. To avoid hematoma use 38- or 36-gauge needles (diameter, 0.18 or 0.20 mm, respectively). The depth for needling ranges from 2 to 5 mm.

Clinical Notes The H19 infraorbital is always the first tender acupoint on the face because the infraorbital nerve is the largest cutaneous nerve in this area. In addition to homeostatic decline, all symptoms related to the face and the head may further sensitize this acupoint and increase its size. Thus the sensitivity and size of the point provide useful information about the severity or chronicity of the symptom. The common symptoms that may aggravate this acupoint are cranial neuralgias; all kinds of headache; facial, myofascial, and temporomandibular disorders; pain of dental and intra-oral origins; ocular and periocular pain; pain in the ear; sinusitis; cold; allergy; and facial paralysis. The H19 infraorbital acupoint should be used for all these symptoms. It should be noted that pain caused by cancer of the head and neck also sensitizes this acupoint.

H23 Supraorbital This acupoint is formed right on the supraorbital notch, which is the passage for the supraorbital nerve (see Figure 5-2). This cutaneous nerve from the ophthalmic branch (V1) of the trigeminal nerve extends to the top of the head. The method of needling this point is similar to the H19 infraorbital.

Clinical Notes Because the supraorbital nerve is smaller than the infraorbital nerve, the H23 supraorbital becomes tender after the H19 infraorbital does (see Chapter 1). For example, the H19 infraorbital is always tender in a patient with a slight headache. If the headache lingers for some time, the H23 supraorbital becomes tender, too. If the headache continues to deteriorate, other points in the face, such as the mental nerve (V3), the zygomaticofacial nerve (V2), and the zygomaticotemporal nerve, also appear tender. More tender points indicate that the symptom is more chronic and more severe and requires more treatments.

When treating patients with facial problems such as temporomandibular pain, chronic sinus pain, or facial paralysis, other points innervated by the facial nerve (VII) (Figure 5-3) should be carefully palpated and selectively needled according to the individual symptom.

H2 Greater Auricular This acupoint is located just behind the earlobe and on the anterior border of the sternocleidomastoid muscle (see Figure 5-3).

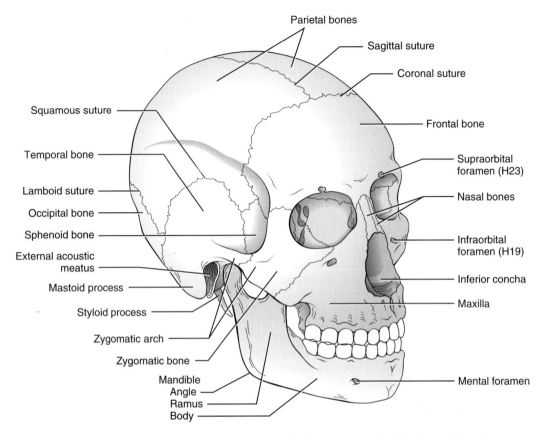

Figure 5-2   Locations of acupoints H23 supraorbital and H19 infraorbital. (Modified from Jenkins D: *Hollinshead's functional anatomy of the limbs and back,* ed 8, Philadelphia, 2002, WB Saunders.)

The greater auricular nerve is one of the four branches from the cervical nerve plexus (CNP, C2-4). The anterior rami of C2 to C4 interconnect to form the cervical nerve plexus. The CNP lies deep below the internal jugular vein and the sternocleidomastoid muscle. Four cutaneous branches from the CNP emerge around the middle of the posterior border of the sternocleidomastoid muscle.

The greater auricular nerve curves over and ascends obliquely toward the earlobe and the angle of the mandible. This nerve bundle surfaces through the investing fascia just below the earlobe and divides into branches to supply the skin on the inferior part of the ear and the area extending from the mandible to the mastoid process. The three acupoints formed by the CNP are shown in Figure 5-3.

Clinical Notes   The H2 greater auricular is tender in almost every patient. Needling this point, however, often causes bleeding because the external jugular vein descends just beside the greater auricular nerve. If the external jugular vein is observed to be prominent throughout its course, this is a sign of raised venous pressure resulting from heart problems, and this point should not be needled to avoid an accident such as a venous air embolism. A fine 36- or 38-gauge needle (diameter, 0.20 or 0.18 mm) may be used to needle this point. The needling depth is about 5 to 8 mm.

Several acupoints on the neck are formed by three other nerves derived from the CNP. These nerves are the (1) lesser occipital nerve, which forms an acupoint located on the insertions between the sternocleidomastoid and the trapezius muscles on the occipital bone; (2) the transverse cervical nerve, which curves around the middle of the posterior border of the sternocleidomastoid and then passes transversely to the anterior border of the same muscle (several acupoints are formed over the anterior triangle of the neck); and (3) the supraclavicular nerve, which divides into medial,

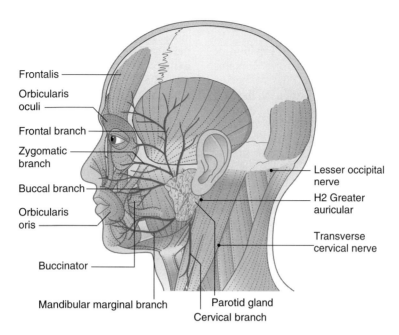

Frontalis

Orbicularis oculi

Frontal branch

Zygomatic branch

Buccal branch

Orbicularis oris

Buccinator

Mandibular marginal branch

Lesser occipital nerve

H2 Greater auricular

Transverse cervical nerve

Parotid gland
Cervical branch

Figure 5-3   Acupoint H2, greater auricular, and diagram of the facial nerve (VII) and two less important acupoints: the lesser occipital nerve and the transverse cervical nerve. (Modified from FitzGerald M, Folan-Curran J: *Clinical neuroanatomy and related neuroscience,* ed 4, Edinburgh, 2002, WB Saunders.)

intermedial, and lateral branches. These nerves send small branches to the skin of the neck and then emerge from deep fascia just superior to the clavicle to supply the skin over the anterior aspect of the chest and shoulder. When needling tender acupoints in this area, a practitioner always should pay attention to the direction and depth of the needling so as not to puncture the lung. A safe needling method is suggested later in this chapter.

H7 Greater Occipital   This acupoint is located at the base of the occipital region, 2 or 3 cm from the midline (see Figure 5-1). This acupoint can be palpated easily because it is tender in more than 95% of patients. The dorsal rami of the C2 spinal nerve form the greater occipital nerve. This nerve emerges between the posterior arch of the atlas (C1) and the lamina of the axis (C2), below the small muscle obliquus capitis inferior. It then surfaces to supply the skin of the occipital region.

   Clinical Notes   The H7 great occipital is frequently used because many symptoms can be traced to the problems of the neck. Neck-related problems are discussed in detail in Chapter 9. For effective treatment, we usually use needles of

gauge 34 (diameter: 0.22 mm). The depth varies from 2 to 4 cm, depending on the thickness of the patient's neck tissues.

H3 Spinal Accessory   The spinal accessory nerve (XI) originates from both cranial roots (nucleus ambiguus in medulla) and spinal roots (C1 to C6), and it contains both afferent (sensory) and efferent (motor) fibers. The branch of the spinal accessory nerve enters the trapezius muscle at the point over the shoulder bridge in the middle of the front edge of the upper trapezius muscle (see Figure 5-1). This acupoint is a neuromuscular attachment point.

   Clinical Notes   The H3 spinal accessory appears tender in more than 98% of the population. We use a needle no more than 2.5 cm long and insert the needle perpendicularly to the skin. Practitioners should be extremely careful when needling this point because the apex of the lung is just below this point. We suggest four needling methods in Chapter 9. A practitioner can choose the method he or she is most comfortable with or explore other safe methods. Another branch of the spinal accessory nerve also innervates the sternocleidomastoid muscle, but the acupoints formed in that muscle are less important.

Other Facial Acupoints   Two cranial nerves, the trigeminal nerve (V) and the facial nerve (VII; see Figure 5-3), are involved in the formation of facial acupoints. The trigeminal nerve contains both sensory (afferent) and motor (efferent) nerves and is responsible for general sensations in the skin of the face and front of the head as well as controlling the chewing muscles. The two types of facial muscles are the muscles of mastication (chewing) and the muscles of facial expression. Two important muscles of mastication, the temporalis and masseter muscles, are innervated by the motor nerves of the trigeminal nerve. The acupoints formed in those two muscles are essential in treating some headaches and facial symptoms such as temporomandibular joint syndrome (TMJ) and facial paralysis.

The five branches of the complicated facial nerve innervate 20 known muscles of facial expression and other structures, including the tongue. Injury to the facial nerve or some of its branches leads to paresis (weakness) or paralysis (loss of voluntary movement) of all or some of the facial muscles on the affected side. The injuries may be caused by chilling the face, inflammation, middle ear infection, fractures, tumor, and other disorders. Proper needling of the affected muscles helps to reduce inflammation and accelerates healing in many facial symptoms, including Bell's palsy.

Homeostatic Acupoints on the Upper Extremity

The upper extremity is the organ of manual activity. It consists of two parts: the shoulder (junction of the arm and the trunk) and the free arm. The free arm includes four parts: the arm (brachium, between the shoulder and the elbow), the forearm (antebrachium, between the elbow and the wrist), the wrist (carpus), and the hand.

The bones of the upper extremities comprise the clavicle (collar bone) and the scapula (shoulder blade) in the shoulder, the humerus in the arm, the radius and ulna in the forearm, the eight carpal bones in the wrist, the five metacarpal bones in the hand, and 14 phalanges in the digits (fingers). More than 50 large and small muscles are attached to the bones of the upper extremities.

The large nerve network of the brachial plexus supplies the upper extremities. The brachial plexus is formed by the union of the ventral rami of nerves C5 to C8 and most of the ventral ramus of T1 (Figure 5-4). To supply the upper extremities, these five rami interconnect to form three nerve trunks: upper (C5-6), middle (C7), and lower (C8 and T1).

Each trunk splits into anterior and posterior divisions. All the posterior divisions unite to become the posterior cord, which has two major nerves, the axillary and radial nerves. The anterior divisions form the lateral cord and the medial cord. The lateral cord becomes the musculocutaneous nerve, and the medial cord the ulnar nerve. The union of fibers from both the lateral and the medial cords forms the median nerve. The small branches from the upper trunk and the three cords supply the shoulder (back and front); the five major terminal nerves are made up of the three cords innervating the free arm. Six primary homeostatic acupoints are located in the upper extremities: one on the chest, two on the shoulder, two on the forearm, and one on the hand. Here we discuss only the major nerves that give rise to the primary homeostatic acupoints.

The Lateral Cord   Two primary HAs are formed by two terminal branches, the lateral pectoral nerve on the pectoralis major muscle and the lateral antebrachial cutaneous nerve on the lateral elbow.

The Posterior Cord   The radial nerve branches into two nerves, the deep and superficial radial nerves on the forearm. Each of the two nerves contributes a primary HA (H1 and H12) at its branching location. Two primary HAs on the posterior shoulder muscles are supplied by the posterior branches of the superior trunk from the brachial plexus, the dorsal scapular nerve (H13), and the suprascapular nerve (H8).

H17 Lateral Pectoral   As one of the small terminal branches of the lateral cord, the lateral pectoral nerve (C5-7) pierces the clavipectoral fascia and enters the pectoralis major muscle at the spot about 4 to 5 cm inferior to the middle point of the clavicular bone (collarbone) (see Figure 5-1). A commonly used acupoint is formed at this neuromuscular attachment point.

Clinical Notes   This acupoint is commonly used for chest and upper back symptoms. Needling should be done cautiously because the lung is just below this point. We usually use two needling methods. The first step is to palpate the pectoralis major muscle. Then, in thin patients, use a needle 1.5 cm long and insert it perpendicular to the skin, ensuring that the needle does not puncture the lung; or, in patients with a developed pectoralis major muscle, use a needle 4.0 cm long. Direct the needle horizontally and inferiorly. Be sure that the needle is outside the rib cage so as not to puncture the lung.

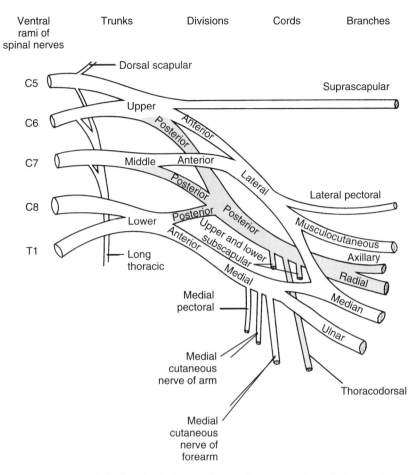

Figure 5-4 Diagram of the brachial plexus. The small nerve to the subclavius, from the upper trunk, is omitted. (Modified from Jenkins D: *Hollinshead's functional anatomy of the limbs and back,* ed 8, Philadelphia, 2002, WB Saunders.)

The lateral pectoral nerve also sends a branch laterally to the medial pectoral nerve, which supplies the pectoralis minor muscle and forms an acupoint. The lateral pectoral nerve is so named because it arises from the lateral cord of the brachial plexus. Note that H17 lateral pectoral acupoint is located medially on the pectoralis major and the medial pectoral nerve is on the pectoralis minor lateral to the H17 lateral pectoral acupoint.

H9 Lateral Antebrachial Cutaneous This acupoint is located at the lateral end of the skin crest at the elbow joint and is easy to detect when the forearm is flexed at a 90-degree angle (Figure 5-5). The musculocutaneous nerve (C5-7) from the lateral cord of the brachial plexus courses along the lateral side of the arm and pierces the deep fas-

cia at the lateral edge of the cubital fossa to become the lateral antebrachial cutaneous nerve. An acupoint is formed at the location where the nerve pierces the deep fascia.

H1 Deep Radial The H1 deep radial can be detected by palpation in more than 99% of the population (see Figure 5-5). The deep radial nerve (C5-8 and T1) is one of the terminal branches from the posterior cord of the brachial plexus (see Figure 5-4). This nerve provides the major nerve supply to the extensor muscles of the upper extremities: triceps, anconeus, brachioradialis, and all the extensor muscles of the forearm. It also supplies cutaneous sensation to the skin of the extensor region, including the hand.

The radial nerve leaves the axilla and runs posteriorly, inferiorly, and laterally between the long

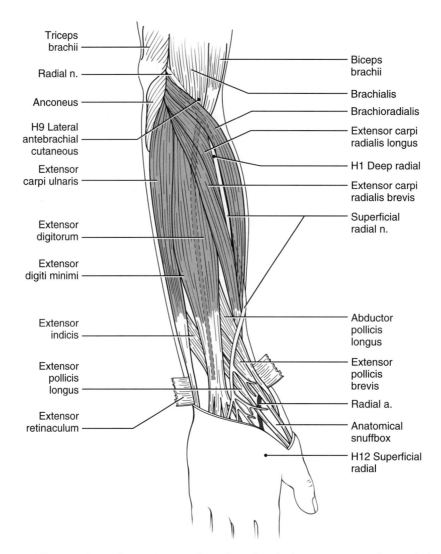

Figure 5-5 Locations of acupoints H9, lateral antebrachial cutaneus; H1, deep radial; and H12, superficial radial. (Modified from Jenkins D: *Hollinshead's functional anatomy of the limbs and back,* ed 8, Philadelphia, 2002, WB Saunders.)

and medial heads of the triceps muscle. It enters the radial groove in the humerus. The radial nerve penetrates the lateral intermuscular septum of the arm and divides into two terminal branches: the deep and the superficial radial nerves. The first tender HA of our body is located at the branching spot, which is about 4 cm distal to the lateral epicondyle between the brachioradialis muscle and the extensor carpi radialis longus muscle. Here the deep radial nerve is accompanied by the radial artery and vein and their tributaries. As the deep radial nerve runs distally to the wrist from this point, it sequentially gives branches to nine muscles.

Clinical Notes The H1 deep radial is the first acupoint to become tender in our body, and it can be used in every treatment to improve homeostasis; however, its clinical value rests more in diagnosis. Remember that the efficacy and prognosis of acupuncture therapy depend first on the self-healing capability of the body. As homeostasis declines, the self-healing potential drops, and more tender points gradually display along the deep radial nerve distally from the H1 deep radial. Thus the number of tender points appearing on the deep radial nerve provides quantitative information about the body's homeostasis and self-healing potential. The diagnostic method is detailed in Chapter 6. The H1 deep radial acupoint can be needled all the way down to the bone below.

H12 Superficial Radial   After branching from the deep radial nerve just below the elbow, the superficial radial nerve runs under the brachioradialis muscle and emerges to the surface at the distal portion of the radius. This nerve starts branching first at the anatomical snuff box and then on the web between the thumb and the index finger. The acupoint H12 superficial radial is located on the second branching spot.

H13 Dorsal Scapular   The dorsal scapular nerve branches from the ventral ramus of C5 and descends from the cervical region down to the medial border of the scapula. It innervates three muscles: the levator scapulae, the rhomboid major, and the rhomboid minor. This nerve enters the levator scapulae muscle about 1 cm superior to the base of the spine of the scapula (Figure 5-6). The

H13 dorsal scapular acupoint is formed at this neuromuscular attachment.

Clinical Notes   The H13 dorsal scapular is used in all symptoms related to the head, neck, shoulder, arm, and upper back. All the three muscles—the levator scapulae and the rhomboid major and minor—are innervated by the dorsal scapular nerve and are sore or tender in most patients. These muscles should be treated in most patients; however, the needling is tricky because the lung is directly under this acupoint and under both the rhomboid muscles. We suggest the following needling methods, but the practitioner should ensure that the needle is always outside the rib cage.

1. In a thin patient, use a 2.5-cm long needle, and direct the needle horizontally and either inferiorly or laterally to ensure that the muscle is properly needled while the needle is still outside the rib cage. If this is difficult, the alternative method is to use four or five

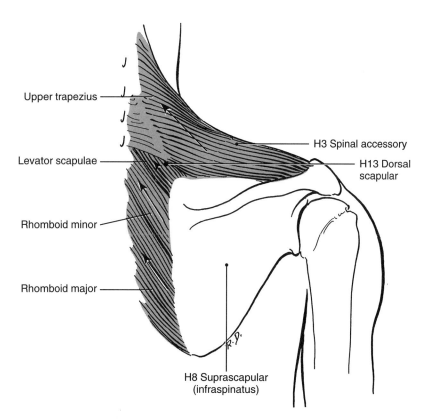

Figure 5-6   H13, dorsal scapula, is located about 1 cm superior to the base of the spine of the scapula. (Modified from Jenkins D: *Hollinshead's functional anatomy of the limbs and back,* ed 8, Philadelphia, 2002, WB Saunders.)

needles 1.5 cm long and needle this point perpendicularly. This method is less effective but safer in dealing with thin patients.

2. In patients with average musculature, needle this point perpendicularly with a needle 2.5 cm long.

3. For more effective treatment, raise the scapula by laying the forearm of the patient under the back with a 90-degree flexion. Direct a 4-cm-long needle laterally to needle this point (see Figure 10-30, p. 181). The same method can be used to needle both the rhomboid muscles and the subscapularis muscle, which lies on the costal surface of the scapula.

H8 Infraspinatus   This acupoint (Figures 5-1 and 5-6) is so named because it is located right on the infraspinatus muscle. The infraspinatus and the supraspinatus muscles are all innervated by the same nerve: the suprascapular nerve.

The suprascapular nerve receives fibers from C5 and C6 and arises from the posterior division of the superior trunk of the brachial plexus. It supplies the suprascapular and infrascapular muscles and the shoulder joint. This nerve descends down from the neck, divides a muscular branch to the supraspinatus, and curves around the scapular notch to reach the infraspinatus. The nerve enters the muscle underneath at the center of the infraspinatus fossa and the acupoint forms at this neuromuscular attachment. It is not difficult to palpate this tender point because it is in the center of the infrascapular fossa.

Clinical Notes   Finding this point is easy and needling can be done safely because it is right on the scapular bone, but caution is still needed. If a patient positions his or her arms above the shoulder, the scapulae move laterally and the lung is exposed. For the sake of safety, the acupoint must be palpated on the infraspinatus fossa of the bone.

Some patients have a thicker infraspinatus muscle, and so the needle should be directed perpendicular to the acupoint and inserted all the way to the bone. For patients with a thin infraspinatus muscle, the needle can be tilted at a proper angle according to the thickness of the muscle.

Homeostatic Acupoints on the Lower Extremities

The primary functions of the lower extremities are locomotion, bearing weight, and maintaining equilibrium. The lower extremity consists of four major parts: the hip, the thigh, the leg, and the foot. Eight primary HAs are on the lower extremity: one on the hip, one on the thigh, five on the leg, and one on the foot.

The lower extremity, its bone, joints, muscles, and skin are innervated by nerves from both the lumbar nerve plexus (LNP) and the sacral nerve plexus (SNP). All the spinal nerves have dorsal and ventral rami. Only ventral rami of the lumbar and sacral spinal nerves are interconnected to form the LNP and SNP. Collectively we call them the lumbosacral plexus (LSP) (Figure 5-7). Just like the brachial plexus, the LSP divides to give off the anterior and the posterior divisions. The posterior divisions form the two major nerves: the femoral and the common fibular nerves. The anterior divisions form the two major nerves: the obturator and the tibial nerves. The tibial nerve gives two terminal branches: the medial plantar and the lateral plantar nerves. The common fibular and tibial nerves compose the sciatic nerve on the thigh region.

In the leg region, the saphenous nerve is the longest branch of the femoral nerve. Branches from the tibial nerve (medial) and the common fibular nerve unite to form the sural nerve. We discuss here only the terminal nerves that contribute to forming the primary HAs in the lower extremities.

H16 Inferior Gluteal   The H16 inferior gluteal is located in the center of the gluteal region (see Figure 5-1). The inferior gluteal nerve arises from the posterior divisions of the ventral rami of L5, S1, and S2. It leaves the pelvis through the inferior part of the greater sciatic foramen and inferior to the piriformis muscle, accompanied by the gluteal artery. This nerve enters the gluteus maximus muscle deeply from underneath.

Clinical Notes   This acupoint is tender in all patients with lower back pain, sciatica, or piriform muscle syndrome. Usually we use 5- to 8-cm-long needles to needle this acupoint all the way down to the bone below.

In many patients with chronic lower back pain and lower extremity pain, more tender points can be found around the H16 inferior gluteal acupoint on the gluteus medius and minimus muscles. These tender points should be treated along with the H16 inferior gluteal acupoint.

H18 Iliotibial   This acupoint can be palpated on the lateral surface of the thigh, about halfway between the hip and the knee on the iliotibial tract (see Figure 5-1). Possibly the sciatic nerve sends cutaneous branches to innervate the iliotibial tract.

Clinical Notes   The H18 iliotibial is used in treating lower back and lower extremity problems.

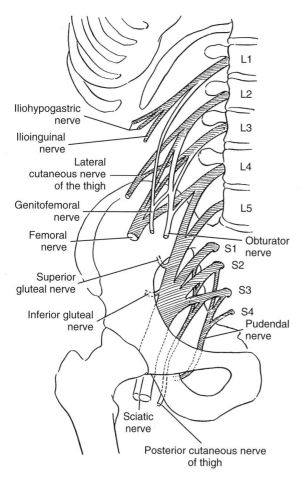

Iliohypogastric
nerve

Ilioinguinal
nerve

Lateral
cutaneous nerve
of the thigh

Genitofemoral
nerve

Femoral
nerve

Superior
gluteal nerve

Inferior gluteal
nerve

L1
L2
L3
L4
L5
S1
S2
S3
S4

Obturator
nerve

Pudendal
nerve

Sciatic
nerve

Posterior cutaneous nerve
of thigh

Figure 5-7 Diagram of the lumbosacral plexus. (From Jenkins D: *Hollinshead's functional anatomy of the limbs and back,* ed 8, Philadelphia, 2002, WB Saunders.)

It should be noted that as the symptoms become worse or chronic, more tender points appear on the iliotibial tract. These secondary or tertiary points should be palpated and needled to achieve better and faster results. The needling depth can be all the way to the bone.

H11 Lateral/Medial Popliteal These acupoints are located either on the lateral side of the tendon of the semitendinosus muscle (H11 medial popliteal) or on the medial side of the tendon of the biceps femoris (H11 lateral popliteal) (see Figure 5-1). The tenderness of these points can be palpable in most patients on the lateral side, the medial side, or on both sides.

The innervation of these points is unclear. The femoral cutaneous nerve (L2-4) is around the H11 medial popliteal; the H11 lateral popliteal is close to the common peroneal nerve (L4 to S2). The ten-

derness of these two acupoints is possibly related to those two nerves.

Clinical Notes These acupoints are palpable in more than 93% of patients. They may appear laterally or medially or on both sides, and therefore the H11 lateral/medial popliteal is treated as one acupoint. In patients with back or sciatic problems, this acupoint is definitely sensitive. A 4-cm-long needle is suggested for needling this point perpendicularly. Alternatively the needle can be tilted slightly toward the midline of the popliteal fossa. Many patients may feel a tingling sensation moving along the peroneal nerve down to the ankle if the H11 lateral popliteal is needled.

H4 Saphenous The H4 saphenous is easily palpable on the medial side of the knee below the medial condyle of the tibia (see Figure 5-1). This point is tender in almost every patient.

The H4 saphenous is formed at the site where the saphenous nerve emerges from the deep fascia. The saphenous nerve is a cutaneous branch of the femoral nerve that descends through the femoral triangle. This nerve accompanies the femoral artery and vein, and its branches supply the skin and fascia of the anterior and medial surface of the knee and leg as far as the medial malleolus.

The femoral nerve, from which branches the saphenous nerve, is the largest branch of the lumbar plexus (L2-4). The femoral nerve forms in the abdomen and enters the lower extremity through the pelvis to the midpoint of the inguinal ligament. After passing distally in the femoral triangle, the femoral nerve divides into several terminal branches to supply the hip and knee joints and the skin on the anteromedial side of the leg.

Clinical Notes   The H4 saphenous is useful for both the treatment and evaluation of prognosis, like the H1 deep radial on the forearm. As homeostasis declines, more tender points gradually appear along the saphenous nerve distally from the H4 saphenous. Thus this nerve provides quantitative information about healing potential and treatment prognosis. This acupoint, alongside the H1 deep radial, constitutes the basis for the method of quantitative evaluation of patients.

H24 Common Fibular (Peroneal)   The H24 common fibular is located just anteroinferior to the head of the fibula (see Figure 5-1). The common fibular nerve is one of the two terminal branches of the sciatic nerve. The finger-width sciatic nerve, the largest nerve in the body, is formed by the ventral rami of L4 to S3. It leaves the pelvis through the greater sciatic foramen and runs inferolaterally deep to the gluteus maximus. As it descends in the midline of the thigh, this nerve is overlapped posteriorly by the adjacent margins of the biceps femoris and semimembranosus muscles. In the lower third of the thigh, it divides into the tibial and the common fibular nerves.

The common fibular nerve enters the popliteal fossa following the medial border of the biceps muscle. It leaves the fossa by crossing superficially the lateral head of the gastrocnemius muscle. It then passes behind the head of the fibula, winds laterally around the neck of the bone, pierces the peroneus longus muscle, and divides into two terminal nerves: the superficial and the deep fibular nerves. The H24 common fibular is formed at the branching site.

Clinical Notes   The H24 common fibular is a terminal branch from the sciatic nerve, which justifies using it to treat all symptoms related to the lower back and sciatic nerve. The common fibular

nerve, like the deep radial nerve and the saphenous nerve, has a linear course down the leg medial to the fibular bone. More tender points will appear on the common fibular nerve distal from the H24 common fibular as body homeostasis declines.

H10 Sural   This acupoint is palpable around the middle of the posterior aspect of the leg, between the two heads of the gastrocnemius muscle (see Figure 5-1). As mentioned, the sciatic nerve contains two nerves, the common fibular and the tibial. These two nerves separate before they enter the popliteal fossa, where the common tibial nerve forms a branch termed the lateral sural nerve, and the tibial nerve forms the medial sural nerve. These two branches descend and unite between the two heads of the gastrocnemius muscle to form the sural nerve. The sural nerve pierces the deep fascia around the middle of the posterior leg where the acupoint is formed. The sural nerve is then joined by the fibular communicating branch of the common fibular nerve.

The sural nerve supplies the skin on the lateral and posterior part of the inferior third of the leg. It enters the foot posterior to the lateral malleolus and supplies the skin along the lateral margin of the foot and the lateral side of the fifth digit.

H6 Tibial   The H6 acupoint is palpable on the medial aspect of the leg, about 6 to 8 cm above the medial malleolus (see Figure 5-1). The tibial nerve is the larger terminal branch of the sciatic nerve (L4 to S3). The tibial nerve descends through the middle of the popliteal fossa, straight down the median plane of the calf, deep to the soleus muscle, and it supplies all the muscles in the posterior compartment of the leg. In addition, the tibial nerve gives off a cutaneous branch to form the sural nerve. The tibial nerve comes close to the medial skin about 6 to 8 cm above the medial malleolus, where the important H6 tibial acupoint is formed. From this point the tibial nerve courses down and passes deep to the flexor retinaculum between the medial malleolus and calcaneus. Here the tibial nerve divides into the medial and lateral plantar nerves and the calcaneal branches, which supply the skin of the sole and heel.

Clinical Notes   The H6 tibial is tender in almost every patient. This point is superficial in patients with thin leg muscles. For more effective needling for these patients, a 4-cm-long needle can be tilted downward to make better contact between the needle and tissues.

H5 Deep Fibular (Peroneal)   The H5 deep fibular (peroneal) acupoint is located about 2 cm proximal to the web between the great and second toes (see Figure 5-1). It appears tender in almost every patient.

As mentioned (see H24, common fibular), the deep fibular nerve is one of the two terminal branches of the common fibular nerve. The deep fibular nerve descends down the leg and gives off branches to the arteries, the ankle joint, and other articulations. This nerve becomes cutaneous about 2 cm proximal to the web between the great and second toes, where the acupoint is formed.

Homeostatic Acupoints on the Back

The back has five primary HAs. The general neuroanatomic plan of back acupoints is detailed in the section on paravertebral acupoints.

H20 Spinous Process of T7   This acupoint is located right on the spinous process of T7 (see Figure 5-1). The tenderness at this point is palpable in 80% of patients. The tissues of this acupoint are mainly innervated by small branches from the posterior primary ramus of the seventh thoracic spinal nerve.

Two methods can be used to locate this acupoint. In the first method, the spinous process of C7 is palpated. The spinous process of the seventh cervical vertebra is the most prominent at the base of the neck. From C7 palpation down to T7 can be performed. The second method is faster: this acupoint is level with the inferior angle of the scapula; so the scapula and its inferior angle can be located first.

Neuroanatomically it is still not clear why this acupoint becomes more sensitive than most other body points. We suspect that T7 is located at the lower edge of the scapula and so serves as a mechanic pivot between the upper thoracic spine and lower thoracic spine. Because of the scapula, the intervertebral joints from T1 to T6 are less bendable. As a mechanic pivot, T7 is most vulnerable to mechanical wear.

Clinical Notes   A 3-cm-long needle can be inserted perpendicularly downward until resistance is felt. From T1 to T9, the spinous process of T7 is always the first tender point. The second tender spinous process is usually T5. As homeostasis declines, more tender points appear on the spinal processes from T1 to T9. Thus the number of tender spinous processes from T1 to T9 provides quantitative information showing the homeostatic status of a patient. Manual palpation of the spinous processes from T1 to T9 should routinely be included in examinations.

H21 Posterior Cutaneous of T6   The H21 posterior cutaneous acupoint is located about 3 cm lateral from the spinous process of C6 (see Figure 5-1). It is tender in 80% of our patients. This acupoint is supplied by the cutaneous branch and the medial branch of the posterior primary ramus of the T6 spinal nerve. A 2.5-cm-long needle should be tilted toward the midline and inserted to a depth of about 2 cm.

H15 Posterior Cutaneous of L2   This acupoint is tender in about 90% of patients (see Figure 5-1). In most patients it lies on the lateral border of the lower back muscle (erector spinae), level with the narrowest part of the waist. In patients with much subcutaneous fat, a practitioner can palpate the lowest edges of the rib cage on both sides and draw an imaginary line between them. This point lies on the crossing point of this line and the lateral border of the erector spinae muscle. An experienced practitioner can easily locate the spinous process of L2 and find this acupoint quickly by palpating the erector spinae muscle in the lumbar region.

This acupoint is supplied by the cutaneous branch of the primary posterior ramus of L2. The posterior primary ramus of each spinal nerve gives off two terminal branches, the medial and the lateral. In the thoracic region the medial branch is cutaneous and the lateral branch is muscular. In the lumbar region the medial branch is muscular and the lateral branch is cutaneous. Thus in the lumbar region it is important to palpate to locate the tender spot.

Clinical Notes   This point is usually tender in about 90% of patients, especially in those with lower back, leg, and gynecologic problems. A 4- to 5-cm needle is inserted, slightly tilted to the midline. The depth varies from 3 to 5 cm.

H22 Posterior Cutaneous of L5   To locate this point, it is better to locate the H15 posterior cutaneous of the L2 or spinous process of L2 first and then palpate down to locate the spinous processes of L4 and L5. This point is located about 3 cm from the spinous process of L5 (see Figure 5-1) on the bulge of the erector spinae muscle. In some people this point is closer to L4 and in others it is closer to L5. This point is innervated by the muscular branch of the posterior primary ramus of the spinal nerve of L5.

Clinical Notes   This point is important in the treatment of lower back pain. The needling methods are the same as for the H15 posterior cutaneous point of L2, but the needle should be inserted perpendicularly downward.

H14 Superior Cluneal   This point is located at the highest point of the iliac crest (see Figure 5-1). First the iliac crest should be palpated to locate this acupoint, which is tender in about 90% of patients. The lateral branches of the posterior primary rami of the first three lumbar nerves unite to form the superior cluneal nerves. The superior cluneal nerves take an oblique downward course to the buttock region and emerge from the deep fascia just superior to the iliac crest. These nerves supply the skin on the superior two thirds of the buttock.

Clinical Notes   A 5- to 7-cm-long needle is inserted perpendicularly just superior to the iliac crest. In case of severe lower back and leg pain, a large area around the iliac crest may be tender and painful, and three to five needles can be used. Some needles can be directed inferiorly into the gluteus medius muscle, which is attached to the external surface of the ilium.

SYMPTOMATIC (OR ASHI) ACUPOINTS AND THEIR SPINAL MECHANISMS

Needling HAs is the source of the nonspecific effect of acupuncture therapy, that is, improving or restoring homeostasis. Needling SAs provides the specific effect because it inoculates lesions into sensitized soft tissues, which directly accelerates local recovery.

HAs themselves can become SAs. For example, the lower back HAs H15, H14, H22, and H16 are always tender in patients with lower back pain. In these cases HAs are also SAs.

We needle local tender acupoints to desensitize them because these sensitized points usually generate pain. These points, consisting primarily of sensitized sensory nerve fibers, appear randomly on the injured part of the body.

The body of a sensory neuron is housed in the dorsal (posterior) root ganglion (DRG), which is outside the spinal cord (Figure 5-8). This sensory neuron sends the nerve fiber peripherally to the skin or muscle and an axon centrally to the spinal cord gray matter. Pain is perceived by the brain if the peripheral nerve fibers are sensitized by pathological factors and send nociceptive signals to the brain.

The spinal cord gray matter contains different neurons and is divided into three parts: the dorsal (posterior) horn, the lateral horn, and the ventral (anterior) horn (Figure 5-9). The neurons in the dorsal (posterior) horn form a synapse with the axons from the sensory neuron of the DRG.

The dorsal horn neurons may inhibit, facilitate, and relay the sensory signals to the lateral horn and the ventral horn or to other segments of the spinal cord and to the brain. The processed signals from the dorsal horn neurons modulate the physiologic activities of the neurons of the lateral and ventral horn.

The lateral horn neurons control the autonomic physiology of internal organs, blood vessels, and glands. The ventral horn neurons are motor neurons that control muscle activity. The brain centers, after being activated by the ascending signals from sensory neurons, may send signals to the segment to manipulate spinal cord neurons. This anatomic picture shows that the signals from the sensory nerve fibers will influence lateral horn neurons, ventral horn neurons, other spinal segments, and the brain.

The lateral horn neurons regulate the autonomic activity of the organ systems, blood vessels, joints, muscles, and skin. For example, as a result of vasoconstriction the skin may become pale and cold. The muscle may show a diminished ability to stretch because of trophic changes caused by low blood circulation. Lack of sufficient blood circulation means low nutrition and oxygen supply to the joints. As a result of the trophic changes of the ligaments the joints will have a restricted range of motion.

The motor ventral horn controls muscle movement. It is important to keep in mind that the sensitized sensory fibers will, in their turn, sensitize the motor neurons, which will cause muscle shortening or stiffness of the muscles (see Chapter 3). The shortened muscles on the back can lead to blocked vertebral joints, resulting in stiffness of the neck and back, or they can create injuries to other shortened skeletal muscles and restrict the power of normal movement.

Every tender acupoint contains sensitized sensory nerve fibers. If the sensitivity of the sensory nerve increases persistently for an extended period, the sensitized nerve will sensitize the neurons in the lateral horn and anterior horn of the spinal cord in retrograde fashion.

This spinal sensitization causes increased sympathetic activity, which affects the motor nerves and the postganglionic nerves. This process leads to vasoconstriction (constriction of the blood vessels) and muscle tension. Once this vicious circle is established, the local nerve fibers become more sensitive and influence more nerve fibers and other soft tissues and finally result in the local tissues reacting abnormally to mechanical, thermal, and chemical stimuli (see Chapter 3).

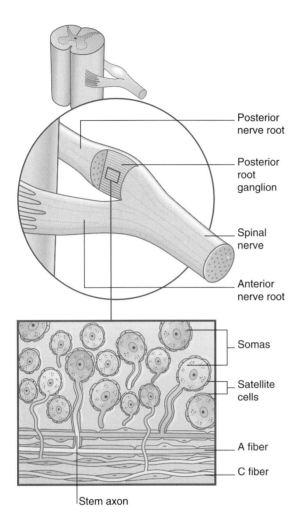

Posterior
nerve root

Posterior
root
ganglion

Spinal
nerve

Anterior
nerve root

Somas

Satellite
cells

A fiber

C fiber

Stem axon

Figure 5-8 Dorsal (posterior) root ganglion is located outside the spinal cord. The bottom figure shows the internal organization of bodies of the sensory neurons in the dorsal root ganglion. (Modified from FitzGerald M, Folan-Curran J: *Clinical neuroanatomy and related neuroscience,* ed 4, Edinburgh, 2002, WB Saunders.)

This pathologic phenomenon is named hyperalgesia (painful sensation) or hyperesthesia (sensation of discomfort). *Local tender points are created by the acute onset of diseases/injuries or chronic diseases.*

The disease- or injury-related tender points are defined as *symptomatic,* or *local* acupoints according to their physiologic nature. Now we will explain why the acupoints have different names. For example, injuries on the upper extremity, such as tennis elbow and carpal tunnel syndrome, create tender points on the upper extremity. These points are SAs or local points in comparison with HAs, which are distributed systemically all over the body.

These SAs of the upper extremity can be traced through the pathway of their peripheral nerve to spinal segments C5 to T1. These acupoints are neurosegmentally related to spinal segments C5 to T1.

Treatment Protocol

The treatment protocol is based on the mechanism of segmental sensitivity. In healthy people with only acute symptoms, a few sessions of needling SAs are enough to cure the symptoms. In chronic pain patients, more treatment sessions are needed to desensitize both peripheral nerve fibers and corresponding segmental neurons in the spinal cord. This desensitization is achieved by needling SAs, PAs, and HAs.

Healthy people may have only a few tender homeostatic acupoints with minimal sensitivity, and the neurons in their spinal cord may be barely sensitized. If acute symptoms develop, the number and sensitivity of the local tender acupoints will increase. At this acute stage, the peripheral nerve fibers of the acupoints become sensitized but the neurons in the corresponding segment of the spinal

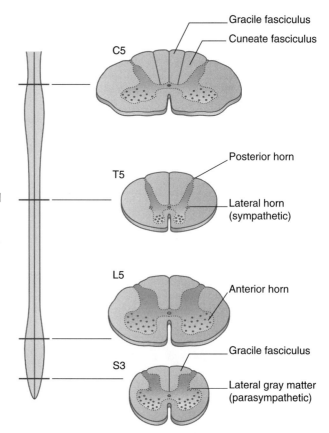

Figure 5-9   Organization of the dorsal (posterior) horn, lateral (sympathetic) horn, and ventral (anterior) horn in the spinal cord. (Modified from FitzGerald M, Folan-Curran J: *Clinical neuroanatomy*, ed 4, Edinburgh, 2002, WB Saunders.)

cord are still not sensitized. For such patients a few acupuncture sessions will desensitize the peripheral nerve fibers and the symptoms will be permanently cured.

If local tenderness (sensitivity) persists, the sensitized acupoints will increase in both size and sensitivity, eventually causing more tender points to appear in their vicinity. Now the symptom is spreading and entering the chronic stage. As the chronicity persists, the peripheral tender acupoints gradually sensitize the neurons in the same segment of the spinal cord as already discussed, and possibly even sensitize HAs all over the body, as we see in patients with chronic pain.

Thus, to treat chronic symptoms, we needle both SAs and HAs. The needling will activate the spinal segmental (SAs) and supraspinal (HAs) mechanisms (see Figure 3-2, p. 33). In other words, to treat chronic pain, we need to desensitize both peripheral nerves and the spinal cord. This is why chronic pain requires more acupuncture treatments than acute pain.

After the symptoms of chronic pain improve, the desensitized neurons of the spinal cord and the peripheral nerve fibers are still susceptible to resensitization when exposed to any pathologic factors such as repetitive injuries or internal diseases. It is possible that the resensitized spinal cord neurons can resensitize the peripheral nerve fibers of the same spinal segment. This explains why chronic pain symptoms may improve but are likely to relapse after a time.

In severe cases of chronic pain, such as fibromyalgia, the tender points can be palpable all over the body. This fact shows that a large number of peripheral nerves have been extensively sensitized for a long time. The chronic process of fibromyalgia not only oversensitizes numerous neurons in multiple segments of the spinal cord, but it also oversensitizes the neurons of the pain-modulation centers in the brain. Oversensitization of the pain-modulation centers of the brain will limit or impair the mechanisms of central pain inhibition in the spinal cord and brain and finally jeopardize the self-healing process.

Now it is clear why acupuncture sometimes produces "miracles" in reasonably healthy persons experiencing acute pain: a few needles and two to four sessions can cure the problems permanently. More treatment sessions will be required to reduce symptoms in chronic pain patients, and the symptoms are likely to recur after some time. For a few patients with severely impaired homeostasis, acupuncture therapy provides little or no relief no matter how many treatments are offered. The difference between these three groups of patients (strong, average, and weak responders to acupuncture) is that the neurons responsible for pain perception in their spinal cords and brains have different pathologic sensitivities.

Neuroanatomically and neurophysiologically, peripheral neural segmentation is not simple because segmentation involves sensory nerves, motor nerves, and autonomic nerves. The three types of peripheral nerves of the same spinal segment may go to different tissues and organs in different portions of the body. In addition, an increased nociceptive activity in one part of a segment also affects other parts of the same segment, thereby expanding segmental symptoms, such as referred pain and hyperalgesia, and autonomic symptoms, such as vasomotor and trophic changes. For example, a long-lasting painful shoulder is more likely to give neck troubles. When the neck is troubled, the shoulder and lower back should be treated at the same time. This implies that treating a local problem requires both local and distal acupoints. A practitioner will achieve better and faster results if he or she is able to relate the SAs to their segmental origin in the spinal cord and understand how to find and use homeostatic (distal) acupoints to increase the efficacy of symptomatic (local) acupoints. Fortunately, after a meticulous analysis of the neuroanatomic data, we have found a clinical protocol that resolves this complexity.

The following are some examples of SA formation. The respiratory symptoms from allergy, lung infection, or asthma will make acupoints tender on the front of the chest and the upper back. These points are often innervated by the cutaneous and muscular nerves from anterior and posterior rami of the spinal nerves of T1 to T8 (see Figure 5-13). An acute or chronic gastritis gives tender points just below the front rib cage on the rectus abdominis muscle and on the back along T5 to T11. If an athlete sprains an ankle, tender or even painful points appear around the injured ankle area, which is innervated by the fibular and tibial nerves derived from L3 to S3. Tennis elbow and carpal tunnel syndrome are related to the brachial plexus from C5 to T1. All these points are caused by either exogenous injuries or endogenous diseases, and they are locally restricted. If, however, the treatment of the pathologic condition is delayed, that is, if the SAs persist for some time, more tender points may develop far from the original symptomatic points. For example, some acute lower back pain produces tender points only on the lower back area or the gluteal region. If not properly treated, new tender points may appear on the thighs or legs and acute lower back pain will become chronic lower back pain, which will require more treatments to alleviate and may be subject to a relapse.

The appearance of symptomatic points is an individualized process because no two patients are identical in terms of their body types, genetic makeup, medical history, how they were injured or became ill, their lifestyle, and their tolerance to needling.

To decide which SAs should be prescribed for current treatment, a practitioner needs to obtain the patient's medical history, especially the data from medical examinations, including laboratory tests and MRIs; all the injuries sustained by the patient; and related events. If the case is suitable for acupuncture therapy, visual examination should be performed first.

With the patient undressed and standing in a relaxed way, the practitioner can check the muscle balance on both sides and the spine morphology. Such visual data may help find symptomatic points. Subsequently a thorough examination by manual palpation of the body should be performed. This process enables a practitioner to determine the following:

1. Where and what structures are involved in the injuries or related to the symptoms
2. Where the symptomatic points are located
3. The physical and psychological status of the patient (some patients are psychologically and physically less tolerant to needling)
4. The possible prognosis for treatment (see Chapter 6)

More clinical techniques and procedures are detailed in Chapter 6.

NEUROANATOMY OF THE PARAVERTEBRAL POINTS

After finding the SAs, we need to trace their spinal segments to find corresponding PAs. The purpose of needling the corresponding PAs is (1) to facilitate the peripheral and spinal desensitization, (2) to relax the neck and back muscles to remove stress from the roots of the spinal nerves such as radiculopathy, and (3) to better balance autonomic activity.

Every spinal nerve divides into two primary rami: posterior (dorsal) and anterior (ventral) (Figure 5-10). The anterior primary ramus gives two branches: the lateral cutaneous and the anterior cutaneous nerves. Each cutaneous nerve separates into two end branches to supply side and anterior parts of the same dermatome.

The posterior primary ramus also separates into two end branches: lateral and medial. In the thoracic region, the lateral branches are muscular and the medial branches are cutaneous. Each end branch may form an acupoint when it penetrates the fascia to supply the skin. Thus a spinal nerve may form six tender acupoints in its dermatome at the locations

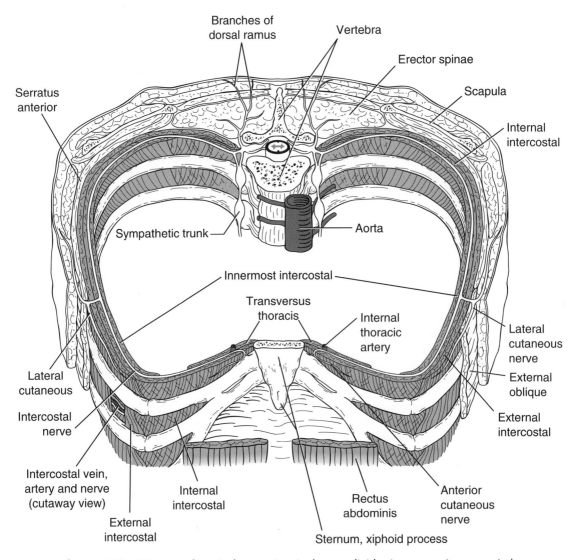

Figure 5-10   Diagram of a spinal nerve. A spinal nerve divides into two primary rami: the dorsal (posterior) ramus and the ventral (anterior) ramus. The short dorsal (posterior) ramus, with its two end branches, innervates the muscles and skin of the back. The ventral (anterior) primary ramus travels within the body wall to innervate the skin and muscles on the lateral and anterior parts of the body. Please note that there are two lateral end cutaneous branches and two anterior cutaneous end branches separating from the anterior primary ramus. (Modified from Jenkins D: *Hollinshead's functional anatomy of the limbs and back,* ed 8, Philadelphia, 2002, WB Saunders.)

where each of the branches penetrates the fascia. From the cervical region to the sacral region of the spine, there are 33 pairs of spinal nerves.

All facial acupoints are formed on the cranial nerves, and all body acupoints are associated with the spinal nerves. Once the spinal nerve leaves the intervertebral foramen, it divides into two major branches: the anterior primary ramus and the posterior primary ramus (see Figure 5-10).

Most symptomatic and homeostatic acupoints are formed on the terminal branches of the anterior primary rami. A posterior primary ramus goes to the back and divides into two terminal branches: the medial branch and the lateral branch. In the thoracic region, the medial branch supplies the skin and the lateral branch supplies the muscles. The posterior primary ramus also sends small branches to innervate the vertebral joints. In general, there is a total of 33 posterior primary rami from the neck to the sacral region: 8 from cervical vertebrae (C1-8), 12 from thoracic vertebrae (T1-12), five from lumbar vertebrae (L1-5), 4 from sacral vertebrae (S1-4), and four (or three in some cases) from the coccygeal bones (Figure 5-11). The coccygeal spinal nerves are very small and are needled only in treating pain in the coccygeal regions.

Paravertebral acupoints are physiologically different from both SAs and HAs. We select and needle SAs and HAs because they are pathologically tender and sensitive. We select and needle PAs because they are located close to the nerve roots of the SAs. These acupoints are not necessarily sensitive or tender during the acupuncture session. Both PAs and SAs are innervated by the spinal nerve fibers of the same spinal segment(s). Needling PAs desensitizes SAs through the physiologic segmental reflex.

For example clinical evidence shows that successful results have been obtained by needling only PAs while treating patients diagnosed with complex regional pain syndrome (CRPS, previously called *reflex sympathetic dystrophy* [RSD]). In addition, in many healthy people who come for routine health maintenance treatments, needling PAs also provides a destressing effect.

Clinical Notes Different techniques are used to needle PAs because the related anatomy of each part of the vertebral spine is different in each patient. The needling methods described in the following section provide general guidance to follow during acupuncture treatment. A practitioner has room to explore his or her own methods as long as safety and efficacy are taken into consideration.

The techniques described here apply to patients of "average" body size and placed in the prone position. For thinner or larger patients, the length of the needle as well as the depth and direction of needling should match the appropriate body anatomy to avoid accidents and to produce desirable results.

Locating the PAs starts with palpation of the midline (the spinous processes). The precise location of the acupoints is not critical, as already explained, but locating the point at the same level with the spinous process of the corresponding vertebra is preferable because this point may be closer to the primary ramus of the spinal nerve. Both sides of the spine should be needled to ensure that muscles on both sides are relaxed, which helps to realign the vertebral joints and provides enough stimulation signals to be sent to the nerve endings. The points to be needled are located usually 2 to 3 cm (about 1 inch) away from the midline.

Instructions for Needling Different Paravertebral Acupoints

Cervical Vertebrae (C2-7) We use needles 4 to 5 cm long (34-gauge, 0.22-cm diameter) and palpate and locate the points situated about 2.5 cm from the midline. The direction of the needle is perpendicular to the skin. The patient is lying in a prone position, and the needle should be lightly pushed down until it touches the bony structure below the skin. Two to three acupoints may be selected on each side of the spine. If a palpated region is painful, this means that a muscle(s) or a joint structure is affected and the painful region should be needled. Once the needle touches the bone, slight manipulation of the needle, such as rotating the needle back and forth or "pistoning" the needle up and down, helps reduce the pain. The needles are kept in place for about 5 minutes.

Thoracic Vertebrae (T1-12) Great care must be taken not to puncture the lung. To palpate the point about 2 to 3 cm away from the midline (the spinous process), use needles 2.5 cm long and direct the needles toward the midline. The needling depth can be 2 to 2.5 cm. Either three or seven points may be selected on each side for a treatment. Needles may be kept in place for 10 to 15 minutes.

Lumbar Vertebrae (L1-5) Most people have tender points in this area. A practitioner may locate the two primary acupoints, H15 posterior cutaneous of L2 and H22 posterior cutaneous, as described previously. Two or four points may be selected on each side. Needles 4 to 6 cm long are used in this region.

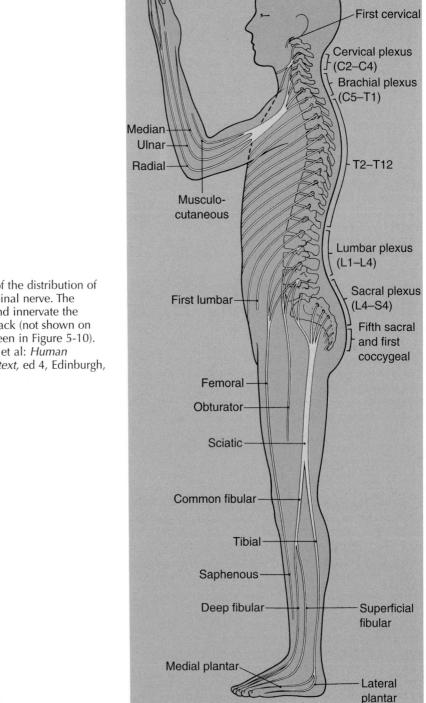

Figure 5-11   Diagram of the distribution of the anterior rami of the spinal nerve. The posterior rami are short and innervate the muscles and skin of the back (not shown on this diagram but can be seen in Figure 5-10). (Modified from Gosling J, et al: *Human anatomy: color atlas and text,* ed 4, Edinburgh, 2002, Mosby.)

Sacral Vertebrae   All the points are located over the sacrum bone. This area is safe and a practitioner can apply any preferred needling method in this area. Acupoints in this region can be needled all the way down to the sacral bone.

PRINCIPLES OF USING SPINAL SEGMENTATION IN ACUPUNCTURE THERAPY

The innervation of skin, muscles, bones and even viscera is segmented in terms of the supply of the spinal nerves. Understanding the basic principles of this spinal segmentation will help select proper PAs to match corresponding SAs.

How to Select Paravertebral Acupoints

PAs are selected to match the corresponding SAs according to spinal segmentation. For symptoms of the upper extremity, needle PAs from C4 to T1. For lower-extremity disorders, use PAs along L2 to S3. PAs along T1 to T7 are used for problems of upper back and chest and PAs from T8 to L1 for problems of the abdominal region (Figures 5-11 to 5-13).

Segmentation of the Body Structure

The following description of body segmentation is aimed at helping the practitioner match SAs with their corresponding spinal segments. Please note that for purposes of clinical acupuncture the precise segment is not critical because the innervated field of one spinal nerve overlaps with the innervated fields of both neighboring spinal nerves.

The segmental innervations of the skin, muscles, viscera, and bones are referred to as dermatome, myotome, viscerotome, and sclerotome, respectively. Segmentation of the neural supply presented in the following section is intended simply as an aid to understanding the segmental relationship between local points (SAs) and their corresponding spinal segments.

Segmental Innervation of the Skin: Dermatomes

In the trunk the cutaneous segmentation is in the form of dermatomes, which are arranged in regular bands from T2 to L1 (Figure 5-12). A few body marks can help with remembering the dermatomes: T2 is at the sternal angle, T10 at the level of the umbilicus, and L1 in the region of the groin. As mentioned, there is considerable overlap between neighboring dermatomes of the trunk. Thus, for clinical simplicity and efficacy, it is important to treat both affected dermatomes and their neighboring dermatomes. For example, if postherpetic neuralgia is associated with T5 and T6, the PAs of dermatome from T4 to T7 should be needled together.

Segmental Innervation of the Musculature: Myotomes

The segmental innervation of muscles of the trunk has a strictly segmental pattern from T1 to L1. The posterior rami supply the thoracic and lumbar muscles (spinal extensors), and their anterior rami innervate the intercostal muscles, abdominal flank muscles, and the rectus abdominis in a regular segmental fashion.

The segmental pattern of the muscles in the extremities is more functionally arranged. The groups of muscles that act for similar primary functions are often innervated with adjacent spinal nerves. For example, elbow flexor muscles are supplied by C5 and C6, whereas the elbow extensor muscles are innervated by C7 and C8.

For clinical practicality and efficacy, acupuncture practitioners do not need to remember which single muscle is supplied by which single segmental nerve, but we do need to know what portion of the segments are related to the particular muscles. For example, elbow flexors are innervated by C5 and C6, extensors by C7 and C8. When we treat any elbow pain or even any upper-extremity problems, we simply needle PAs from C4 to T1. Table 5-1 is designed for this purpose. Readers may consult textbooks of neuroanatomy to study myotomes in more detail.

Segmental Innervation of the Skeletal System: Sclerotomes

Some patients seek acupuncture therapy for pain on the bones that may involve the inflammation of the periosteum. One common example is the pain on the shin bone (tibia). Knowledge of the segmental supply by the spinal nerves (sclerotomes) helps to select the proper PAs. Readers will find that the principle of using sclerotomes is actually very similar to that of myotomes (Table 5-2).

Segmental Innervation of the Internal Organs: Viscerotome

Some patients complain that their pain is related to internal organs such as stomach, kidneys, or gallbladder. Whereas the visceral pain can be relieved by acupuncture, these patients should be referred to

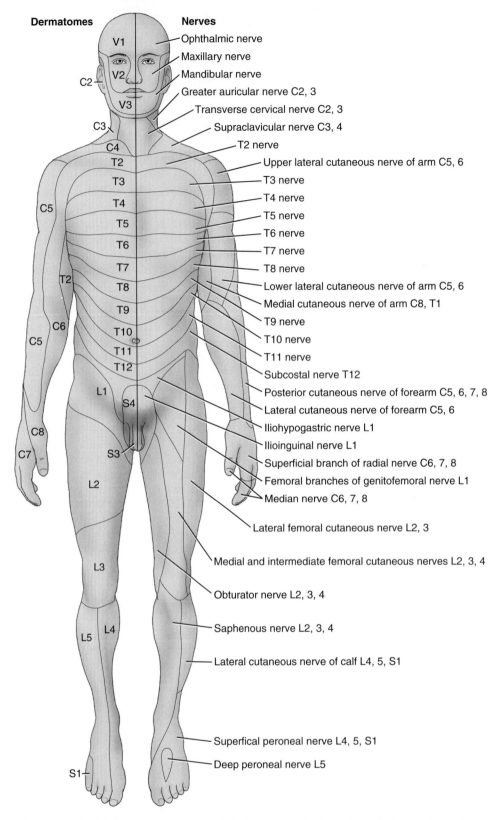

Dermatomes

V1
V2
C2
V3
C3
C4
T2
T3
C5
T4
T5
T6
T7
T2
T8
C6
T9
C5
T10
T11
T12
C8
L1
S4
C7
S3
L2
L3
L4
L5
S1

Nerves

Ophthalmic nerve
Maxillary nerve
Mandibular nerve
Greater auricular nerve C2, 3
Transverse cervical nerve C2, 3
Supraclavicular nerve C3, 4
T2 nerve
Upper lateral cutaneous nerve of arm C5, 6
T3 nerve
T4 nerve
T5 nerve
T6 nerve
T7 nerve
T8 nerve
Lower lateral cutaneous nerve of arm C5, 6
Medial cutaneous nerve of arm C8, T1
T9 nerve
T10 nerve
T11 nerve
Subcostal nerve T12
Posterior cutaneous nerve of forearm C5, 6, 7, 8
Lateral cutaneous nerve of forearm C5, 6
Iliohypogastric nerve L1
Ilioinguinal nerve L1
Superficial branch of radial nerve C6, 7, 8
Femoral branches of genitofemoral nerve L1
Median nerve C6, 7, 8
Lateral femoral cutaneous nerve L2, 3
Medial and intermediate femoral cutaneous nerves L2, 3, 4
Obturator nerve L2, 3, 4
Saphenous nerve L2, 3, 4
Lateral cutaneous nerve of calf L4, 5, S1
Superfical peroneal nerve L4, 5, S1
Deep peroneal nerve L5

Figure 5-12 Adult dermatome pattern. (Modified from Abrahams P, Hutchings R, Marks S: *McMinn's color atlas of human anatomy*, ed 4, London, 1997, Mosby.)

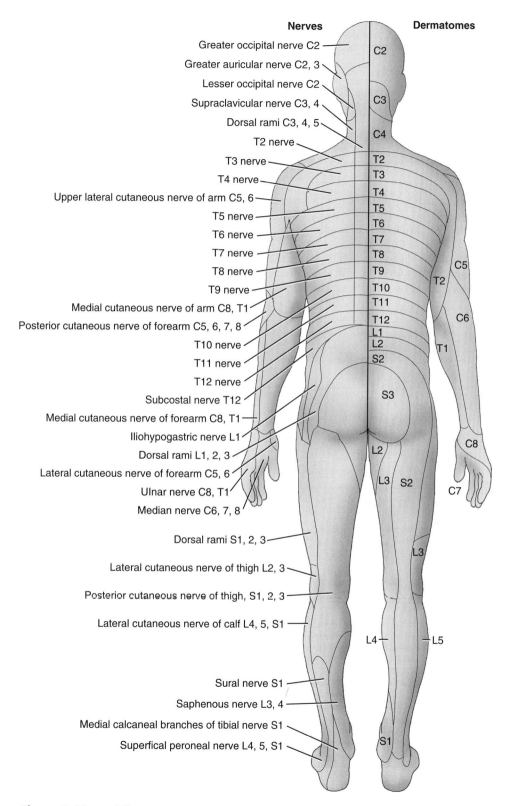

Nerves

Dermatomes

Greater occipital nerve C2

Greater auricular nerve C2, 3

Lesser occipital nerve C2

Supraclavicular nerve C3, 4

Dorsal rami C3, 4, 5

T2 nerve

T3 nerve

T4 nerve

Upper lateral cutaneous nerve of arm C5, 6

T5 nerve

T6 nerve

T7 nerve

T8 nerve

T9 nerve

Medial cutaneous nerve of arm C8, T1

Posterior cutaneous nerve of forearm C5, 6, 7, 8

T10 nerve

T11 nerve

T12 nerve

Subcostal nerve T12

Medial cutaneous nerve of forearm C8, T1

Iliohypogastric nerve L1

Dorsal rami L1, 2, 3

Lateral cutaneous nerve of forearm C5, 6

Ulnar nerve C8, T1

Median nerve C6, 7, 8

Dorsal rami S1, 2, 3

Lateral cutaneous nerve of thigh L2, 3

Posterior cutaneous nerve of thigh, S1, 2, 3

Lateral cutaneous nerve of calf L4, 5, S1

Sural nerve S1

Saphenous nerve L3, 4

Medial calcaneal branches of tibial nerve S1

Superfical peroneal nerve L4, 5, S1

C2

C3

C4

T2
T3
T4
T5
T6
T7
T8
T9
T10
T11
T12
L1
L2
S2

S3

C5

T2

C6

T1

C8

C7

L2

L3 S2

L3

L4 L5

S1

Figure 5-12, cont'd

Table 5-1 Segmental Innervation of Muscles	
Musculature of the Body Region	**Segments of the Spinal Cord**
Upper extremity (including shoulder)	C4-T1
Lower extremity (including hip)	T12-S3
Trunk	
Diaphragm	C1-5
Other trunk and abdominal muscles	Regular segmental pattern from C5-S2

internists. However, knowledge of segmental innervation of internal organs helps to select correct PAs to relieve pain or muscle spasm of the internal organs (Figure 5-13).

Figure 5-13 shows that most important internal organs are innervated by both cervical and thoracic nerves (including kidneys). Thus it is important to needle the cervical PAs when treating disorders of these organs.

SUMMARY

Changes in homeostasis, chronic diseases, and acute injuries convert latent acupoints into passive

Table 5-2 Segmental Innervation of the Skeletal System	
Bones of the Body Region	**Segments of the Spinal Cord**
Cervical vertebrae	C1-8
Upper extremity (including shoulder)	C4-T1
Lower extremity (including hip)	T12-S3
Trunk	
Costae	Regular pattern from T1-12
Thoracic and lumbar vertebrae	Regular segmental pattern from T1-5

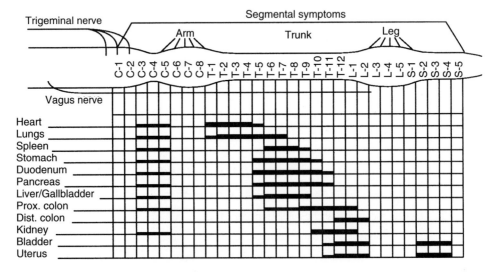

Figure 5-13   Segmental innervation of the internal organs. This diagram shows that neck injury can affect many internal organs. (Modified from Filshie J, White A: *Medical acupuncture,* Edinburgh, 1998, Churchill Livingstone.)

or active acupoints. The three types of acupoints used in pain management are symptomatic (SAs), homeostatic (HAs), and paravertebral (PAs).

As homeostasis declines, HAs appear nonsegmentally all over the body in predictable sequential order and locations. SAs are associated with external injuries or internal diseases. The third type of acupoints, PAs, help to desensitize SAs, balance the activities of the autonomic nervous system, relax back muscles, and relieve radiculopathy. For effective treatments, all three types of acupoints should be properly combined because each type provides different therapeutic effects.

The 24 primary HAs are used to treat *all* symptoms because these points improve homeostasis, which normalizes and maximizes the self-healing physiology. All other HAs may develop in some patterns related to or around these 24 primary HAs. By knowing the locations of the 24 HAs, we can predict where to find other HAs needed for a particular treatment.

SAs are used to treat specific symptoms. Their appearance is usually local, individualized, or seg-mentally (in some cases of internal disease) related to a particular portion of the spinal cord. A practitioner should carefully palpate the body to locate these points for each treatment.

PAs should be selected to facilitate the therapeutic efficacy of the SAs. The selected PAs and SAs should be innervated by the spinal nerves of the same spinal segments.

In pain physiology, acute symptoms sensitize only peripheral neurons, whereas chronic diseases sensitize both peripheral sensory and central spinal neurons. Acute symptoms can be easily desensitized with a few local treatments. Chronic diseases require more holistic treatments to desensitize both peripheral and central neurons, and the pain symptoms are susceptible to relapse as a result of resensitization, even after improvement is achieved.

Reference

1. Dung HC: *Anatomical acupuncture,* San Antonio, Texas, 1997, Antarctic Press.

CHAPTER 6

Quantitative Acupuncture Evaluation and Clinical Techniques

INTRODUCTION: QUANTITATIVE EVALUATION PREDICTS THE EFFICACY OF ACUPUNCTURE THERAPY

To be a good clinical procedure, an acupuncture evaluation of patients should be simple, precise, reliable, and reproducible by any practitioner. In traditional Chinese medicine (TCM) the goal of qualitative evaluation (pulse, tongue, and tongue coating) is to determine the nature and the cause of the symptoms according to ancient pathologic concepts: (1) the diseased organ or organs (*Zang fu*) and related channels (meridians) and (2) the nature of the imbalance (*yin* or *yang*, hot or cold, excessive or deficient).

The coating of the tongue and the character of the pulse reflect qualitative features of the body's pathophysiology but do not always provide stable, reliable information. For example, the tongue coating may change after food intake and the pulse is altered after drinking, walking, or emotional disturbance.

In addition, the art of qualitative diagnosis is subtle and complex. Years of training are required for a practitioner to learn the 28 different pulses and their combinations and the numerous types of coatings. Thus qualitative diagnosis is a time-consuming, highly empirical procedure that is difficult to master and unnecessary in acupuncture pain management.

The goal of the quantitative method presented in this book is to evaluate the self-healing capacity of each patient and to predict the effectiveness of acupuncture therapy for each individual case. Two pathophysiologic factors affect the efficacy of acupuncture: the individual self-healing potential of each patient and the severity and "healability" (the healable nature of the disease[s]) of the afflicting symptom(s) or disease(s) itself. These two factors affect the efficacy of treatment and the time required for each patient to heal. Therefore, when making an evaluation, acupuncture practitioners must take these factors into account to understand whether and to what degree a patient can recover from his or her specific pathologic symptoms or diseases.

The following clinical example can help us to understand the nature of acupuncture therapy.

Four patients (not necessarily in the same age group) were afflicted with essentially the same pain symptom. After receiving four acupuncture treatments using the same treatment protocol, patient A and patient B experienced total pain relief, patient C experienced a reduction of pain up to about 50%, and patient D did not feel any improvement from the treatments.

Five months later patient A was still experiencing no pain; patient B experienced some pain, which was totally relieved after two additional acupuncture treatments; patient C experienced a return of most of the pain symptoms and needed four additional acupuncture treatments to maintain control of the pain; and patient D experienced little or no benefit from acupuncture therapy despite having continued the treatments for 5 months.

Statistically, patient A represents 28% of the patient population who can completely self-heal; patient B, 34%; patient C, 30% (B and C can partially self-heal); and patient D, 8% (can slowly, or not all, self-heal) (Table 6-1).

This example clearly illustrates that the efficacy of acupuncture treatment depends primarily on (1) the degree of the patient's self-healing potential and (2) the healability of the afflicting symptoms or diseases.

A good acupuncture evaluation should provide information concerning treatment efficacy and give an answer to the following questions for a specific patient:

1. Is the symptom treatable (responsive to acupuncture treatment)?
2. If it is treatable, how many treatments are needed?

Group	A	B	C	D
Number of passive HAs carried by a patient	<24	24-52	53-79	>80
Percentage of patient population (%)	28	34	30	8
No. of treatments required for pain relief	4-8	8-16	16-32	>32
Time lapse before recurrence of same pain	Years	Months to years	Weeks to months	Days to weeks

**Table 6-1
Patient Classification**

Modified from Dung HC: *Anatomical acupuncture,* San Antonio 1997, Antarctic Press, p 226.

3. Will the symptom return after initial relief is achieved?
4. When will the symptom return or relapse?

Our method of quantitative acupuncture evaluation (QAE) determines the healing potential of each patient and provides answers to these questions. QAE is an easy method to learn, as well as being time-saving, reliable, and reproducible by any practitioner.

QUANTITATIVE ACUPUNCTURE EVALUATION

The results of QAE allow practitioners to predict the efficacy, duration, and prognosis of the treatment. Any pathologic insult or disease tends to reduce the patient's self-healing potential and impairs homeostasis. The impaired or declining homeostasis transforms latent (nonsensitive) acupoints into passive (tender) acupoints. The homeostasis of each patient reflects his or her body's ability to repair the damage evidenced by pathologic symptoms.

Thus the number of tender homeostatic acupoints (N_{HAs}; see Chapter 5) shows the interaction between the self-healing potential (HP) and the severity of the symptoms (SS). This relationship can be roughly expressed in the following linear formula:

$$N_{HAs} = f \frac{SS}{HP}$$

This formula expresses the condition that the number of HAs is proportional to the severity of the symptoms (SS) and inversely proportional to the self-healing potential (HP); f represents a factor that varies for each individual.

A healthy person maintains optimum homeostasis, which results in the best self-healing and produces a fast, complete cure of most pain symptoms. Such a person will have only a few tender acupoints. If a healthy person suffers from acute pain symptoms, they can usually be relieved by two to four acupuncture treatments.

When chronic disease or chronic pain is affecting the body, homeostasis declines, the healing potential is reduced, and additional tender HAs gradually appear in a predictable sequence and in predictable locations. Patients with chronic pain usually need 8 to 16 acupuncture treatments to achieve pain relief. The same symptoms may return after about 4 to 6 months, and then additional acupuncture treatments will be needed to keep the pain under control for another 4 to 6 months.

If homeostasis deteriorates beyond a certain physiologic limit, the mechanism of self-healing is severely impeded. No matter how many treatments are administered, these patients will feel little or no relief.

Dr. H.C. Dung classified patients into four groups (see Table 6-1) according to their self-healing potential and treatment prognosis, after studying more than 15,000 cases.

Classification of patients is important because it allows prediction of the efficacy, duration, and prognosis of acupuncture therapy. To classify patients into groups, it is not necessary for a practitioner to count every passive HA in the body. Because HAs appear in an anticipated sequence and at highly predictable locations, it is sufficient to check a few landmark acupoints to obtain a clear picture about the group to which a patient belongs at the time of the treatment.

The selected landmark acupoints for patient evaluation are the H1 deep radial on the forearm (Figures 6-1 and 6-2) and H4 saphenous (Figure 6-3). The deep radial nerve and the saphenous nerve are similar to one another. Both emerge from deep tissues at similar locations just below the elbow and knee and start to branch to innervate other muscles.

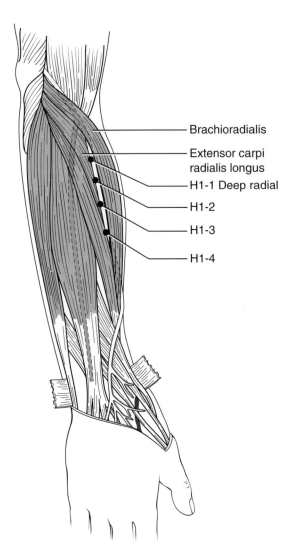

Brachioradialis

Extensor carpi radialis longus

H1-1 Deep radial

H1-2

H1-3

H1-4

Figure 6-1   Acupoint used for quantitative evaluation. H1 deep radial is the first tender acupoint appearing in every person. As homeostasis declines, more tender points (H1-2, H1-3, and H1-4) gradually develop along the deep radial nerve distally from H1. So the number of tender points appearing on the deep radial nerve provides reliable information about the level of homeostasis; this information reflects the patient's self-healing potential. (Modified from Jenkins D: *Hollinshead's functional anatomy of the limbs and back,* ed 8, Philadelphia, 2002, WB Saunders.)

radial nerve) and H4-2, H4-3, H4-4 (located on the saphenous nerve). Thus the total number of points is 16 bilaterally.

The two points, H1 and H4, are tender in almost all patients. When the self-healing potential of a patient declines, the second points, H1-2 and H4-2, appear tender. If the self-healing potential continues to decline, the third points, H1-3 and H4-3, also become sensitive. When the self-healing potential is minimal, the fourth acupoints, H1-4 and H4-4, become tender.

When examining a patient we palpate all these 16 diagnostic points on the forearms and legs on both sides of the body. Using the results of this examination we can classify our patients into four groups, as shown in Table 6-2.

By combining data from Tables 6-1 and 6-2, we can predict the efficacy, duration, and outcome of acupuncture treatments. Statistical analysis shows

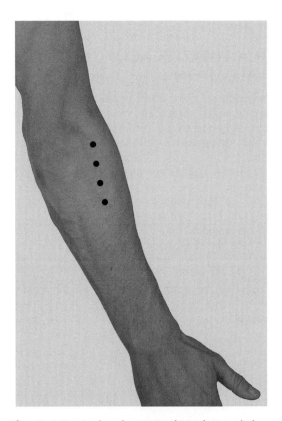

Figure 6-2   Surface location of H1 deep radial and its derivative tender points H1-2, H1-3, and H1-4 used to evaluate the self-healing potential. (Modified from Lumley J: *Surface anatomy: the anatomical basis of clinical examination,* ed 3, Edinburgh, 2002, Churchill Livingstone.)

Figures 6-1 and 6-3 show that more HAs can appear distally to both H1 and H4. These additional points are located along the deep radial and saphenous nerves, about 2 to 3 cm apart. We call these points H1-2, H1-3, H1-4 (located on the deep that about one third of patients belong to group A (28%). The effects of acupuncture can seem miraculous for this group. Group D accounts for about one tenth of patients (8%), and these are least able to benefit from acupuncture therapy. Most patients, about 64%, belong to groups B and C and represent an average or slightly below average health level. Acupuncture treatments can successfully control chronic pain for patients in groups B and C for some time. In some cases the pain will recur in about 4 to 6 months (see Table 6-1); some patients may enjoy longer pain relief if they take appropriate measures for health maintenance. The mechanism of pain relapse was explained in Chapters 3 and 5. Age and genetic factors may influence the self-healing potential. The age of most group A patients is below 40, and most group D patients are above 60 years of age. Nevertheless it is not uncommon to see older patients in group A and younger patients in group D. We should not assume that older patients are necessarily sick or weak.

When checking acupoints, the practitioner must be able to apply correct and consistent pressure to each acupoint, which is not a difficult skill to learn. As a general rule, apply 2 to 3 pounds of thumb pressure on each diagnostic point. Applying insufficient pressure may cause underestimation of the tenderness of the acupoint, and applying excessive pressure may cause overestimation of the sensitivity of the acupoint.

The following simple guidelines facilitate the evaluation procedure:

1. The practitioner should adjust the thumb pressure to the pain threshold level of each patient. For example, when pressure is applied to H1-1 and H4-1, some patients will jump because of intolerable pain, whereas others will feel only a little tenderness. The practitioner should adjust the level of thumb pressure accordingly.
2. Less experienced practitioners can use the color change in their thumbnail as an indicator. When pressing acupoints H1-1 and H4-1, simply look at the nail of the thumb: when the pink color turns to white, the pressure is about 2 to 3 pounds. Care must be taken when treating patients who have a lower tolerance for pressure.

CLINICAL TECHNIQUES

The following section describes how to apply the quantitative evaluation method to acupuncture treatment.

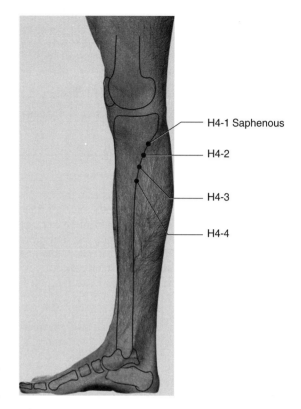

H4-1 Saphenous

H4-2

H4-3

H4-4

Figure 6-3 Surface location of H4 saphenous. The saphenous nerve is a cutaneous branch of the femoral nerve and supplies the skin of the medial side of the leg and foot. Just below the medial condyle of the tibia, the saphenous nerve emerges from the deep fascia and forms an important acupoint H4 saphenous. As homeostasis declines, more tender points appear along the course of the saphenous nerve distal from the H4 location. Thus these tender points on the saphenous nerve, if they appear, provide valuable information about the degree of homeostasis. These points, in order from proximal to distal, are termed H4-1, H4-2, H4-3, and H4-4. The distance between two points is about 2 to 3 cm (varying according to the length of the leg). (Modified from Lumley J: *Surface anatomy: the anatomical basis of clinical examination,* ed 3, Edinburgh, 2002, Churchill Livingstone.)

Definition of Efficacy of Acupuncture Treatments

Acupuncture efficacy is measured by (1) the number of treatments needed for maximal relief and (2) the duration of the pain relief. It depends on the interaction between a patient's self-healing potential and the severity and nature of the symptoms. In Tables 6-1 and 6-2, we classify pain patients into

Table 6-2 Classification of Patients According to 16 Evaluation Points (H1-1, -2, -3, -4) + (H4-1, -2, -3, -4)				
	No. of Tender Points			
	0-4	**5-8**	**9-12**	**12-16**
Patient group	A	B	C	D

four groups: A, B, C, and D. Accordingly we can classify acupuncture efficacy into four groups: excellent for group A, good for group B, average for group C, and poor for group D. Different groups need a different number of treatments and experience different durations of pain relief.

With two to four treatments, patients in group A enjoy complete pain relief for at least 1 year or even for years if proper preventive measures are taken.

Group B patients need about four to eight treatments to obtain pain relief of about 4 to 6 months' duration or longer if they adopt appropriate preventive maintenance.

Acupuncture treatments achieve average efficacy in group C patients. Patients in this group need more than eight treatments to obtain pain relief for an average of 5 months. After the symptoms relapse these patients need another session of acupuncture treatments to keep the pain under control for another 5 months (5 ± 1 months). Patients in this group can upgrade to group B by continuing preventive acupuncture treatments even after the pain symptoms are relieved.

Acupuncture generally demonstrates poor efficacy in group D patients. Acupuncture treatments may offer patients in this group pain relief for only a few days. Our clinical evidence shows that, with help from other supportive procedures such as diet, exercise, massage, and change of lifestyle, some of the group D patients may upgrade to group C. Sometimes remarkable results can be achieved for group D patients who demonstrate a strong desire to be healed and who are well supported by their practitioner and family members.

Collecting Information to Evaluate a Patient's Healing Potential

In acupuncture therapy for soft tissue pain, understanding the full capacity of a patient's self-healing potential is more important than understanding the mechanism and nature of the pathologic symptoms or diseases afflicting that patient. This is why acupuncture is able to treat with success symptoms that originate from what might be labeled *mechanism unknown* by health care professionals.

Thus QAE is not meant to differentiate diseases or to investigate the mechanism of diseases. The goal of QAE is to provide the information necessary for evaluating the self-healing potential of a patient and the projected efficacy of acupuncture treatments.

Before making a plan for acupuncture treatment, a practitioner should create the patient's complete medical profile, and to do this the following information should be obtained.

Current Pain Symptoms   What current pathologic symptoms is the patient experiencing? Where are the symptoms located on the body? How have the pain symptoms developed over time?

Medical Examinations   Blood pressure should always be recorded. Patients with blood pressure lower than 120/70 may have a needle reaction during the first few sessions (see later discussion). A practitioner needs to pay attention to the patient's previous medical history, laboratory tests, and diagnoses.

Medical Interventions Used to Treat Pain Symptoms   By *medical interventions* we mean all conventional and alternative procedures and modalities. Acupuncture therapy by its nature does not conflict with any other medical modalities, but some medical procedures might reduce the effectiveness of acupuncture therapy. For example, addictive medications such as morphine will reduce acupuncture efficacy for pain relief. Blood-thinning medications may cause excessive bleeding or produce bruising during acupuncture treatments. Mild or moderate bruising produces no harmful consequences, but the practitioner should prevent any bleeding from occurring in the joint capsule.

Medical History   Medical history includes all medical problems, beginning from childhood, such as accidents, severe diseases, surgeries, hormonal problems in women, and any family history related to the symptoms experienced by the patient. Sometimes patients unintentionally ignore important information. For instance, a patient might forget having had whiplash from a low-speed car accident 20 years ago because he or she felt good a week afterwards. This ignored minor event could be the cause of current symptoms.

It is important to collect precise information about any surgical procedures the patient has undergone. Pain symptoms can be more difficult and time consuming to treat when they persist after surgery. This is because surgery alters some of the neuroanatomic structure, whereas acupuncture works best when applied to intact body anatomy.

Even if there are medical problems that are not directly related to the pain symptoms they can play an important role because they can diminish the efficacy of the acupuncture treatments. The more health problems that are found in a patient, the less self-healing potential can be expected; also more treatments will be needed, the pain relief will have a shorter duration, and the likelihood will be higher that the current symptoms will return.

Lifestyle and Profession Special attention should be given to the patient's lifestyle, personal habits, and occupational hazards. The practitioner's ability to accurately project the efficacy of acupuncture treatments will be directly affected by the reliability of this information.

Contraindications and Complications During or After Acupuncture Needling Correct acupuncture treatment produces no clinical side effects. Some adverse physiologic reactions occur because of human error or the unpredictable reaction of a patient. In acupuncture such adverse reactions are few and can be prevented and avoided when acupuncture treatments are given by a cautious and well-trained professional.

In the following section we describe possible negative reactions to acupuncture needling and the skills required for handling and preventing accidents.

Syncope or "Needle Fainting" Dr. Chen, of the Center for Traditional Chinese Medicine of Veterans General Hospital in Taipei, Taiwan, reported 55 syncope events in 28,285 clinical acupuncture visits (0.19%).[1] These data are similar to our own clinical evidence. According to Dr. Chen's statistical analysis, 28,285 visits account for about 3,235 patients, with each patient having an average of eight acupuncture treatments. Thus an acupuncture practitioner may encounter one syncope event in about every 500 treatments; in other words about 2% of patients in an acupuncture clinic will experience syncope. Fortunately syncope, or "needle fainting" as it is called in China, can be predicted and prevented.

In most cases syncope or "needle fainting" refers to the sudden loss of consciousness as a result of temporary low blood supply to the brain. Syncope occurs within 2 to 10 minutes of initial needle insertion. When only a few needles are inserted into the body, a syncope-prone patient complains of feeling dizzy and light-headed, the eyes become crossed, the muscles become rigid, and syncope follows.

Syncope usually happens in the early phase of the treatment; however, older patients may develop syncope in the middle or even at the end of the treatment. Close care should be taken throughout the course of a treatment when dealing with older patients.

Handling Syncope

When a patient experiences syncope during acupuncture treatment, the practitioner should remain calm and use the following procedures:

1. Immediately remove all needles from the patient. Have the patient lie down on his or her back with the head lower than the feet by elevating the feet on a cushion. This position helps to maintain the blood flow to the brain. If the patient is going to vomit, position the person on his or her side to prevent choking.
2. Needle the following regions: the middle part of the philtrum, just below the nasal septum on the vertical groove in the median portion of the upper lip (Figure 6-4), and the tip of the index or middle fingers.

This procedure is clinically proven and effectively brings the patient back to consciousness. The physiologic mechanism of this centuries-old prescription is still unclear; possibly needling these points increases blood pressure.

Usually this type of needling terminates syncope quickly, almost immediately. As a rule, after "needle fainting" a patient feels tired and experiences slight discomfort all over the body, partly caused by psychological panic. If the patient does not wake up in a few minutes, an emergency call to a hospital is advised, although the acupuncture literature has never recorded a syncope of such prolonged duration.

Prevention of Syncope During Acupuncture Treatment

Acupuncture syncope happens mostly to patients when needles are inserted in the body in a seated or upright position. Prone, supine, or side positions of the body during acupuncture treatment are the most secure.

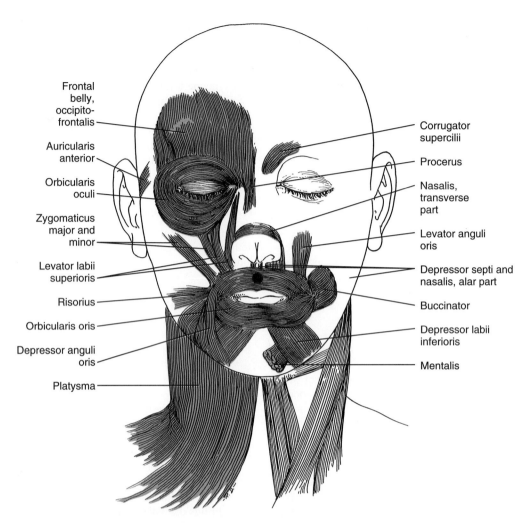

Figure 6-4   The point on the philtrum to be needled in cases of syncope. It is just below the septum of the nose. (Modified from Jenkins D: *Hollinshead's functional anatomy of the limbs and back,* ed 8, Philadelphia, 2002.)

The following types of patients are more likely to experience syncope, and practitioners should always be prepared when treating patients in these categories:

1. A new patient without previous acupuncture experience or one who has not had acupuncture treatments for more than 6 months. Acupuncture provides a new stimulus to the physiologic activity of these patients, and their bodies need to adjust to this new modality.
2. Young, healthy, athletic males who may have a strong vasovagal reaction to needling.
3. Thin, middle-aged women with blood pressure lower than 120/70.
4. Older or weak patients who have a low energy level and multiple medical problems. In this group of patients, syncope may occur at any time during the acupuncture treatment.
5. Patients who are hungry, dehydrated, or exhausted after intense physical activities, or who eat just before the treatment.

As a preventive measure, inform new patients that they should eat no more than a light meal at least 1 hour before acupuncture treatment.

Bleeding and Bruising Caused by Needling

The estimated probability of bleeding from needling is about 10%, and the estimated probability of bruising after needling is less than 10%. Bleeding and bruising at needling sites do not cause any adverse effects to the patient's health. As a preventive measure, a practitioner should avoid needling visible veins or palpable arteries below the skin surface, although ancient practitioners purposely needled the pulsing arterial points to treat diseases.

Bleeding caused by needling produces a tiny drop of blood on withdrawal of the needle and can be stopped by pressing with a cotton swab. Bruises caused by needling may take 5 to 7 days to disappear. Before a patient's first acupuncture treatment, a practitioner should explain to the patient the possibility that harmless bleeding or bruising may occur.

Patients who have capillaries close to the skin surface, who have blood vessel problems, or are using a blood-thinning medication may experience bleeding or bruising more often. In this case the practitioner may press a cotton ball to the needle site immediately after withdrawing the needles. The practitioner should avoid needling directly on the joint capsule.

Pneumothorax

If an acupuncture needle perforates the pulmonary pleura (the serous membrane investing the lungs and lining the chest wall), the needle may cause a local lesion to the pleura or in some cases to the lung. As a result air could penetrate the lesion-damaged tissue of the thoracic wall and accumulate in the pleural cavity, which prevents lung expansion and results in difficult breathing accompanied by chest pain. This condition is called *pneumothorax*. Special attention to thoracic anatomy is needed (see Chapter 9 and Figure 9-12, p. 137) to avoid pneumothorax when needling points on the anterior, lateral, or posterior thorax.

No medical record exists to indicate that pneumothorax caused by needling has led to a life-threatening condition, but improper acupuncture needling will produce a severe traumatic effect on the patient. If an acupuncture needle perforates the pleura, the patient may suddenly feel pain radiating from the needling site. Usually the patient starts coughing about 30 minutes later and experiences short breaths, pain in the chest area, and tingling or numbness in the arms. When pneumothorax is suspected, the patient should be hospitalized for emergency aid. To prevent pneumothorax, we suggest using needles 25 to 30 mm (about 1 inch) long for paravertebral points (see Chapter 5) and 15 mm long for the lateral and anterior thorax.

When needling acupoints such as the H3 spinal accessory and H13 dorsal scapula (see Chapter 5), we recommend the following procedure: insert a needle (40 mm long) skin deep, and then grasp and hold up the muscle tissue between the fingers and the thumb. After the muscle is raised, continue inserting the needle until it reaches the nodule in the muscle and then immediately withdraw the needle without loosening grasp of the tissue. This safe procedure can be repeated a few times to achieve better muscle relaxation. This needling method should be performed only by experienced practitioners who are familiar with the gross anatomy of this region. Inexperienced practitioners may use an alternative procedure by inserting a few shorter needles (25 mm long) around H3 and H13 to achieve desirable results.

Special care should be taken when treating patients with a thinner body wall, especially patients with a spine problem, such as scoliosis, or a history of heavy smoking, because these patients have thinner, less elastic, weaker thoracic muscles. They may require more time to recover from the needle-induced lesions.

Acupuncture lesions may produce possible pneumothorax symptoms even after treatment. The hole from a needle-induced lesion in less elastic muscles may reopen when patients in the high-risk group simply breathe or do physical exercises. For safety reasons, when needling PAs in the thoracic region of patients in the high-risk group use only shorter needles tilting to the midline.

Needling Reaction

Physiologic reactions to acupuncture needling can be observed in some patients. The reaction may appear during treatment *(immediate reaction)* or a few hours after treatment *(latent reaction)*.

Immediate Reaction An immediate reaction manifests through the phenomena of syncope, sweating, brief hot or cold flashes, and in rare cases an anxiety attack. Among these reactions, only syncope needs a special procedure as described.

Latent Reaction About 10% of patients feel more pain within 24 or 48 hours after acupuncture treatment. This pain may be "wandering" or appear in a new location. For instance, a patient complaining of lower back pain might experience shoulder pain, knee pain, or a headache for 1 or 2 days after acupuncture treatment.

This latent reaction occurs mostly in two different groups of patients: very healthy (group A) or very unhealthy (group D). The reaction in group A is referred to as a *positive latent reaction* and the reaction in group D as a *negative latent reaction.* A majority of patients experience none of these temporary side effects.

In older or weaker patients with multiple chronic health problems, the negative latent physiologic reaction can be induced by overstimulation from needling. During the first few treatments of weaker or older patients, no more than 10 needles should be used to avoid a negative latent reaction. After patients adjust to the needling and become physically stronger, more needles can be introduced if necessary.

The negative latent reaction can be explained as follows. Each acupuncture needle creates a tiny lesion or trauma to the soft tissues, including peripheral nerve endings. The healing of the needle-induced lesions is an energy-consuming process. A physically weak body with multiple injuries or symptoms can accept only a limited number of new needle-induced lesions because a weak body does not have enough healing energy to heal many of them. Patients who experience a negative latent reaction are mostly women 40 years of age or older.

Another group of patients, mostly young, healthy, athletic males in their twenties or thirties, may feel more pain within 24 hours after their first acupuncture treatment. This positive latent reaction does not indicate overstimulation but is a *positive* sign showing that the patient is having a strong response to acupuncture therapy. This type of patient usually requires fewer treatment sessions and recovers faster than most other patients.

What to Do When a Patient Experiences a Latent Reaction   A latent reaction, whether negative or positive, is not dangerous and can be easily relieved. When a patient experiences a latent reaction, a practitioner may insert a few needles in the painful area for about 5 to 10 minutes to cause the pain to subside. Usually we use one or two needles in a patient experiencing a negative latent reaction and four needles in a patient experiencing a positive latent reaction. Mild and light massage or moist heat also can help to calm down latent reaction pain.

More than 30% of patients feel tired and fatigued for a day after the treatment. This tiredness forces patients to sleep more and to perform fewer physical activities. Subsequent to the fatigue phase, patients usually experience a feeling of improvement and relief of symptoms. Thus the fatigue phase should be interpreted as positive body language convincing the patients to conserve the energy needed for healing of the symptoms after stress is removed.

A few patients complain of soreness at needle sites for 2 to 5 days after treatment. We suggest two explanations for this phenomenon. The first possibility is that needling interrupts the contracture structure deep in the muscle and/or other tissues and causes an antiinflammatory reaction. The needle-induced lesion continues to stimulate the tissues for a few days after the needle is removed. The second possibility is that a needle may perforate the deep blood vessel slightly and cause tiny internal bleeding, which stimulates the tissues for a few days. Usually massage or moist heat will reduce the soreness.

Drowsiness

Most patients feel relaxed or sleepy during treatment. Immediately after treatment, a few patients feel a little drowsy, possibly because of temporary lower blood pressure. These patients should lie down and rest until their drowsiness is gone and before they drive a car or go home.

Skin Reaction

Small red spots on the skin commonly appear at needle sites. The redness is most likely caused by local histamine release in reaction to the needle-induced lesion. This transient erythema lasts from a couple of minutes to 2 or 3 days after treatment. The erythema disappears once the needle-induced lesion heals. There is definitely neuroimmune reaction at the needling sites.

Pregnancy

Pregnant women frequently consider acupuncture to reduce lower back pain and treat other problems. Classic acupuncture texts list several acupoints that might induce abortion during the first trimester or even later. These acupoints are the H12 deep radial and H6 tibial (see inside cover). Some practitioners in China believe that needling any point in the body of a pregnant woman when she is 30 years old or older may induce abortion. A practitioner should fully understand the risk when working with pregnant patients.

Needling Skill

We highly recommend using disposable needles with individual guide tubes to minimize any possibility of infection. To insert this type of needle, hold the tube with one hand and lightly and swiftly tap the top of the tube with a finger of the other hand. Subsequently a practitioner can continue to insert the needle by either "pistoning" up and down or rotating clockwise and counterclockwise. These manipulation techniques help to relax the muscle contracture (see Chapter 3) and increase stimulation. Some patients might not tolerate the manipulation and will experience excessive pain, in which case the practitioner should use a finer needle and insert it with minimal twisting or rotating.

How Many Needles Should Be Used for Each Treatment?

Understanding the needling mechanisms and the physiologic strength or weakness of a patient permits a practitioner to decide how many needles should be used during an acupuncture treatment.

Each needle creates a microlesion in the tissues. In most patients it takes 2 days or longer for the needle-induced lesions to be replaced by fresh cells, and this process takes longer in weak patients. Thus, as indicated earlier, acupuncture-induced healing is an energy-consuming process.

Because the healing of needle-induced lesions usually takes longer for weaker and older patients because of their low energy level and low self-healing potential, a practitioner should use fewer needles during acupuncture treatments for these patients. As a reaction to overneedling, some patients may feel tired after treatment; they may feel soreness on the needled spots, or experience more pain for 1 or 2 days.

Healthier and younger patients have enough energy to heal the needle-induced lesions faster, and a practitioner could use more needles during an acupuncture treatment for these patients. As a rule of thumb, up to 30 needles can be used in one session.

For first-time patients without any previous experience of acupuncture treatments, fewer acupoints should be needled because these patients' bodies need time to adjust to this new modality. A patient should be treated as a first-time patient if he or she has not received acupuncture treatments for longer than 6 months.

To provide effective acupuncture treatments, practitioners are encouraged to modify the protocol and to adjust it to each patient's level of homeostasis, severity of pain symptoms, and tolerance to needles.

Frequency of Acupuncture Appointments

A successful acupuncture therapy should be administered with proper treatment "dosage" and treatment timing. Acupuncture "dosage" refers to the number of needles used in each treatment and to the timing of treatment. "Underneedling" may slow the healing process in most patients, whereas "overneedling" may cause strong "postneedling" reaction in a few patients.

For most patients, about 2 days are needed to heal the needle-induced lesions. For weaker and older patients, more than 2 days will be needed to heal the same lesions. Sufficient time should be allowed to heal the needle-induced lesions between treatments, especially for weak and older patients. Therefore the timing of acupuncture appointments depends on the following three factors.

General Health Healthier patients need about 2 or 3 days between treatments, whereas weaker and older patients need 4 to 7 days between treatments. Keep in mind that the success or efficacy of acupuncture therapy depends not only on the skills of the practitioner but also on the general health of the patient.

Number of Needles Used During Treatment The more needle-induced lesions that are made during an acupuncture treatment, the longer the time required between treatments.

Severity of Pain Symptoms A severe symptom usually requires more treatments. When working with weaker patients who are experiencing a severe pain symptom, sufficient postneedling recovery time between treatments should be allowed. In practice a healthy patient can receive a treatment every day or every 2 to 3 days, whereas a weak or older patient needs 4 to 7 days between treatments. In China, weaker patients may receive daily treatment with minimal needling.

Types of Pain Relief

Three types of recovery are observed:

1. *Immediate relief.* This can usually be expected in young, healthy patients (group A) with simple acute pain symptoms.
2. *Cumulative relief.* Most patients feel some improvement after each treatment (groups B

and C), and major or complete relief can realistically be expected after several treatments.

3. *Delayed relief.* Sometimes pain reduction is not obtained from the first few treatments but may be suddenly experienced 2 to 3 weeks after the first treatment.

If a patient has not experienced pain relief after the first four to six treatments, allow the patient to stop treatments for a week before resuming treatment again. Patients usually feel an improvement during the break.

Treatment Protocol

Acupuncture therapy by its nature (nonspecific) does not directly treat any particular symptoms or diseases; rather, it activates the process of self-healing for "healable" symptoms or diseases, either completely or partially. Our treatment protocol reflects the nature of acupuncture therapy and is clinically proven to be effective and applicable to every pain patient.

As we know, no two patients are identical. They have different homeostasis states, medical histories, lifestyles, and genetic makeup. The treatment protocol should be adjusted to the needs and health of each patient.

Our Integrative Neuromuscular Acupoint System (INMAS) protocol is standardized to be applicable to all pain symptoms and is individualized to be adjustable for each patient and each treatment. Please note that even the same patient could be treated differently at different sessions.

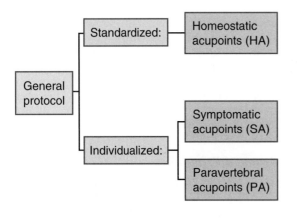

Explanation of the General Protocol

The general protocol consists of two parts: the standardized protocol and the individualized protocol.

1. *Standardized protocol.* The standardized protocol uses all or some of the 24 HAs for all pain symptoms (Chapter 5).

2. *Individualized protocol.* The individualized protocol uses symptomatic acupoints (SAs) and paravertebral acupoints (PAs), which are adjustable to each patient's pain symptoms.

The following is a technical description of the general protocol and presents clinical examples of its practical applications.

Body Positions During Acupuncture Treatment

The body positions used during treatment depend on the location of the symptoms and the patient's condition. Some patients, for example, cannot lie prone. A practitioner can decide whether to use one body position—prone, supine, or on the side—for a whole treatment, alternating for each successive treatment, or to use two or three positions in one treatment.

Use the prone position first in cases of pain in the neck, shoulder, back, hip, or knee. Note that knee pain often involves back muscles. For facial, elbow, or abdominal problems the supine position is preferable during the first treatment.

The sitting position should be used with discrimination and only for patients who cannot lie down. A practitioner should be alert and remember that a patient with lower blood pressure (lower than 120/70) may be susceptible to syncope while in the sitting position.

Standardized Protocol for the Prone Position

The patient lies comfortably in the prone position. The practitioner, using a finger or a thumb, palpates all 13 accessible HAs. All HAs are bilateral except H20 spinous process of T7. The forearms are not included.

Head (2):	H2 great auricular, H7 greater occipital
Shoulder bridge (1):	H3 spinal accessory
Shoulder (2):	H8 infraspinatus, H13 dorsal scapula
Upper back (2):	H20 spinous process of T7, H21 posterior cutaneous of T6
Lower back (3):	H14 superior cluneal, H15 posterior

cutaneous of L2, H22 posterior cutaneous of L5

Lower limbs (3):
H10 sural, H11 lateral popliteal, H16 inferior gluteal

Clinical Notes During the treatment of a patient from one of the healthier groups (groups A, B, and some of group C), all 13 HAs can be needled, a total of 25 acupoints bilaterally (H20 is not bilateral).

When treating a weak or older patient, a practitioner should use fewer needles, as mentioned already, usually less than 20. The principle for selecting HAs in weak patients is as follows: All HAs should be needled in the main area of pain, but only the most tender HAs are needled in other regions. For example, when treating a weak patient with lower back pain, all lower back HAs (H14, H15, H16, and H22) should be needled first. Then the practitioner should palpate the lower extremities and find one or two more tender HAs and needle them. One or two HAs may also be selected in the neck, shoulder, and upper extremities, but these regions can be ignored if the patient is too weak to accept more needles. Weak patients need more treatments than those who can tolerate more needles at one time.

Standardized Protocol for Supine Position

The patient lies comfortably in the supine position. Using the thumb or other finger, the practitioner palpates the 11 accessible HAs.

Face (2):
H19 infraorbital, H23 supraorbital

Upper limbs (3):
H1 deep radial, H9 lateral antebrachial cutaneous, H12 superficial radial

Chest (1):
H17 lateral pectoral

Lower limbs (5):
H4 saphenous, H5 deep peroneal, H6 tibial H18 iliotibial, H24 common peroneal

Clinical Notes When treating a patient from one of the healthy groups (groups A, B, and some of group C), all of the previously mentioned 11 HAs can be needled, bilaterally a total of 22 HAs. Sometimes it is necessary to avoid using the facial acupoints H19 and H23 because the feeling of needles being inserted into the face makes some patients uncomfortable.

For older or weaker patients, the same principles apply as were described in the previous section.

Individualized Protocol

The individualized protocol combines SAs and PAs to customize acupuncture treatments to the patient's needs and pathologic symptoms.

Locating Symptomatic Acupoints As explained in Chapter 5, HAs appear in a similar pattern in every patient. Each HA also serves as a "road map" for locating SAs. Finding and treating the right SAs greatly enhances the efficacy of the treatment. The following is an explanation of the general procedure of locating SAs.

Most symptomatic SAs emerge around local HAs. SAs are affected by a patient's individual pain symptoms and therefore have an individual pattern. Some SAs are predictable, and some are not.

Example 1: Locating SAs When Treating "Tennis Elbow" A patient complains about "tennis elbow" symptoms (lateral epicondylitis). In this case, tender acupoints can be found at or distal to the lateral epicondyle of the humerus, to which the common extensor muscles of the forearm are attached. The locations of some tender SAs are predictable: they appear around the lateral side of the elbow.

The individual pattern of each personal injury also creates some unpredictable tender SAs. For the treatment of tennis elbow, the areas around the cubital fossa, the radial or ulnar side of the forearm, the wrist, and the hand should be carefully palpated to locate individual SAs.

In cases like this, a practitioner can apply the following procedure to locate SAs, whether predictable or unpredictable:

1. Locate the three HAs on the upper limb: H1 deep radial, H9 lateral antecutaneous, and H12 superficial radial.
2. Palpate the vicinity of H9. Tender points (SAs) are most likely to be found at the lateral epicondyle; some SAs may appear around the medial epicondyle.
3. Palpate H1 and its surrounding areas. Search the pathway of the deep radial nerve all the way to the wrist. Usually several tender points (SAs) will be found in the muscles of the forearm.
4. Palpate the hand around H12 to locate possible SAs. After locating all the SAs in the elbow, forearm, wrist, and hand, a decision

of how many SAs should be needled can be made according to the needling tolerance of the patient.

Example 2: Locating SAs in Patients With Lower Back Pain   A patient complains of "lower back pain" symptoms. With the patient lying in a prone position, locate and palpate all seven lumbar and leg HAs: H15 posterior cutaneous of L2, H14 superior cluneal, H22 posterior cutaneous of L5, H16 inferior gluteal, H18 iliotibial, H11 lateral popliteal, and H10 sural. Tender SAs might be located around any of these HAs:

1. In the lumbar area, around H15, H14, and H22
2. In the area between H14 and H16
3. In the area around H18 (in the iliotibial band or other muscles)
4. In the calf muscles around H10

Once all the SAs around these HAs have been located, the practitioner must decide, according to the condition of the individual patient, whether to needle all SAs or only the most tender ones in every treatment.

Selecting PA Acupoints   The location of SAs dictates the selection of the PAs, as was explained in Chapter 5. In general, the following principles are used to select the PAs:

1. Cervical PAs (C1-C4 or C5) for facial or head pain symptoms
2. C4-T1 PAs for pain symptoms located in the upper limbs
3. T1-T7 PAs for symptoms related to the lungs and the heart
4. T5-T12 PAs for stomach or other digestive system problems
5. L1-S4 PAs for problems related to the lower limbs and the organs located in the abdominal cavity, including the reproductive organs and the urinary tract

Practical Application of the General Protocol

The following examples show how to apply the protocol and modify it for different patients. The treatment begins with the quantitative evaluation and palpation of HAs and SAs to locate the most tender acupoints. Then, based on information collected from the patient, the practitioner decides how to modify the protocol according to the indi-

vidual pain pattern, homeostasis, and needling tolerance of the patient.

Below are examples of how to modify the protocol.

Example 1: Chronic Neck Pain

Evaluation and Prognosis   A patient reports having had neck pain for more than 6 months, referring especially to tenderness in the areas around the transverse processes on both sides of C4 to C6. Use QAE to evaluate the patient and palpate all HAs as well as the painful neck area. The patient belongs to group B. Four to eight acupuncture treatments will be needed.

1. Protocol for prone position
   Acupoints prescribed:
      HAs: All the 13 points that are accessible in this position.
      SAs: One to three needles in the tender area on each side of the neck, according to the needling tolerance of the patient.
      PAs: One to three needles on each side along C4-C6, according to the needling tolerance of the patient.
2. Protocol for supine position
   Acupoints prescribed:
      HAs: All that are accessible in this position.
      SAs: None in the neck, but check upper extremities because neck pain frequently projects pain to the shoulder and forearm.
      PAs: None.
3. Protocol for side position
   Acupoints prescribed:
      HAs: All that are conveniently accessible in this treatment position.
      SAs: One to three needles in the tender area of the neck, according to the needling tolerance of the patient.
      PAs: One to three needles on each side along C4-C6, according to the needling tolerance of the patient.

In each treatment, the practitioner can use one or more positions. The patient may receive treatment once or twice a week.

Clinical Notes   Treatments should be continued until the pain subsides. As more relief is experienced, time between treatments can be extended to 2 to 3 weeks. After maximal relief is achieved, regular maintenance treatments will be needed. The patient should understand that (1) chronic pain may recur even after it appears to have been relieved and (2) regular acupuncture maintenance not only prevents a recurrence but also promotes healthy body function.

Example 2: Acute Neck Pain

Evaluation and Prognosis A generally healthy patient reports an acute neck muscle sprain. Tender areas are palpable around the right transverse processes of C4 to 6. The patient belongs to group A, with few tender HAs on the body. Only local HAs, PAs, and SAs will be used. Two to four acupuncture treatments will be enough to provide complete pain relief.

> Treatment 1, Day 1
>   Position: Prone
>   Acupoints prescribed:
>   HAs: H7, H3, H13, and H8
>   SAs: Three needles on each side of the neck
>   PAs: C3-5, three needles on each side of the body
> Treatment 2, Day 3
>   Repeat treatment 1
> Treatment 3, Day 7
>   Repeat treatment 1
> Treatment 4, Day 11
>   Repeat treatment 1

Clinical Notes This case is an example of treating a healthy patient with a simple acute symptom. Local treatment is sufficient to provide complete relief. The second treatment is just 2 days after the first treatment. Usually, in cases like this, the first two treatments drastically reduce pain symptoms, and the pain will be completely relieved subsequently.

Example 3: Chronic Lower Back Pain

Evaluation and Prognosis The patient experienced lower back pain for more than 6 months. MRI showed no pathological changes. Use QAE to evaluate the patient and palpate all 24 HAs. Lower back pain frequently projects pain to the neck and shoulder; therefore HAs in these areas also should be treated. Tender SAs appear in the area between H14 and H16. The patient belongs to group B. Four to eight treatments will be needed. Palpate all 24 HAs to locate the primary pain area.

> Protocol for prone position
>   Acupoints prescribed:
>   HAs: All HAs that are accessible in this position. If the patient cannot tolerate much needling, only HAs in the lower back and legs are needled. For cases with even lower tolerance, only four HAs

(H15, H22, H14, and H16) in the lower back area are needled.
SAs: Needle the most tender point(s) or the area around H15, H14, H16, and H18. SAs in the neck area, if they appear, should be needled too.
PAs: In this case, H15 and H22 are both HAs and PAs. In some patients, palpation will reveal tender or painful points in the sacral area, and these should be needled.

Repeat the same treatment every 3 to 5 days. After pain relief is experienced, the treatment can be administered weekly or biweekly.

Clinical Notes When a patient experiences pain in the lower back area, the five local HAs (H15 posterior cutaneous of L2, H22 posterior cutaneous of L5, H14 superior cluneal, H16 inferior gluteal, and H18 iliotibial) are usually tender and can be classified as both HAs and SAs at the same time. When pain symptoms are severe or chronic, more tender points will appear around each of the five HAs and down to H11 and H10. Practitioners should locate these HAs first and should carefully palpate the surrounding area of each HA to find additional tender points. These new points may differ from one patient to another, some being found around H22, some around H14, and some around H18, H11, or H10. These new tender points should be needled.

The practitioner can decide whether the patient should alternate between prone and supine positions. In this example, the prone position in each treatment is sufficient to achieve pain relief. If patients also have symptoms in front, such as in the knee, both prone and supine positions can be used alternately or even in the same treatment.

Example 4: Shoulder Pain for More Than 6 Months

Evaluation and Prognosis A patient reports pain in the left shoulder area for more than 6 months. The left H8, H13, H3, H7, and H17 are tender. Painful areas are palpable around the transverse processes of C2 to C5 and on the front deltoid muscle. The patient belongs to group B and has no other pain symptoms. Four to eight treatments will be needed to provide pain relief.

> Treatment 1, Day 1
> Position: Lying on the right side
> Acupoints prescribed:
>   Because the patient lies on the right side, only some HAs are accessible, and these should be used.

HAs located on the left side: H2, H7, H3, H13, H8, H15, H14, H16
SAs:
1. On the left lateral side of the neck, around the transverse processes of C4 to C6: Two needles are used in this area.
2. The anterior, lateral, and posterior deltoid: one needle in each area.
3. Palpate the whole upper extremity. If SAs are found, they also should be needled.

PAs: From C4 to T1: Three needles on each side, six needles total.

Repeat the treatment once or twice a week, according to the patient's condition.

Clinical Notes Because the patient complains of localized pain in the left shoulder area, the neck and the left arm should also be examined and treated as a preventive measure, because the problem with the shoulder may provoke pain in the neck and arm. This patient belongs to group B and has no other symptoms, so repeating the same procedure will be sufficient to relieve the pain.

SUMMARY

The therapeutic efficacy of acupuncture depends on the patient's self-healing potential and on the ability of the practitioner to activate it. As a rule, healthy people have a greater healing potential. As symptoms or diseases become severe, the self-healing potential is impaired and the healing process is slowed.

When health or homeostasis declines, acupoints transform from the latent phase (nonsensitive) to the passive phase (sensitive) in an anticipatable sequence and HAs appear in predictable locations. Thus the number of passive HAs is a quantitative indicator of the degree of homeostasis in the body.

Based on the number of tender HAs, we can statistically differentiate patients into four types of homeostasis/self-healing potential: 28%, excellent (group A); 34%, good (group B); 30%, average (group C); and 8%, poor (group D). Patients in each group react to acupuncture differently (see Tables 6-1 and 6-2).

From an understanding of the nature of acupuncture therapy, we have been able to develop a universally applicable treatment protocol for all peripheral pain symptoms. The protocol has both standardized and individualized components.

The standardized part of the protocol is based on the 24 HAs, and the individualized part includes SAs and PAs. The SAs should be carefully searched for because they appear in different places for every patient. Local HAs provide the "road map" for finding local SAs. The location of SAs is in turn a direct guide to which PAs should be used (segmental mechanism, see Chapters 3 and 5).

The entire procedure presented in this chapter for selecting, combining, and prescribing acupoints is practitioner-friendly and standardized but is flexible enough to address each patient's individual needs. The treatment protocol simultaneously (1) promotes homeostasis and enhances self-healing potential and (2) treats particular pain symptoms.

As noted, by its neurophysiological nature acupuncture therapy is *nonspecific*. Through the use of SAs and PAs, we are able to make it *specific* for particular symptoms and patients as well.

Reference

1. Chen F, et al: Clinical study of syncope during acupuncture treatments, *Acupuncture and Electro-therapeutics Research* 15:107-119, 1990.

CHAPTER 7

The Psychology of Acupuncture Therapy: Placebo and Nocebo Effects in Acupuncture Pain Management

INTRODUCTION

Pain, especially chronic pain, results in psychological and physical dysfunction. The expression of pain is a personal characteristic and is influenced not only by abnormal neurophysiologic processes, as discussed in previous chapters, but also by environmental and cultural factors, as well as psychological aspects such as personal experiences, learning, beliefs, and expectations related to the pain and its treatment. All these factors are woven together to form the individual psychological characteristics of a pain patient, and have a significant influence on the efficacy of treatment. In addition, practitioner-patient interactions can exert powerful positive or negative effects on the outcome of treatment.

Once the pain impulses from the peripheral sensory receptors reach the neural networks of the brain, what happens is no longer a purely sensory neurophysiologic mechanism. The perception becomes a complex cognition of the sensory information from the injured tissue, and the processing cannot be independent of the patient's unique and individual psychological background. Here the pain perception enters a higher level of the hierarchy of biological organization: the psychological. If acute pain is still an element at the neurophysiologic level, chronic pain has been incorporated into the psychological organization. Thus patients with chronic pain show special psychological characteristics in their pain symptoms, in the areas of pain perception, emotion, cognition, expectancy, assigning meaning, and decision making.

Interactions between the factors of neurophysiology and cognitive psychology can produce positive placebo effects or negative nocebo effects. If the interaction favors self-healing, the patient experiences positive placebo effects. If the interaction promotes an internal environment of self-destruction, negative effects occur. Changes in pain over time reflect complex interactions between physiologic processes and psychological syntheses and environmental factors.

A pain patient views his or her pain as a personal experience. The quality and intensity of this experience are influenced by the patient's unique history, by the meaning he or she gives to the pain-producing situation, and by his or her state of mind at the moment. All these factors modify the actual patterns of pain impulses that ascend from the body to the brain and travel within the brain itself. In this way pain becomes a function of the whole person, including his or her current thoughts and fears as well as hopes for the future.

The same injury can have different effects on different people or even on the same person at different times. Psychological variables may intervene between the stimulus and the perception of pain and can produce different expressions of the pain and a different response to the same medical treatment.

For decades pain professionals have been puzzled by the phenomena of placebo and nocebo effects. In fact these effects are expressions of self-healing or self-destruction that result from interactions between neurophysiology and cognitive psychology. In some patients, both placebo and nocebo effects affect application of every medical modality—drugs, surgery, psychotherapy, acupuncture, physical therapy, biofeedback, manipulation, and massage in every treatment. Thus these effects are inevitable processes that must be taken into account in every field of medical practice. If the psychological condition of the patient and the mechanism of placebo and nocebo effects are properly understood, the practitioner and the patient can work together to exploit these factors for better pain relief.

OVERVIEW OF THE PSYCHOLOGICAL ASPECTS OF PAIN

The study of the psychology of pain is a rapidly growing field that has developed from behavioral and cognitive psychology. Its fundamental assumptions, although still neuroscientifically based, differ markedly from those of medical disciplines that are based on neurophysiology, such as neurology, psychiatry, and anesthesiology. *Neurophysiology* is concerned with biological organization and the chemical and physical laws that relate to the structure and function of the nervous system, whereas *psychology* is a complex of physiologic, cognitive, emotional, and social factors.

Cognition is a self-organizing process that gives coherence to an individual's life and sense of self, extending across various external settings and through long periods of time.[1] Cognition, for our immediate purposes, consists of the perception of events in the internal (bodily) and external environments, along with the higher-order rational processes of reasoning and decision making. An intensive dialogue between neurophysiology and cognitive psychology is needed to achieve the level of integration that the study of pain management requires, and such an integration will be a path toward better pain management.

Clearly pain is both an important mechanism of biological protection and an aversive psychological experience toward tissue trauma, inflammation, or disease. The following section briefly describes the psychological processes of patients with chronic pain.

Attention

Attention refers to the selective filtering of information from the internal and external environments.[1] A pain patient cannot concentrate his or her attention on normal work and the ordinary routines of life because the pain frequently or constantly intrudes on awareness.

Pain diminishes when attention is intentionally directed toward other events, such as exciting games, books, or films. Distraction of attention, however, is effective only if the pain is steady or increasing in intensity at a slow rate.

Imagery

Our sensory information always creates some sort of image; for example, thinking about a family member may draw the visual image of this person from the memory. Listening to an old melody may bring back an image of a past event. Awareness of pain is one of many types of psychological image that recall for us a kind of aversive experience associated with bodily injury, trauma, or inflammation. Pain as a personal image can be described as a mental representation of the actual sensory activity associated with an injurious external event.[2]

Expectation

A patient with acute pain may expect the pain simply to go away. A patient with chronic pain gradually becomes hypervigilant for pain and will try to determine whether the pain will worsen, whether it might be associated with some sort of tumor, or perhaps whether the pain is the inevitable result of an inherited genetic disposition. Positive expectation helps the patient respond to medical treatment, whereas negative expectation can induce psychological disorganization and physiologic self-destruction.

Meaning

Most pain patients attempt to attribute their pain to some physical cause, such as rheumatoid arthritis, or speculate about the origin of the tissue trauma and its effect on their immediate and long-range well-being. In some cases this search for a physical cause is difficult or impossible because medical enquiry is unable to identify it. Some patients develop a negative attitude toward personal relationships during this process of seeking the meaning of their pain because they believe that they are "victims." This negative attitude impedes a patient's ability to respond to medical treatment and rehabilitation.

If the cause of the pain can be determined, it will influence pain perception and the effectiveness of treatment. For example, a stomach pain may become persistent if the sufferer learns that stomach cancer occurs often in his or her family history; if medical examination excludes the possibility of cancer, the stomach pain may soon stop.

Sensory and Emotional Disturbances as Causes of Anxiety

Pain feels unpleasant, causes fatigue, impairs sleep, interferes with memory, distracts concentration, and disrupts organized action and thought. Chronic pain often becomes the theme around which the patient organizes thinking and action. Chronic pain patients may preferentially recall negative ideas and feelings. Pain can interfere with a person's ability to see clearly and evaluate his or her situation and the factors that may be causing stress. The results are anxiety, depression, irritability, social withdrawal, and a tendency to expect the worst. All these psychological behaviors increase the intensity of the perceived pain.

Schemata

A *schema* is a normally unconscious pattern of concepts, assumptions, images, affects, and associations that reflects a person's experiences and influences his or her perception of the present and expectations for the future.[3] Thinking of a university brings a host of associations for those who studied in a university environment: the campus, buildings, young students, professors, and laboratories, for example. This schema is formed by activating a learned network of associations. It does not bring to mind the focused image of a particular teacher in a particular class; rather, it is a nonspecific frame of reference that the brain has collected from many aspects of the personal background.

When thinking about pain, the patient activates a complex schema that involves past pain experiences and medical history, present fear, the possible meaning of the pain, the social consequences of pain, future expectations, and more. This pain schema definitely promotes interaction between cognition and sensory pain signals.

The idea of the schema explains how the human brain can generate its own patterns of awareness and imagery from past experiences. The schema can be retrieved selectively from the memory, modified by the new experience, and put back into storage. This process of schema formation constantly builds and remodels one's view of the world. Therefore pain is no longer a passive experience of tissue trauma; rather, it becomes a complex organization that involves multiple dimensions of cognitive psychology.

Most doctors view a patient's description of pain as directly reflecting a sensory experience that provides an important basis for diagnosis. This view is usually accurate when dealing with acute pain. In the case of chronic pain, it is more helpful to view it as a cognitive schema that involves multiple determinants and complex patterns of association. Thus the treatment of chronic pain requires the practitioner to understand not only the neurophysiologic cause of the symptoms but also the psychological associations, such as past experiences, present circumstances, and expectations for the future.

Some Pain Behaviors Seen in Acupuncture Clinics

A patient with pain who is seeking help in the form of acupuncture therapy comes to the clinic as an individual with a unique background and psychological organization; so his or her symptoms become individualized. Each patient presents a different picture of pain. To make the best treatment decision, a practitioner should understand both the neurophysiological basis and the psychological aspects of the pain presented by each patient.

Behavior 1 We learn early in life that after an injury, such as broken skin on the knee, the pain will persist for a couple of days. A child may cry to attract attention and may solicit help after hurting a knee; he or she feels better after the parents offer attention and help. This situation shows that pain can be considered unbearable when help is unavailable, but it diminishes or vanishes when relief is at hand.

Many patients suffer from pain for several days but feel better on the day before they go to the office for treatment. The practitioner should understand that this remission can be a real sign of the beginning of natural healing, but it also can be a temporary relief obscured by psychological factors. Complete treatment should still be administered.

Behavior 2 After one or two treatments, the patient usually feels much better and may regard the result of treatments as "miracles." Acupuncture sometimes provides fast pain relief, especially in healthy patients who are experiencing acute symptoms (mostly group A patients, see Chapter 6). If this type of "miracle" appears in patients suffering from chronic pain, the practitioner should not be overly optimistic. Chronic pain represents a long-term pathologic change of tissues, such as sensitization of neurons in the spinal cord, and thus for chronic pain there is no quick fix. The "miracle" can be enhanced by psychological elements, such as expectation, strong personal willpower, distraction, and social factors such as family support.

Often a patient with chronic pain has tried many other modalities and failed to get significant results. Acupuncture therapy is new, is "mystical," and may be positively introduced to the patient through the media, articles, or friends. Often the first treatment produces positive effects such as a good night's sleep, which the patient may not have had for a while. All these factors arouse in the patient great expectations related to acupuncture treatment. In a case like this, however, the patient may soon feel that the old pain is returning, and therefore that the efficacy of acupuncture is decreasing.

Acupuncture is effective in relieving pain sensation, but healing takes time. The practitioner should understand the true nature of the healing process and work to prevent drastic psychological fluctuations so that the patient's expectations will be realistic.

A comparable situation is when a new medication is much more effective than the existing ones because it has just come to the market and both doctors and patients are overly enthusiastic about it. After a while, the perceived efficacy of the new drug declines and its real efficacy can then be more objectively evaluated.

Behavior 3   The blood pressure of some patients sometimes increases when measured in a physician's office. The perceived intensity of pain may increase in the presence of a physician or spouse. This is often seen in patients who have other significant stressors and problem areas in their lives.

If a patient is suspected to belong to this category, another modality, such as psychotherapy, is advised. Recognition that psychological processes influence pain is important for the development of psychological techniques to fight pain.

Importance of Pretreatment Education

Pretreatment education is important during acupuncture therapy. It helps patients to cooperate with the practitioner and thus get more effective treatment.

Simply giving patients information about their pain tends to make them focus on the discomforting aspects of the experience, and their pain is magnified rather than reduced. When patients are taught skills to cope with their pain, such as relaxation, self-treatment, or distraction strategies, they feel that they have some control over the pain and therefore it is felt as less severe.

Most patients expect passively that the practitioner can completely or partially solve their problems and that they will regain their health from the treatment that he or she provides, but active participation of the patient is far better than passive treatment alone.

There is no quick solution to chronic pain. The process of battling it is not a straight line: there are ups and downs. During treatment the pain may become more intense for a short time if the patient is a strong responder. This is good sign, showing that the patient may be healed faster, but the reaction may frighten the patient to the point of stopping treatment. Sometimes, in the case of weaker or older patients, treatment may be followed by more pain or fatigue for 1 or 2 days. Practitioners have to explain to patients that there may be a flare-up reaction to the needling. They should suggest where such pain might arise, how severe it might be, and how long it might last, and they should reassure the patient that such pain is normal after a needling treatment, and that there are steps that can be taken if it happens (e.g., the practitioner can put one or two needles in a painful area to relieve the pain or show a patient how to relax by using breathing and other relaxation strategies). Patients who receive these instructions come to believe that they have better control of the pain, and so will have less anxiety and more confidence to continue treatments. This process is a good psychological preparation and thus reduces the uncertainty and anxiety associated with both the pain and the treatment. It is essential to provide the patient with the knowledge and skills to cope with the pain and anxiety.

The Patient's Personality

The perception of pain and outcome of the treatment are profoundly influenced by the patient's personality. Anxiety, neurosis, or a predisposition to becoming overemotional in daily life may greatly impede the effectiveness of healing.

Patients who expect complications and problems ("catastrophizers") experience more pain. On the other hand, people who have a predisposition to successfully manage life's stresses tend to use any available strategy—and invent their own when necessary—to manage specific threats to their psychological equilibrium. In the case of the catastrophizer a successful outcome will require the practitioner to call on appropriate techniques and skills.

PLACEBO OR NOCEBO EFFECTS: PSYCHOLOGICALLY INDUCED SELF-HEALING OR SELF-DESTRUCTIVENESS

Biological survival requires the interaction of both physiologic homeostasis and psychological integrity, and the phenomenon of self-healing is a vital factor for survival. Without self-healing, no biological entity can recover from even a minor injury. In fact, recovery and rehabilitation after all medical procedures, especially those of allopathic medicine such as surgery and drugs, depend on the self-healing capability of the individual. This varies from one person to another, which is a reason why any medical modality, including acupuncture, may produce varying results when used for the same pathophysiologic disorder. When we understand the trigger mechanism and the role of self-healing in biological survival, the placebo and nocebo phenomena are no longer mysterious.

Currently *placebo* is defined as "an intervention that is designed to simulate medical therapy but is not believed to be a specific therapy for the target condition," or "an inefficacious treatment believed efficacious at the time of use." The placebo effect is also described as "a change in a patient's illness attributable to the symbolic import of a treatment rather than its specific pharmacologic or physiologic properties."[4] A study showed that about 35% of postoperative patients reported marked pain relief after being given a placebo.[5] This is a strikingly high proportion because morphine, even in large doses, relieves severe pain in only about 70% of patients.

The *nocebo effect* has been defined as "the causation of sickness (or death) by expectations of sickness (or death) and by associated emotional states."[6]

Placebo and nocebo effects can be found in every treatment and in every modality, whether surgery, drug, acupuncture, psychotherapy, chiropractic manipulation, physical therapy, or massage. An understanding of placebo and nocebo effects can help practitioners improve the efficacy of their treatments and patient satisfaction.

Thus the outcome of acupuncture treatment depends on the following:

1. The patient's physiologic condition, including health status and the severity of symptoms
2. The use of proper treatment methods by the practitioner
3. Psychological interactions between the practitioner and patient that might induce placebo or nocebo effects (Box 7-1)

Placebo

When a drug or medical procedure is referred to as a placebo, there is an implicit negative connotation. This is a misconception that should be reevaluated. Of course the placebo effect should be filtered out when evaluating a new drug or medical procedure, but it is an indispensable part of clinical practice, and every practitioner should understand and use it to benefit those patients who are placebo responders. It is unfortunate that this misunderstanding of the placebo effect is particularly prevalent with respect to acupuncture. In the following section, we examine some placebo studies and explain the mechanism underlying each case.

Case 1: "Sham" Transcutaneous Electrical Nerve Stimulation Therapy   Despite the chronic nature of their pain (an average duration of 4

Box 7-1

Factors that Influence Acupuncture Efficacy

1. Self-healing potential of patients (better and faster results can be achieved in healthier patients. Healthier patients maintain better self-healing potential).
2. Severity of symptoms (better and faster results can be achieved in patients with less severe symptoms. Less severe symptoms are more healable or reversible).
3. Specific acupuncture effects (selection of the most effective acupoints especially SAs and correct needling technique such as proper depth of the needling).
4. Placebo and nocebo effects (psychological interactions between the practitioner and patient).

---

years), patients with back pain showed improvement in measurements of pain severity, pain frequency, and ability to function. On average the scores improved by 20% to 40% after sham (meaning in this case "unplugged") transcutaneous electrical nerve stimulation (TENS) plus hot packs.[7]

Case 2: Mystery of the Drug Placebo Effect
Drs. Ronald Melzack and Patrick D. Wall cited a placebo case in their book *The Challenge of Pain*[8]:

> A surprising recent discovery about placebos is that their effectiveness is always about 50% of that of the drug with which they are being compared, even in double-blind experiments.[9] That is, if the drug is a mild analgesic such as aspirin, then the pain relief produced by the placebo is half that of the aspirin. If it is a powerful drug such as morphine, the placebo has greater pain-relieving properties, again about 50% of that of morphine. How is this possible?

Case 3: "Sham" Surgery   One classic double-blind, randomized study[10] showed substantial and sustained improvement in angina pectoris after sham surgery (skin incision alone). In this study, 6 months after the operation, 63% of genuinely operated patients and 56% of falsely operated patients had substantial improvement. Benefits were not limited to decreased pain; they also included a reduction in drug use and increased tolerance of exercise.

In other more recent placebo experiments involving the effect of "sham" surgeries on lower back pain and osteoarthritis of the knee, the results showed exactly the same pattern as in this classic experiment.

Case 4: "Sham" Acupuncture In classic acupuncture practice it is believed that "sham" acupoints cannot be effective. However, one study that used acupuncture for chronic pain concluded that needling sham points seemed to work for 33% to 50% of patients, whereas true points were effective in about 55% to 85% of cases. There was no statistical significance between the results for true and sham acupoints.[11] The same study found another puzzle, that although sham acupuncture works in 33% to 50% of patients with chronic pain, it does not work at all in cases of acute laboratory-induced pain.

Of these four examples, only case 2 represents a "pure" placebo effect. The other three cases show the effects of specific treatments but it is a misinterpretation to describe them as placebo effects.

Analysis and explanation of these four placebo cases are provided in the next section.

Mechanism of the Placebo Effect

The remarkably powerful effect of a placebo in no way implies that a patient who responds to a placebo does not have a real medical problem. In Chapter 6 we discussed quantitative evaluation of patients. Based on the number of tender acupoints, we classified patients into four groups:

Group A: 28% of patients. Pain can be eliminated with an average of 4 treatment sessions. Usually this group of patients will respond immediately to any medical intervention, including over-the-counter medications or massage.
Group B: 34% of patients. Pain can be relieved for about 5 months after 8 to 16 treatment sessions (average of about 8 treatments).
Group C: 30% of patients. Pain can be reduced for about 5 months after 16 to 32 treatment sessions (average of about 12 to 16 treatments).
Group D: 8% of patients. Very weak or no response to acupuncture treatments.

The number of tender acupoints in the body is the result of the interaction between physiologic homeostasis and psychological integrity. These classifications indicate that patients have different healing potential and thus respond to treatment differently. Because placebo responders show some improvement, it is a sign that there is self-healing,

regardless of whether it is temporary or longer lasting. This finding clearly indicates that self-healing could be achieved without any real intervention from outside. Placebo responders are most likely to belong to group A, B, or C.

In Case 1 we saw that 20% to 40% of patients responded to sham TENS plus hot packs. Clinical evidence shows that the application of hot packs alone does reduce pain in some patients, so it is not a placebo but stimulates self-healing, especially in group A and some group B patients.

Case 2 is seemingly puzzling; the placebo response rate is 50% that of either aspirin or morphine. The explanation is simple. Placebo responders will respond to placebo pills because their self-healing potential is capable of being activated psychologically without *any* medications, regardless of what drugs are used as control—aspirin, morphine, or others.

Case 3 is a comparison between true surgery and sham surgery. The results are not difficult to understand if one is familiar with acupuncture therapy. In China acupuncture is traditionally used with some success to treat cardiovascular problems, including angina pectoris, high blood pressure, and stroke. If the pathologic damage of angina pectoris is slight or mild, the stimulation of needling can relax the smooth muscle and myocardium through the mechanism of cutaneous-visceral reflex. Chinese doctors even invented a special procedure to implant foreign material like sheep gut into acupoint locations, especially on the arms, to prolong the effect of the cutaneous-visceral reflex. The skin incision functions like acupuncture-induced lesions (see Chapter 3). In case 3, therefore, the sham surgery in fact is not sham; rather the body's self-healing mechanisms respond to stimulation produced by the sham surgery, which, like acupuncture, activates self-healing through stimulating sensory nerves in the area of the surgery. Such a response might equally have followed the use of acupuncture or possibly other modalities as well.

Case 4 is discussed in Chapters 3 and 4. Neurophysiologically there are no sham acupoints because acupuncture therapy is the central nervous system's (CNS) response to stimulation of sensory nerves, and sensory nerves are distributed all over the human body, except in nails and hair. What are called true acupoints nevertheless provide more significant therapeutic results because they are located on the major nerve trunks. That is why true acupoints provide higher efficacy than sham acupoints.

Laboratory-induced pain is not the same as real clinical pain. Most clinical pain involves sensitized nerves, injured tissues, and inflammation, and as it persists it may change the physiologic homeostasis and the psychological integrity of the patient. Laboratory-induced pain is a type of localized sensory stimulation to which the brain tries constantly and rapidly to adjust. Soon the laboratory-induced pain is ignored by the brain like long exposure to a bad odor in a room. Thus psychologically and physiologically, persons with laboratory-induced pain are no different from pain-free persons. Nevertheless laboratory experiments provide the basic data for understanding pain mechanisms and the principles of pain management.

Now it is clear that the placebo effect is a process of self-healing activated either by psychological suggestion alone or by a combination of psychological suggestion and physiologic stimulation. The effect also occurs in subjects whose self-healing potential is suppressed by psychological factors such as anxiety. We should not exclude the possibility that even some persons with very intractable health problems may experience short-term placebo effects under some psychological conditions.

The placebo effect provides a remarkable form of therapy for some medical problems involving psychological factors that may be partially or completely self-healing. It can be effective not only for pain but also for anxiety and depression and a variety of other medical complaints in which psychological factors play a role. Practitioners may use a placebo to influence cognitive processes as well as to treat injured areas of the body. It is prudent for practitioners to seek to maximize any of the self-healing effects of a placebo that can contribute to the relief of the pain and suffering of their patients.

Acupuncture Therapy Is Not a Placebo Effect

Like other medical modalities, acupuncture therapy induces placebo effects in some patients but by itself it is not a placebo. The reason is obvious. The effectiveness of acupuncture treatment, especially in the field of pain management, is predictable. The degree of effectiveness of a placebo is unpredictable, and whether a particular patient will benefit from the placebo effect is unpredictable as well. In an acupuncture session that uses the Integrative Neuromuscular Acupoint System (INMAS) and its quantitative method of evaluation, we can reliably differentiate patients into four response groups and can predict the effectiveness of the treatment. This will be true for any practitioner who uses the INMAS method.

Placebo Responders

As discussed already, potential placebo responders are patients who maintain a fairly good or at least minimal level of self-healing capability, although this capability may be reduced for psychological reasons or suppressed from time to time.

Some researchers have suggested that placebos are more effective for severe pain than for mild symptoms, and that the effect is stronger when patients are under great stress and anxiety. Experiments show that a reduction in anxiety may result in a partial reduction of the placebo effect.[12] Thus the placebo effect is more powerful in people who have chronic generalized anxiety (personality-trait anxiety), although even in such people placebos are more effective when pain levels are high rather than low. Apart from trait anxiety levels, no consistent differences have been found to distinguish between placebo responders and nonresponders.

Placebo effects appear more in patients with severe or chronic problems because they tend to have more psychological problems, such as habitual anxiety, than do patients with mild or acute pain symptoms.

Placebo effects also vary according to the kind of pain. Most kinds of pain are relieved by placebo treatment in 35% of patients; however, as many as 52% of people suffering from headaches are helped by placebos. This may be due to the particularly strong role of anxiety in headache patients. Clearly the placebo effect is produced by suggestion, personality predispositions, and other psychological factors.[13] However, practitioners should not be overly optimistic about placebo effects because patients tend to get less and less relief from repeated administration of placebos.

Clinical Inducement of Placebo Effects: Practitioner-Patient Interactions

Placebo effects are induced by practitioner-patient interactions, but we are not able to predict who will be a placebo responder before administering treatment. Understanding the factors that are relevant to both patient and practitioner will help to maximize the placebo effects.

Characteristics of Placebo Responders
Placebo effects appear mostly in patients who maintain fairly good self-healing potential, with this potential being temporarily suppressed by psychological factors such as anxiety. In addition all placebo responders share some common characteristics:

1. They have a positive attitude and confidence toward practitioners and treatments.
2. They have good expectations of the treatment.
3. They cooperate with practitioners, adhere to the treatments, and follow instructions.
4. Their anxiety decreases after treatment is administered.

Practitioner's Attitude   The practitioner plays a powerful psychological role in inducing placebo effects. Methods and skills may include the following:

1. Convey a positive attitude toward the patient. Talk to the patient with warmth and friendliness.
2. Show a genuine interest in the patient's story and deep sympathy, empathy, and concern about his or her situation.
3. Perform an earnest and careful evaluation and physical examination.
4. Convey an air of confidence in handling the case.
5. Elicit and address the patient's worries, concerns, and goals so the patient will know that you understand the whole picture. This decreases the patient's worries and fears.
6. Convey "realistic optimism and prognosis" about the treatment. Encourage the patient to adhere to and participate in the treatment process, such as following an exercise routine.
7. During a follow-up visit, let the patient know that you have reviewed previous medical records and history and have up-to-date knowledge with which to make correct medical decisions.
8. Display diplomas, board certifications, awards, and professional memberships so the patient can know that you have the appropriate medical qualifications.

The psychological interactions between the practitioner and patient may also enhance the effect of the treatment. Several studies have shown that placebo effects and the effects of treatment can interact. One study[14] demonstrated that a standard dose of morphine was only 54% effective in placebo nonresponders, but was 95% effective in placebo responders. Clearly the drug effects are dramatically enhanced in persons who are fortunate enough to be placebo responders.

Nocebo Effects

As mentioned at the beginning of this chapter, nocebo effects have been defined as the cause of sickness (or death) by expectations of sickness (or death) and by associated emotional states.[6] The following two cases show nocebo effects.

Nocebo effects are psychologically induced physiologic destructiveness. It is important for practitioners to understand the nocebo possibility in patients and to take appropriate measures to prevent nocebo responses from potential responders.

Case 1   Headaches were reported by 70% of college students who were told that a (nonexistent) electric current was being passed through their heads.[15]

Case 2   A double-blind study was designed to evaluate a method of testing for food allergies. The food substance was injected into the experimental group subjects, and the control group subjects were injected with a saline solution. Twenty-seven percent of those given the food substance and 24% of those given saline experienced symptoms of nose itching or watering, burning eyes, plugged ears, tight or scratchy throat, dizziness, sleepiness, and depression.[16]

Psychogenic Pain

When psychological factors appear to play a predominant role in inducing pain symptoms, the pain may be regarded as psychogenic. Such patients have elevated scores on the scales for hysteria, depression, and hypochondria. Chronic pain is usually the cause rather than the result of neurotic symptoms. The relief or improvement of the chronic pain may help to reduce psychogenically triggered symptoms, although other modalities may be needed to achieve a better outcome.

SUMMARY

A practitioner should always keep in mind that patients' pain problems represent a pathologic process in which physiologic and psychological factors intertwine. Environmental and cultural factors can also influence the outcome for some pain patients. Changes in pain symptoms over the treatment period reflect complex interactions between physiologic processes and psychological organization. Thus, to achieve the maximal outcome, the treatment of pain should always consist of both a pathophysiologic procedure (pathologic evaluation, acupoint selection, and the application of needling technique) and psychological management, including placebo inducement, patient education, and nocebo reduction.

Self-healing potential, which varies from person to person, is a mechanism of biological survival. Without self-healing potential, no species or individual can survive. Self-healing capability can be suppressed by physiologic trauma and psychological disorganization. In some cases the pain or other persistent medical problems caused by psychological factors may play a major role in suppressing the self-healing process. If the psychological interference is cleared, the self-healing process will be recovered or accelerated.

The placebo effect is the process of self-healing that results from reducing psychological suppression, whereas a nocebo effect is induced by psychological disorganization. *Aspects of practitioner-patient interactions can have positive (placebo) or negative (nocebo) effects on patient treatment.* Placebo effects indicate that some patients can be successfully treated without specific medical procedures. A practitioner will achieve better treatment results if he or she is able to harness the power of the placebo mechanism.

References

1. Chapman CR, Turner JA: Psychological aspects of pain. In Loeser JD, et al, editors: *Bonica's management of pain*, Philadelphia, 2001, Lippincott Williams & Wilkins.
2. Hebb DO: *Essay on mind*, Hillsdale, NJ, 1980, Lawrence Erlbaum.
3. Williams JMG, et al: *Cognitive psychology and emotional disorders,* ed 2, Chichester, NY, 1988, Wiley.
4. Brody H: Placebo effect: an examination of Grunbaum's definition. In White L, Tursky B, Schwartz GE, editors: *Placebo: theory research and mechanisms*, New York, 1985, The Guilford Press.
5. Beecher HK: *Measurement of subjective response*, New York, 1959, Oxford University Press.
6. Hahn RA: The placebo phenomenon: scope and foundations. In Harrington A, editor: *The placebo effect: an interdisciplinary exploration*, Cambridge, Mass, 1997, Harvard University Press.
7. Deyo RA, et al: A control trial of transcutaneous electrical nerve stimulation (TENS) and exercise for chronic low back pain, *N Engl J Med* 322:1627-1634, 1990.
8. Melzack R, Wall PD: *The challenge of pain,* London, 1996, Penguin Books.
9. Evans FJ: Expectancy, therapeutic instructions, and the placebo response. In White L, Tursky B, Schwartz GE, editors: *Placebo: theory research and mechanisms,* New York, 1985, The Guilford Press.
10. Cobb LA, Thomas GI, Dillard DH, et al: An evaluation of internal-mammary-artery-ligation by a double-blind technique, *N Engl J Med* 260:1115-1118, 1959.
11. Vicent CA, Richardson PH: The evaluation of therapeutic acupuncture: concepts and methods, *Pain* 24:1-13, 1986.
12. McGlashan TH, Evans FJ, Orne MT: The nature of hypnotic analgesia and placebo response to experimental pain, *Psychosom Med* 31:227-246. 1969.
13. Gracely RH, Dubner R, Deeter WR, Wolskee, PJ: Placebo and naloxone can alter postsurgical pain by separate mechanism, *Nature* 306:264-265, 1983.
14. Lasagna L, et al: A study of the placebo response, *Am J Med* 16:770-779, 1954.
15. Schweiger A, Parducci A: Nocebo: the psychologic induction of pain, *Pavlov J Biol Sci* 16:140-143, 1981.
16. Jewett DL, Fein G, Greenberg MH: A double-blind study of symptoms provocation to determine food sensitivity, *N Engl J Med* 336:542-545, 1990.

CHAPTER 8

Introduction to the Practical Application of the Integrative Neuromuscular Acupoint System

This chapter reviews the most important concepts for successful acupuncture therapy.

THE FOUR PRELIMINARY CLINICAL PROCEDURES

1. A practitioner must be familiar with the complete picture of each patient's medical history, lifestyle, current situation, and the signs and symptoms of their problem.
2. A practitioner should understand the nature of each patient's complaint to the fullest extent possible. For example, if a patient presents with lower back pain, a practitioner will expect different treatment results, depending on whether the pain is related to muscle strain, a herniated disk, radiculopathy, spinal stenosis, referred pain from other problems, or infection of the spinal nerves. Information from the patient's physician can be helpful.
3. A practitioner must objectively evaluate each patient's self-healing potential. This evaluation will help the practitioner to understand whether a patient will be an excellent responder, an average responder, or a nonresponder. With our quantitative acupuncture evaluation method (QAE) (see Chapter 6), this information can be obtained reliably in a short time.
4. Finally, a practitioner must use the Integrative Neuromuscular Acupoint System (INMAS). INMAS includes three types of acupoints: homeostatic acupoints (HAs), symptomatic acupoints (SAs), and paravertebral acupoints (PAs). There are 24 HAs, and these form a standardized protocol that can be easily applied. Selection of the most effective SAs requires a practitioner to have a reasonable understanding of the nature of a patient's symptom(s) and its relation to the *anatomic structure and biomechanics* of the

human body. Once the SAs are selected, the PAs can be easily determined according to the principles of spinal segmentation: dermatome (skin) and myotome (muscle) distribution.

QUANTITATIVE ACUPUNCTURE EVALUATION AND CLASSIFICATION OF PATIENTS

Different patients will have different responses to the same acupuncture treatment. The method of QAE allows practitioners to predict the efficacy, duration, and prognosis of the treatment for each patient.

The degree of homeostasis of each patient represents his or her individual self-healing potential. Any pathologic insult or disease tends to reduce the self-healing potential, impair homeostasis, and transform latent (nonsensitive) HAs into passive (tender) HAs. The number of HAs reflects the body's ability to repair the damage caused by pathologic symptoms. Thus, the number of tender HAs is the result of the interaction between the self-healing potential and pathologic condition of the patient.

After examining a patient, the practitioner should be able to know:

- To which one of the four groups (A, B, C, and D) the patient can be classified according to the number of passive (tender) HAs found (i.e., whether the patient will respond to the treatment and what kind of response can be expected: excellent, good, average or no response).
- The number of treatments the patient needs.
- The possible time lapse before recurrence of the same pain.

Chapter 6 provides the technical details of how to quantitatively evaluate a patient.

INTERACTION BETWEEN THE NEURO-, IMMUNE, ENDOCRINE, AND CARDIOVASCULAR SYSTEMS

Please refer to Chapters 3 and 4 for an explanation of the peripheral and central mechanisms of acupuncture therapy.

The Nervous System and Endocrine System: Endorphin Release

Acupuncture needling stimulates the peripheral nerves, resulting in the synthesis and release of endorphins by the central nervous system. The term endorphin was coined by combining the words "endogenous" and "morphine." Endorphins are a group of opiate-like peptides produced naturally by the body in the spinal cord and brain, where they modulate the transmission of pain signals to reduce the perception of pain by raising the pain threshold. In addition, endorphins work on other body systems, relaxing the cardiovascular system, improving the activity of the immune system, and modifying the endocrine system. All these effects make the patient feel relaxed and speed up the self-healing process.

Acupuncture Needling Normalizes Muscle Physiology

Muscle is the biggest organ in our body and contributes more than 50% of the body weight. It is the most dynamic organ in our body. Please note that here we discuss only the skeletal muscle, not smooth or cardiac muscles. If we do not move our muscles frequently, they become stagnant and lose their ability to function. If we use them improperly, for example, without adequate relaxation between contractions or with excessive repetition, even with sufficient relaxation between contractions, the muscle will become sick and refuse to move any more. This is the built-in self-protection mechanism of muscles.

The sick muscle is painful, spasmodic, tight, swollen, inflamed, fatigued, and starved for energy; it requires more nutrition and an improved oxygen supply to recover. It also requires an increase in blood circulation to remove metabolic toxins, but the tightness of the muscle or the contracture formed in it reduces or blocks the normal blood circulation. This process is a vicious circle of energy crisis in the muscle (see Chapter 3). The sick muscle is no longer responding to the signals from the

brain that try to create the necessary relaxation. If this condition persists, acute muscle pain will become chronic and result in atrophy.

When a muscle gets sick, it becomes tight and will resist any further stretching to protect itself from further damage. If the tightness of the muscle continues, some part of the muscle fiber develops a condition of persistent contraction, which is the center of the energy crisis in the muscle. This persistent contraction of muscle fiber is called contracture. When an acupuncture needle is inserted into the tight muscle or into the contracture of the tight muscle, the mechanical movement of the needle breaks the contracting muscle fibers and pushes tight tissue aside.

Other tissue fibers, including the collagen fibers of fascia and other connective tissues, are also broken by the needling. The broken fibers of the connective tissues are entangled at the surface of the fine-diameter needle. There is a physical affinity between the surface of the acupuncture needle and the broken tissue fibers.

The mechanical movement of the needling (pistoning and rotating, see Chapter 3) pulls, moves, and stretches all the broken fibers and leads to mechanical relaxation of the tissues around the needle. Thicker needles like those of syringes do not create this type of physical affinity between the needle surface and the broken fibers.

The mechanical needling of sensory nerve endings also stimulates the corresponding motor neurons to send signals to relax the tight muscles. We described this physiologic process in Chapter 3. Thus the needling immediately produces the effect of relaxation, both mechanically and physiologically. Once the needle is removed, the needle-induced lesion prevents the re-contraction of the broken fibers. The broken tissues, triggered by the lesion, start either reconstruction or replacement of fibers.

As a result, the mechanical and physiologic effect of needling, including the lesion it produces, relaxes the tight muscle and dissolves the contracture. The needle-induced lesion continues the relaxing function for at least 2 days after the treatment, until the lesion is healed.

Acute minor or mild tightness and contraction can be released with one or two acupuncture sessions. If a large area of tightness and contraction is involved such as in chronic muscle pain, repeated treatments are needed.

Once the muscle is relaxed, the blood vessels restore the normal circulation that supplies nutrition and oxygen and removes the metabolic toxins. The restored energy supply resolves the energy crisis and desensitizes the irritated nerve endings. This is how needling and its lesion activate the healing process of damaged muscle.

Immune System: Antiinflammatory Reaction Induced by Acupuncture Needling

Inflammation is a localized protective response elicited by injury or destruction of tissues. Inflammation will destroy, digest, dilute, or wall off both the invaders and the injured tissues. However, the inflammation from injuries often becomes uncontrollable, spreading, swelling, and resulting in heat, pain, and loss of function of the tissues involved. This uncontrollable inflammation will slow down the healing process and may become chronic if not treated early. Acupuncture needling, by creating a very tiny, limited injury and destruction of tissue, triggers a controllable acute inflammation in the body.

Acupuncture needling is perceived as a foreign invader by the body and the needle-induced lesion as an injury or mechanical trauma to the tissues. The needling also causes a tiny amount of bleeding in the soft tissues, which causes hemodynamic changes including dilation of the arterioles and the opening of new capillaries and venular beds in the area. Once the blood vessels become more active, the leukocytes (white blood cells) move from the blood vessels to the injured tissues to engulf and digest invaders and the debris resulting from this destruction. Thus needle-induced inflammation stimulates the inflammatory response, which triggers the healing process.

When acupuncture needles are inserted into the injured and inflamed tissues, each needling site triggers a tiny, local antiinflammatory reaction that speeds up the inflammatory process. This process is a protective strategy of the body, but becomes disabling if it lasts too long and spreads too far. Usually when several needles are inserted into inflamed tissues, swelling, inflammation, and pain will all subside and healing will be accelerated.

BASIC CONCEPTS OF THE APPLICATION OF INMAS TO CLINICAL PRACTICE

Previously we discussed the physiologic principles of acupuncture therapy, the mechanisms of acupuncture needling, INMAS, and the quantitative acupuncture evaluation (QAE) method. The understanding of these concepts is an indispensable and critical precondition for the evaluation of patients and practical application of INMAS. Without this understanding, an acupuncture practitioner might still achieve a few "miraculous" results, but the treatment would be *half-blind* because one would not know why the miracle happened or whether it would happen again. By understanding the concepts discussed above, a practitioner will not only know why success occurs but will be able to predict in what patients it can be expected, in what patients there might be no response, and why.

To avoid a half-blind acupuncture practice, practitioners need to know how to select the most effective SAs, which will in turn allow them to select the most effective PAs.

There are three steps involved in searching for effective SAs and PAs:

1. A practitioner must start palpating HAs in the symptomatic area first. For example, if a patient complains of neck pain, a practitioner should first examine the HA7 greater occipital in the neck area.
2. A practitioner must carefully palpate the cervical vertebrae on the back and side. Knowledge of the facet biomechanics of cervical vertebrae will help the practitioner to locate the most injured part of the cervical spine as well as affected soft tissues, such as muscles. The most important SAs for treatment are found in these locations.
3. The PAs are then selected according to the SAs. For instance, if symptoms related to neck pain include some numbness in the upper limb, use C5 to T1.

As noted above, understanding the nature and mechanism of the symptoms in conjunction with the anatomy and biomechanics of the affected location will help a practitioner to select the most effective SAs. Therefore, in the following chapters, which discuss specific pain symptoms, we always try to present neuroanatomical and biomechanical descriptions that are relevant to acupuncture treatment of that symptom.

When applying INMAS, a practitioner uses the same protocol to treat different symptoms but with personal variation: HAs are basically the same for everyone but SAs and PAs are different for each patient, depending on the individualized nature of the symptoms. For example, the HA part of the protocol is exactly the same regardless of whether a patient's headache is a migraine headache, a tension headache, or a whiplash-induced headache. However, the SAs are different for each patient, depending on the type of headache. As noted above, understanding the nature and mechanism of the symptoms in conjunction with the anatomy and biomechanics of the affected location will help practitioners to find and select the most effective SAs. The most effective SAs will then determine which PAs to use.

Usually stable, long-lasting pain relief can be achieved after acupuncture treatments alone. In some cases the additional use of other medical modalities will help to accelerate and stabilize the healing process.

It is important to understand the main difference between the conventional medical approach and the approach of acupuncture in treating pain. In conventional medicine a precise diagnosis of the underlying cause of pain is critical to successful pain treatment. All conventional treatment procedures are designed to deal with the specific cause of the pain. Such precise diagnosis is not required for the successful application of acupuncture therapy for pain management. Our basic protocol is used with some individualized variations to treat all kinds of pain. This is possible because, as you will remember, *acupuncture does not specifically target the underlying cause of specific pain symptoms but activates the healing potential of the body, promoting self-healing.*

CHAPTER 9

Back Pain: Neck, Upper Back, and Lower Back

INTRODUCTION

The unique advantages of using acupuncture as a sole or supplementary modality in treating lower back pain and neck pain include:

1. Acupuncture treats the whole body, concentrating on the cause of the problem and not only on the area where the problem is manifested. Thus, pain in the lower back and neck areas as well as referred pain in the upper and lower limbs can be treated simultaneously.
2. By promoting general well-being, acupuncture accelerates and enhances the self-healing potential of the body. Improved healing potential directly reduces local inflammation, the essential physiologic process that causes pain.
3. Acupuncture needling precisely targets and dissolves tension in acupoints, relaxes muscle spasms, eases physiologic stress by balancing the activity of sympathetic and parasympathetic nervous systems, promotes local blood circulation, and reduces swelling and inflammation in strained or sprained muscles, tendons, and joint capsules.
4. The majority of pain specialists share the opinion that musculoskeletal disorders are the most frequent cause of pain and disability in the lower back region, followed by neuropathic problems and peripheral vascular disease.[1] Most musculoskeletal pain symptoms respond very well to acupuncture therapy. Acupuncture needling can effectively reduce inflammation in the neck and back muscles, facet joints, and ligaments.

When the underlying cause of back pain is physiologically recoverable, acupuncture will achieve stable results. When it is not the case, acupuncture can provide only limited pain relief or is not effective at all. For example, some types of spinal stenosis do not respond to acupuncture therapy, and only short-term pain relief can be expected.

Lower back pain and neck pain have become some of the most common problems in modern society, and can affect anyone. Sufferers include office workers, computer programmers, athletes, healthcare professionals, musicians, painters, manual laborers, housewives, teachers, students, and others.

Statistics show that about 150 million Americans suffer from acute or chronic lower back pain and spend an estimated $20 billion to $50 billion a year in treating their problems.[2] At any given time more than 2.6 million adults are disabled by chronic lower back pain. Reliable statistics as to how many Americans suffer from neck pain are not currently available, although one survey found that two thirds of the people surveyed had had significant neck pain at some time in their lives and 22% have neck pain that is bothersome.[3]

Considering the profound impact of lower back and neck pain on our daily activities and on our society as a whole, there is no questioning the importance of studying its etiology and pathology, of trying to provide timely treatment, and of seeking ways to satisfactorily restore the function of the spine and related tissue.

However, the exact triggers of lower back pain and neck pain are still an enigma to doctors and patients alike. Many doctors recognize that X-rays may show no structural or anatomical abnormalities in cases of acute and chronic back pain and that they are mostly useful for ruling out such conditions as tumors or tuberculosis (TB). Even diagnoses made with the use of high-tech equipment such as magnetic resonance imaging (MRI) are known to be inaccurate in 10% to 20% of cases.

An interesting and disturbing study that appeared in 1994 in the *New England Journal of Medicine* found no direct correlation between structural abnormalities revealed on MRI and back pain: among 98 people without back pain, two thirds had spinal abnormalities, including herniated, bulging, or protruding intervertebral disks, disks with minor "degenerative joint changes," and flattened narrowed disks, especially at the L5-S1 level.[4] An investigation based solely on anatomic structure fails to produce an accurate diagnosis in 80% to 90% of patients with lower back disorders (LBD).[5]

These studies demonstrate the extent of our limitations in attempting to understand the syndromes of neck and back pain from the structural and anatomic points of view. It is more likely that a multidisciplinary study of psychogenic and chemogenic factors will be needed to explain the triggers responsible for provoking back pain.

At present all we have is a general understanding that the majority of pain syndromes in the neck and the upper and lower back areas can be attributed to the following factors:

1. Malfunction and structural defects of the spine
2. Problems associated with the spine soft tissues including muscles with their fascial coating, nerves, and connective tissue such as tendons, ligaments, and joint capsules
3. Various biochemical interactions among soft tissues including muscles, nerves, and connective tissue

It is important to note that neck, lower back, and upper back pain are all closely related and are often inseparable because functionally and anatomically all three parts of the spine—the neck, the upper back, and the lower back—are a *single indivisible entity* and should be treated as such if pain occurs anywhere in the neck or back.

Our spinal column performs two very important physiological functions. First, it houses and protects the delicate spinal cord, which processes and transmits messages from the brain to the rest of the body and vice versa. Second, it supports the body's weight and provides the strength and flexibility needed for difficult and possibly "back breaking" functions. The different functions that the spine is asked to perform often conflict with each other and cause pain, and the design of the spinal column is a compromise between them. This compromise makes us prone to mechanical problems in all three parts of the spine, from the neck to the lower back.

However, although neck pain and lower back pain are closely related, the way in which the pain is manifested can be very different.

Functional and mechanical variations in the anatomical structure can serve as an explanation. For example, we can turn our heads by 90 degrees

because the neck part of the spine provides a wider range of motion than the lumbar column. Due to this mobility, when injury occurs from overuse or accidents, the cause of neck pain is likely to be related primarily to traumatized joints and disks in the neck. Anatomically, the lower back part of the spine is more resistant to side rotation and flexion. Thus back pain in this case has been found more often to be due to the traumatization of muscles.

Despite the differences, all parts of the spine are so interdependent that a problem in one structure will affect all the others and can lead to a vicious circle of pain. For example, chronic muscle strain leads to decreased support and protection of the spine joints, which results in joint pain. Joint pain provokes pain in the muscle tissue. Thus, neck pain will trigger lower back pain, which will in turn cause neck pain, which will in turn cause lower back pain, and so forth.

The important clinical feature of the Integrative Neuromuscular Acupoint System (INMAS) in treating neck and lower back pain is that a practitioner should simultaneously treat *(1) both neck and lower back and (2) both spine and limbs*.

The ability of INMAS to implement functional restoration as well as reduction or elimination of pain makes it an effective modality for reducing inflammation in all soft tissues, rebuilding injured muscles, and relieving or controlling most lower back and neck pain syndromes.

Note that clinical experience shows that apart from very mild acute injury, there is no quick fix for the majority of back problems even with very powerful treatment. Clinical case histories often show that quick relief does not turn out to be a cure, and that the pain becomes worse afterward. The pain itself can be stopped immediately by powerful drugs or a few effective acupuncture treatments but this does not mean that the back problems are solved. Recovery of tissue from injuries and restoration of spinal function require substantial healing time and active participation of the patient in the healing process.

BRIEF REVIEW OF THE NEUROMUSCULAR STRUCTURE AND SOFT TISSUES OF THE SPINE

This chapter presents a brief discussion of the neuromuscular system of the spine in order to assist acupuncture practitioners in understanding the possible underlying causes of back pain and to enable them to draw conclusions about the possibility of repairing the trauma. This information will help the practitioner to judge the likely therapeutic efficacy of acupuncture treatment for a given patient: whether acupuncture alone will be sufficient to achieve the desired result, whether the use of acupuncture by itself will be insufficient and other modalities should be involved, and whether the patient should be referred to other medical experts for further evaluation by means of X-rays, MRI, and so forth.

Our spine is a long linkage of bones, disks, muscles, and ligaments that extends from the base of the skull to the tip of the tailbone (coccyx). The spine is a neuromuscular system that is totally subservient to the brain, spinal cord, and nerves. It protects the spinal cord, supports the body by maintaining proper posture, and ensures kinetic activity (movement).

The entire spine (vertebral column) is made up of 34 bony vertebrae (Figure 9-1) and six additional elements: nerves, muscles, tendons, ligaments, disks, and various connective tissues. The

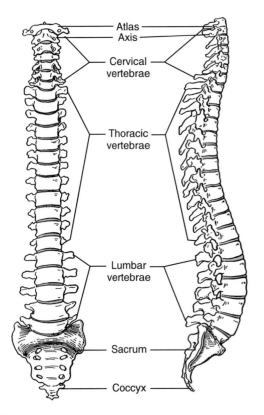

Figure 9-1   The vertebral column as a whole, anterior and lateral views. (From Jenkins D: *Hollinshead's functional anatomy of the limbs and back,* ed 8, Philadelphia, 2002, WB Saunders.)

erect spine consists of four physiologic curves: the cervical and lumbar lordosis (concave to the back) and the thoracic and sacral kyphosis (convex to the back). All of the four curves conform to the center of gravity.

All of these parts contribute to the maintenance of a proper balance, which keeps the body erect, supports the head (which weighs 10 to 15 pounds), and holds the internal organs in an anatomically correct position. The muscular system of the trunk and its fascia ensure the stability of the erect spine and the range of motion of the spine during various physical activities. Co-activation of both flexor and extensor muscles along with a ligamentous structure is a required condition for securing the stable activity of the entire spinal area. Small muscles, tendons, and joint capsules serve as local segmental stabilizers between every two vertebrae.

All of the above mentioned muscles are vital for stabilizing the static and kinetic functions of the spine. A stabilized spine guarantees a smooth, accurate, and rhythmic functioning of the entire body during physical activities. For instance, the incredibly versatile design of the spine enables a gymnast to bend into almost unimaginable positions while a weight lifter can lift hundreds of pounds.

The spine is also in close interaction with the internal organs, and can be deformed by diseases of the internal organs, such as the lung, stomach, heart, or liver. These diseases disturb the balance of the mechanical support system and result in pain of the back. Likewise, an over-kyphotic spine will cause malfunction of the internal organs, especially the lungs. Thus, there is a close pathophysiologic relationship between the mechanical structure of the spine and the internal organs.

Numerous types of neck and lower back pain are triggered by mechanical abnormalities or injuries, inflamed soft tissues, or degenerative diseases, and of course, the pain can be idiopathic, or "origin unknown." *Please note that the INMAS protocol (see Chapter 5) can be used successfully for pain management regardless of which underlying causes produce the pain symptoms as long as the symptoms are physiologically recoverable.*

The Foundation of the Spine: The Coccyx and the Sacrum

An analogy between the spine and a big tree will help to illustrate why many patients experience pain in this area. The trunk of a big tree (like the spine) has to support the canopy (the head) and numerous heavy branches (the upper limbs, ribs, and internal organs) that sprout from the trunk. This construction subjects the trunk to continuous mechanical stress and eventually the stress will affect the root system (the coccyx and sacrum bones).

The root system must be very strong and practically immovable to give adequate stability to the trunk and heavy branches of the tree. In calm weather, the tree ensures its symmetrical balance by having its branches spread in all directions and by evenly distributing gravitational stress among all the roots, which also spread in all directions. When a strong wind tilts the tree to one side, the symmetrical balance is lost and the roots from the opposite side of the tree sustain huge stress, which is many times higher than the weight of the tree (Figure 9-2). Using the physical principle of leverage, we can calculate the stress applied to the root system on the affected side of the tree. For example, if a tree weighs 500 pounds at its center of gravity, the affected part of the root system will sustain a stress of more than 5000 pounds.

The tree analogy explains why the foundation of the spine—the coccyx and sacrum—is so easily stressed and liable to be painful. Bending and twisting in an asymmetric manner are the predominant causes of lower back injury. The leverage described in the analogy with the tree is also applicable to our spine. For example, when a mother bends forward to pick up a 30-pound baby with both hands symmetrically, the stress on the spine and its foundation (sacrum and coccyx) could be 300 pounds. If the mother uses a correct bending posture, such as bending the knee first and staying close to the baby, the stress can be reduced to 100 pounds, which is distributed evenly between the muscles and joints on both sides of the body.

If our right hand picks up a 30-pound package (asymmetric action), the stress on the left sacroiliac joint and lumbar muscles on the left side can be more than 300 pounds, which will be distributed along the whole spine from the neck to the lower back. These are examples of the kind of potentially damaging stressful situations that our spine is exposed to daily, without our conscious awareness, in the workplace, at home, and during sports activities.

To correctly apply INMAS to the coccyx and the sacrum, an understanding of the anatomic structure of this area is important. The coccyx, which is also called the tailbone, is located at the base of the back. It consists of three to five fused bones. If we lose our balance and fall, the coccyx can break and a condition called *coccygodynia* may occur. We will discuss coccygodynia later in this chapter.

Above the coccyx are five more fused bones, the sacrum (S1-S5). The sacrum is a spade-shaped structure that is fixed between the two halves of the pelvis, which is the only structure that connects the spine to the lower limbs. Referring to the tree analogy, the two fused, relatively immovable bones—the coccyx and the sacrum—represent the roots of the tree. The two bones called ilium on either side of the pelvis make a joint on either side of the sacrum, and these are called the sacroiliac joints.

The sacroiliac (SI) joints differ from other joints. They are thicker and stronger and can move only a few millimeters (Figure 9-3). This relative immobility of SI joints stabilizes the spine against gravitational forces. The SI joints are also subject to the tremendous stresses and strains created by the forces of asymmetric imbalance as discussed in the above examples. The SI joints have to support

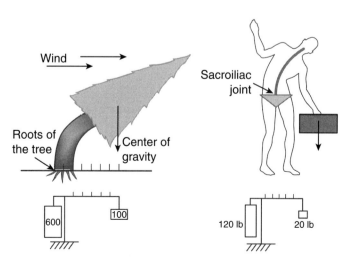

Figure 9-2 Mechanical force sustained at the sacroiliac joint to balance the body is about 3 to 6 times the weight of the luggage if the spine is bent to pick up luggage. A similar mechanical stress occurs at the roots when the wind bends a tree.

the trunk, shoulders, arms, and head and to ensure a full range of motion.

During locomotive activity such as walking, running, carrying weights, raising the arms, or dancing, the joints transfer weight from the spine to the hip bones. The pathological effect of excessive or overextended stress will accumulate in the joints and result in soft tissue disease.

These joints are innervated by the lower lumbar and sacral nerves, as a result of which pathological conditions in the joints can produce lower back pain and sciatica. For example, when the SI joints are inflamed, movement of the spine in any direction causes pain in the lumbosacral part of the spine. Usually the pain is more pronounced at the limit of forward flexion, since the hamstring muscles hold the hip bones in a relatively fixed position while the sacrum is rotating forward as the spine bends down.

INMAS is effective in treating painful symptoms related to the SI joint region. Most SI joint pain is caused by inflammation of the soft tissues such as nerves and ligaments. When needles are inserted into inflamed tissues, the needle-induced

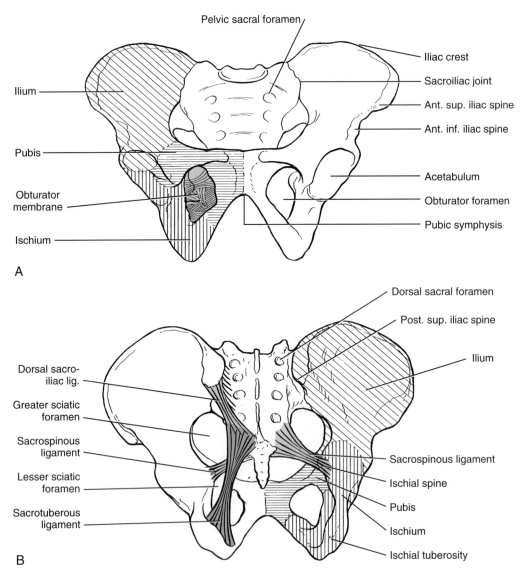

Figure 9-3   Sacroiliac (SI) joints. **A** and **B,** Anterior and posterior views of the SI joints.

Continued

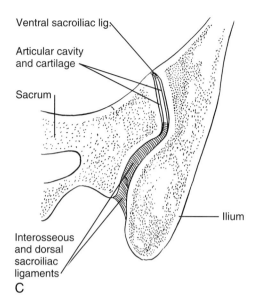

Ventral sacroiliac lig.

Articular cavity
and cartilage

Sacrum

Ilium

Interosseous
and dorsal
sacroiliac
ligaments

C

Figure 9-3, cont'd **C,** Schematic horizontal
section through the SI joints. (From Jenkins D:
*Hollinshead's functional anatomy of the limbs and
back,* ed 8, Philadelphia, 2002, WB Saunders.)

lesions break the blood vessels, thus stimulating
the local defense immune reaction. As a result of
the immune reaction, inflammation of the soft tissues of the SI joint is reduced. The needle-induced
secretion of endorphins from the spinal cord and
the brain reduces the physiological stress caused by
the joint pain, thereby accelerating tissue healing.
Eventually, this process restores normal SI joint
function. The degree of recovery of SI joint function depends on the degree of the injury and the
self-healing capability of the body.

The INMAS protocol for treating SI joints is
provided at the end of this chapter.

Lumbar Spine (L1-L5)

The lumbar part of the spine is situated above the
sacrum. The lumbar spine has five large vertebrae,
and each vertebra has two upper facets (superior
articular facets) that emerge from the top and two
lower facets (inferior articular facets) that descend
from the bottom (Figure 9-4).

The functional unit of the lumbar spine consists
of two adjacent vertebrae with an interposed intervertebral disk. The disk is a hydrodynamic structure that permits weight bearing and ensures the
mobility of the unit itself and the mobility of the
entire vertebral column. The two inferior facets of
the vertebra above are loosely joined to the two
superior facets of the vertebra below. During for-

ward-and-back motion such as in fast dancing, the
facets slide across each other. A side view shows
that the lumbar spine is concave relative to the back
of the body, and this is termed the lordotic curve.

The lumbar spine is located between two different and functionally conflicting parts of the
spine and therefore is always subjected to substantial stress. Below the lumbar spine is the immobilized stability of the sacrum and above it are the
heavy but flexible structures of the thoracic and
cervical spine, which are required to be able to
maintain a full range of spontaneous and rapid
movement. This is why the lumbar spine is constantly engaged in trying to mediate an acceptable
compromise between two conflicting functions,
providing enough of both strength and flexibility at
the same time.

Additional stress on the lumbar spine is created
when a person holds weight in their hands with the
arms extending away from the center of gravity of
the body. In an upright posture the lumbar spine is
supporting the axial compressive forces from the
weight of the head, which is about 10 to 15 pounds,
the weight of the upper limbs, and any additional
loads that the upper limbs are carrying. When this
compressive force is greater than half the body
weight, particularly, the spine becomes unstable.

Because of these factors the lumbar spine is
subject to a greater amount of constant stress than
any other part of the spine, due to:

- The conflicting functions of the immobilized
  sacrum and the flexible cervical spine
- Axial compressive forces of the combined
  weight of the head, upper limbs, and possible additional loads of the upper limbs (e.g.,
  carrying weights)

Thoracic Spine (T1-T12)

The thoracic spine has 12 vertebrae, and each vertebra has a pair of ribs attached to it. The ribs form
a cage that holds open a space for creating a partial
vacuum for inflating the lungs. The rib cage also
protects the heart, lungs, and liver. The upper 10
ribs arise from the spine and are joined at the front.
This allows the spine only a limited range of
motion. Side views show that this part of the back
is slightly concave relative to the front of the body,
and this is termed the kyphotic curve.

The two lower ribs are short and are called
floating ribs. They do not enclose anything, but
they allow a broader range of motion than the first
10 thoracic vertebrae. The joints between the last
thoracic vertebra and the first lumbar vertebra

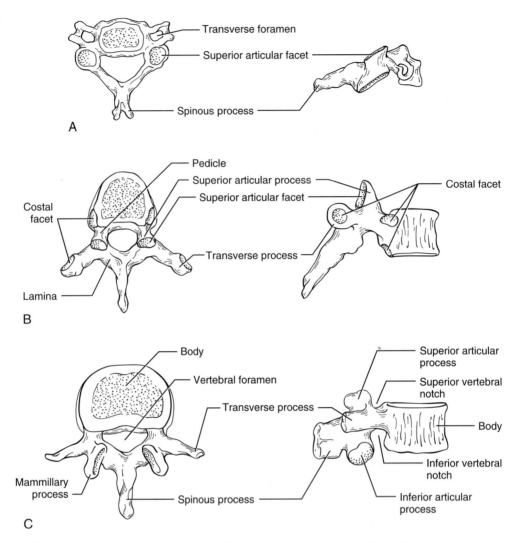

Figure 9-4   Representative vertebrae from the spinal column. **A,** Cervical region. **B,** thoracic region. **C,** Lumbar region.

(between T12 and L1) also facilitate side-to-side rotation of these relatively immobile regions. This rotation implies a significant amount of wear and tear on these lowest two thoracic vertebrae and may result in various pain syndromes and degenerative diseases like osteoarthritis.

Cervical Spine

The cervical spine has seven vertebrae. These vertebrae get progressively smaller as they approach the bottom of the skull (see Figure 9-4). The cervical spine is the upper part of the spine and is capable of a great range of motion, in contrast to the foundation of the spine, the sacrum and coccyx,

which has fused bones and almost immovable sacroiliac joints. For instance, the cervical spine allows the neck to turn 90 degrees in either direction, the ear to almost touch the shoulder, and the head to lean backwards more than 70 degrees.

The cervical spine differs from other parts of the spine in its agile motion and its ability to perform other important tasks; for instance, in addition to supporting the head, the neck provides a passage for air, food, nerves, and blood vessels.

The cervical spine is composed of two major complexes: the upper cervical segment (C1 and C2) and the lower cervical segment (C3 to C7). The occipital bone of the skull sits on the ring-shaped bone C1, which is called the atlas. The joint between them (0-C1), which is the first joint of the cervical spine, is called the atlantooccipital (AO) joint. This joint provides a very important function by anchoring the skull to the spine, and it is therefore necessarily the most immobile joint of the neck spine.

The second cervical vertebra, the axis, is the strongest of the cervical vertebrae. C2 has two large horizontal flat bearing surfaces called the superior articular facets. The atlas, C1, bearing the skull on top of it, rotates on these articular facets.

The distinctive feature of C2 is a blunt toothlike process called the odontoid process, or *dens*, projecting superiorly from the body (Figure 9-5). C1 uses the dens of C2 as its pivot for rotation. The front inner surface of the ring-shaped C1 is attached to the dens of C2, allowing C1 with the skull on top of it to rotate against the dens.

The joint between C1 and C2, called the atlantoaxial (AA) joint, is the most mobile part of the spine. Fifty percent of all cervical rotation occurs at the AA joint.

The first two vertebral joints differ from all other vertebral joints because their main function is to allow head rotation. C1 and C2 are jointed by ligamentous integrity, and not by bony facets as are all other typical vertebrae.

Among all vertebral joints the AO joint is the most immobile, whereas the AA joint is the most mobile. This functional characteristic makes the AA joint more vulnerable to wear and susceptible to pathological conditions like inflammation and arthritis.

The use of homeostatic acupoints (HAs) to implement functional restoration, as well as reducing or eliminating pain, makes it an effective modality in reducing inflammation, rebuilding the function of the joints, and relieving and controlling related pain syndromes.

The facet joint between C2 and C3 is a transitional structure located between the rotation joint above C3 and the flexion-extension joints below C3. The cervical spine from C3 to C7 is organized such that it can rotate and simultaneously flex forward or laterally, or extend backward. The cervical vertebrae have to maintain enough stability to support the head, which weighs 10 to 15 pounds, while providing enough flexibility to perform these motions.

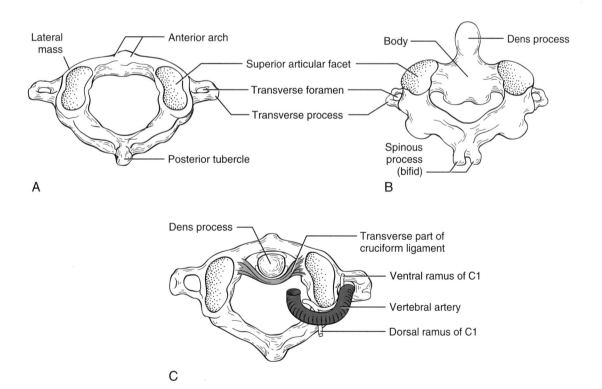

Figure 9-5   Posterosuperior views of the atlas **(A)** and axis **(B)**. **C,** Superior view of the atlantoaxial joint. (From Jenkins D: *Hollinshead's functional anatomy of the limbs and back,* ed 8, Philadelphia, 2002, WB Saunders.)

The peripheral nerve network in the neck region is some of the most complicated nervous wiring in the body. Eight cervical nerves emerge from the intervertebral foramen to form the cervical plexus from C1 to C4, and brachial plexus from C5 to T1. The intervertebral foramen is the passage from which the spinal nerve emerges. The neck is also the passage for the autonomic nervous system, which balances the physiological activities of the majority of the internal organs. Thus, pathological neck problems will affect not only the head and the arms but many different organs ranging from the brain to the large intestine.

A functional unit of the spine consists of two neighboring vertebrae: one above and one below. Examination of what happens to a typical cervical functional unit during a car accident will help to explain how excessive motion of the neck or exposure to sudden external forces can cause neck problems and pain.

In a car accident a sudden external force causes the head to bend forward (forward flexion) and the upper vertebra slides forward about an axis of rotation. The anterior intervertebral disk space narrows, the posterior intervertebral disk space widens, and the intervertebral disk deforms. As a result of this excessive narrowing of the anterior intervertebral space, there may be damage to the cartilage of the anterior joint surface, and the intervertebral disk may be broken and pushed backward. The widened posterior joint may break the joint capsule or even cause tearing of the ligaments. The broken intervertebral disk becomes herniated and the damaged joint surface produces pain and can cause arthritis in the future.

Rotation of the cervical spine is a coupling motion that involves both rotation and lateral flexion. For example, when the head turns to the left, the upper vertebra rotates to the left while its left intervertebral disk space narrows and its right intervertebral disk space widens. When this rotation is caused by violent force, the sudden closure of the left intervertebral disk space will cause damage to the cartilage of the joints, break the intervertebral disk, and force it to the right. Rotation caused by violent force also may cause injury to the spinal nerves: the left intervertebral foramen becomes smaller and pinches the left spinal nerve, and the broken intervertebral disk bulges to the right and pushes the right spinal nerve.

During a whiplash accident, the horizontal force from the back causes the neck to overextend and overflex (Figure 9-6), which causes damage to both posterior and anterior joints. In addition, the translational back-and-forward movement of the

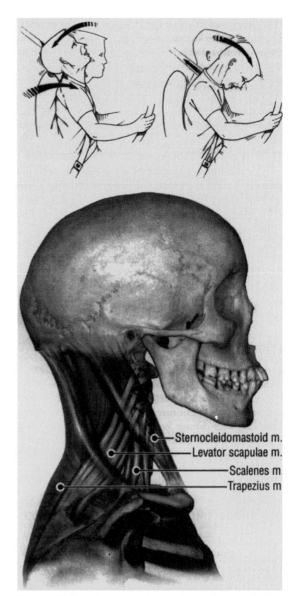

Figure 9-6 Overextension and overflexion during a "whiplash" injury. (From Wall P, Melzack R: *Textbook of pain,* ed 4, Edinburgh, 1999, Churchill Livingstone.)

Labels on figure:
Sternocleidomastoid m.
Levator scapulae m.
Scalenes m
Trapezius m

upper vertebra closes the vertebral canal, which causes injury to the spinal cord. Understanding the basic mechanical structure of the spine and the nature of pathological damage sustained by the spine during an accident is the key to effective acupuncture treatment for back pain.

The INMAS protocol for treating whiplash will be provided in the end of this chapter. Please note that in the case of whiplash, pain symptoms such as neck pain, lower back pain, and upper back pain are all closely related because functionally and anatomically all three parts of the spine—the neck, the upper back, and the lower back—are interrelated structures that should be understood as one whole entity and treated as such.

All the components of the back are so dependent upon each other that a problem in one structure can damage all the others. For example, a mechanical neck injury causes inflammation in spinal joints, which will strain muscles, and chronic muscle strain can contribute to arthritis in the spinal joints. Neck pain and back pain are clinically coupled.

Muscle strain can lead to disk displacement, and displaced disks can further strain the muscles. Motions such as excessive forward flexion, excessive backward extension, or excessive lateral rotation cause injuries to bony joints that involve cartilages, disks, capsules, and ligaments. These injuries strain the muscles, and strained muscles irritate the spinal nerves. All these pathological changes to the basic mechanical structure of the spine produce pain, and eventually this pain can trigger chronic problems such as arthritis and degenerative diseases.

MUSCLE

Strained, overworked muscles are, in up to 80% of cases, the leading cause of all acute and chronic back pain, especially in the lower back.

Muscle is the most dynamic of all the mechanical components of the body. Muscles create energy and are the indispensable providers of the mechanical leverage that moves the bones. Thus, muscles are always in need of sufficient blood circulation to supply energy for movement and to eliminate toxic wastes from energy metabolism.

There is a widespread misconception that the spine is a very strong structure because, for example, a weight lifter can lift hundreds of pounds on his shoulders and in some cultures women habitually carry 40 to 50 pounds of cargo on their heads. In fact, the spine itself can carry only about 5 pounds and most of the work attributed to the spine is performed by the back muscles. The back muscles in turn are helped by the tendons and the ligaments to stabilize the spine and to allow the body to perform a variety of hard physical tasks.

Muscles perform at least three major mechanical functions:

1. Maintaining proper posture while adjusting to gravitational forces during physical activity
2. Moving the bones to allow body movement
3. Absorbing shock and releasing the tension of movement in a controlled way, which prevents damage

Weak back muscles are not able to adequately perform the following functions:

1. Maintenance of the proper spine position
2. Stabilization of the joints
3. Coordination of the full range of motion (since any motion involves several muscles, the activity of the muscles should be coordinated)
4. Absorption of shock and tension resulting from movement.

Inadequate performance of these tasks leads to body weight imbalance or misplacement of the jointed bones, which will result in pain and the onset of tissue inflammation. Weak muscles are not able to support any sudden twist, or sudden change in posture, and will allow a disk to slip out of place, which in its turn can lead to disk rupture and neck and lower back pain syndromes.

Muscles are in a state of minimal contraction when the body posture is erect and static. The spine is maintained erect by muscles, fascia of the muscles, intervertebral disks, ligaments, and joint capsules. All the muscles are covered by a fascial sheath. The erect spine is primarily stabilized by the combined effort of these structures.

When the back muscles as well as the abdominal muscles have to be slightly contracted to maintain erect body posture, the fascial sheaths become taut. Neck and back problems happen when any one of the above mentioned structures experiences fatigue or injury and thus becomes a weak link in the chain.

Strain is a state of overstretching or overexertion of the musculature due to the application of excessive force. Strain disrupts the normal alignment of muscle fibers, ligaments, tendons, joint coverings, and the joints themselves. When strained, these tissues are subjected to microscopic tears that result in pain, bleeding, or inflammation and swelling.

Muscle strain may cause muscle spasms. A spasm is an uncontrollable intensive contraction of a muscle or group of muscles. A spasm increases tension with or without shortening of a muscle. A locally affected strained muscle can cause other muscles to become tight or to go into spasm in order to prevent an injury from spreading from the affected point to other structures.

Usually a spasm has no serious consequence and the pathological effect is not longlasting. However, when a tear caused by strain or spasm is severe or repeated, scar tissue is formed, which weakens the muscles and irritates the nerves, thus provoking pain syndromes. Acupuncture needling is very effective in the treatment of strained tissues and muscle spasms, especially at the acute phase.

A strained muscle or a muscle under spasm undergoes the vicious circle of energy crisis. Injured muscles become tightened. This tightness puts physical pressure on the blood vessels, which results in poor blood circulation. Insufficient circulation results in an insufficient supply of nutrients and oxygen being delivered to the injured muscles. Thus, the energy crisis begins.

As a result of energy deprivation, muscles become tighter and tighter. Then the nerves surrounded by the tightened muscles are subjected to hypoxia (low oxygen) and undernutrition and experience an energy crisis as well. During the energy crisis, metabolic toxins are accumulated in the injured muscles. This vicious circle of energy shortage creates muscle pain.

When needles are inserted into tight, strained, or spasmodic muscles, the needles push the tissues aside and create a microlesion. This process also stimulates a reflex reaction from the motor nerves, which relaxes the tight muscles and manifests as muscle twitching. Once the muscle starts to relax, adequate blood circulation to the injured muscle is restored, the vicious circle is broken, and the energy crisis is resolved. Improved blood circulation brings sufficient supplies of oxygen and nutrients and allows elimination of metabolic toxins. Thus, the muscles and nerves start the process of self-healing.

When the fibers of muscles, tendons, ligaments, or joint capsules are forcibly pulled and actually tear, then strain turns into sprain. A sprain can be a very serious and disabling physical condition. Sprains heal slowly and have a tendency to recur and become habitual. Acupuncture treatment will greatly speed up healing and reduce swelling at any stage, especially at the acute phase of the sprain. This is due to the way that needling and its lesions relax the injured muscles, which are usually tight, swollen, and deprived of nutrition and oxygen, with consequent vasoconstriction. Once the muscles are relaxed, normal blood circulation resumes, which brings the muscle physiology to normal condition. This normalization manifests itself by increased supply of nutrition and oxygen, reduced metabolic wastes, digestion of injured cells, and regeneration of new tissues. In addition, the needling stimulates the central nervous system to secrete neurochemicals such as endorphins, which improve cardiovascular function, and instigate immune reactions, which activate and accelerate the self-healing process.

The degree of muscle involvement may determine how an event is categorized, as a primary or a secondary cause of pain. "Primary muscle pain" means that the pathological condition of the muscles is the major cause of pain. Acupuncture is very effective for treating this type of pain. In cases of acute pain, relief can be achieved almost immediately after the beginning of treatment. In case of chronic pain, more treatments are needed for pain relief. "Secondary muscle pain" means that although the muscles are painful and in spasm, the condition is caused not directly by muscle injuries but by other injured structures such as nerves, joints, or disks, which contribute to the painful symptoms. For example, in the case of arthritis, muscle pain is caused by inflamed joints. More acupuncture treatments over a longer period of time are required to relieve secondary muscle pain because relief depends on healing the primary pain source, such as nerves, joints, disks, or other soft tissues.

Our basic protocol (INMAS) is used with individualized variations to treat all kinds of muscle pain and is provided at the end of this chapter.

As previously mentioned, the front muscles act as antagonists to the back muscles, which means that the front muscles flex the spine, while the back muscles extend it. These forces balance each other in order to maintain stability of the trunk and to secure various kinetic functions of the spine. When the front muscles are fatigued or injured, this balance is disturbed and the ability of the spine to maintain stability and proper posture is diminished. The tired front muscles became shortened and resistant to stretching, forming tender points within the muscle tissue, forcing the back muscles to stretch excessively and preventing relaxation of the back muscles.

Disturbance of this antagonistic balance causes neck, upper back, and lower back pain. This is why in the case of back pain symptoms it is important to carefully examine and to treat the front muscles without delay, namely the pectoralis major and pectoralis minor muscles on the chest as well as the external oblique, the anterior oblique abdominal, the transversus abdominis, and the rectus abdominis muscles.

Weak abdominal muscles often result in back pain. The abdominal muscles do much of the work when lifting or carrying loads, and so when weak abdominal muscles try to relieve the strain on back muscles during such activities, they will sustain further damage. This is why the abdominal muscles should be examined and needled in clinical acupuncture practice when a patient presents with back pain.

The physical condition of the limbs also influences the function of the spine. Thus it is especially important to maintain the flexibility of the powerful hamstring muscle in the back of the leg. When this strong muscle becomes tight, it limits the range of motion of the pelvis, and this can strain the lower back muscles and joints. In cases of back pain, the muscles on the limbs, especially the lower limb muscles of the thighs and legs, should be examined and their tightness relieved by acupuncture, which is a very effective treatment for it. Please note that a relaxed hamstring muscle permits a normal physiologic range of motion of the pelvis and thus allows coordinated movements between the pelvis and all other back muscles.

The Shortened Muscle Syndrome

Muscles become shortened for protective reasons, to prevent further damage to healthy muscle tissue when it is subjected to pathologic factors, such as cold, fatigue, repetitive overuse or overstretching, low oxygen, or deficient blood circulation. When a muscle becomes shortened a domino effect is initiated that can generate many painful conditions. Muscular shortening gives rise to tension in the tissues by pulling tendons and their attachments and by offering resistance to healthy stretching. *Thus, the shortened muscles and the stressed tendons and attachments eventually cause such symptoms as neck and back pain, epicondylitis, tendinitis, and tenosynovitis.* All of these symptoms share the same etiology, although they appear dissimilar and occur at different anatomic sites.

Shortened muscles limit the range of motion of joints. For instance, a pathological condition called "frozen shoulders" is a result of shortening of all the muscles around the shoulder joint in addition to a capsular problem like inflammation. The shortened muscles increase pressure on the articular surface of a joint, which results in joint pain (arthralgia). Muscle shortening is also often responsible for joint misalignment. For example, the shortened muscle (extensor hallucis longus) of the foot causes angulation of the great toe (hallux vulgus) and a painful bunion. Muscle shortening contributes to pathologic conditions of joints, such as restriction of the range of motion and misalignment, and eventually leads to degenerative arthritis and osteoarthritis.

Shortened muscles also put pressure on the nerves and produce an entrapment syndrome. For example, carpal tunnel syndrome is a result of shortening in the pronator teres or pronator quadratus muscles.

The paraspinal muscles, when shortened, draw two adjacent vertebrae closer together, which narrows the intervertebral space and foramen (Figure 9-7). The results are a bulging disk and a compressed nerve root. A vicious circle is gradually built up: shortened muscles cause compressed nerve roots (radiculopathy), and compressed nerve roots lead to further muscle shortening.[4]

Acupuncture treatments can break this vicious circle by using needles to produce a minimal tissue injury, which stimulates the relaxation of muscle stress. The primary goal in the treatment of muscle shortening is relaxation of the affected muscle, and acupuncture needling achieves this goal more swiftly and precisely than any other medical modality. When a fine acupuncture needle pierces a muscle, it pushes aside tissue, disrupts the cell membrane, and inflicts a minute tissue injury, which mechanically creates a brief outburst of microcurrents (injury potentials). The microinjury that results from needling generates relatively long-lasting currents that stimulate the mechanism of repair and regeneration of the affected tissue (see Chapter 3). Thus, acupuncture treatment eliminates the pathological condition responsible for muscle

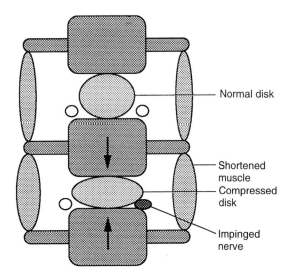

Figure 9-7   Shortened paraspinal muscles across an intervertebral space compress the disk and nerve root. (From Filshie J, White A: *Medical acupuncture: a Western scientific approach,* Edinburgh, 1998, Churchill Livingstone.)

shortening. After treatment a patient feels either no pain or a significant alleviation of pain.

This mechanism explains the efficacy of acupuncture treatment in addressing pain syndromes resulting from radiculopathy or pathological conditions of the joints such as osteoarthritis.

Bursitis

A bursa is a small fluid-filled sac that reduces friction between tissues. Excessive or repetitive use of a joint irritates the bursa and causes it to swell, resulting in pain during movement. The principal symptom of acute bursitis is sudden severe pain resulting in limitation of motion of the affected joints. A chronic bursitis condition may develop if an attack of acute bursitis is left untreated. Acupuncture needling is a very effective modality for treating acute bursitis but its effectiveness decreases proportionally to the degree of development of the chronic stage of the disease. Bursitis causes pain in the bursa and also in the muscles. The affected muscles become shortened and blood circulation is reduced. Needling is able to relax the muscles and increase blood circulation as well as stimulating an immune reaction and thus reducing the inflammation of the bursa.

NERVE TISSUE

The spinal cord is an extension of the brain and contains low-level nerve centers that process some pain sensation. The spinal cord sends out three kinds of nerves into the body: sensory, motor, and autonomic. Sensory nerves bring signals from the skin, muscles, tendons, joints, blood vessels, and organs to the spinal cord and then to the brain. These signals provide vital information about our activities and changes in the outside environment. Pain is the primary response to damage or irritation of nervous tissue.

Motor nerves transmit impulses originating in the brain and spinal cord down to the muscles of the skeleton and inner organs and to the glands in order to initiate and maintain appropriate movement. Autonomic nerves bring physiologic signals to the blood vessels and the internal organs to regulate their physiologic activities.

A nerve bundle may contain only one kind of nerve (sensory or motor nerves) or two or three kinds of nerves (mixed nerves). Normally sensory, motor, and autonomic nerves are interdependent because neither is able to function without the other. When nerves in the spinal cord have been disturbed by tissue damage—such as a pull, bruise,

tear, swelling, or inflammation—they can trigger pain almost anywhere in the body.

Injury to nerves leads either to an involuntary, intense contraction (spasm) of the muscles in the body, the blood vessels, and organs, or to weakness or paralysis of the muscles as a result of insufficient contraction. A spasm causes overstimulation of sensory nerves and undernourishment of muscles because the tightness constricts blood vessels and interrupts the mechanism of nourishment. Weak muscles can easily be overstretched and thus be susceptible to painful tissue damage because this pathological overstretching releases chemicals that irritate the muscles (Chapter 3). Some of the pathophysiologic conditions of the spinal cord are discussed below.

Spinal Stenosis

Lumbar spinal stenosis is defined as a condition involving any type of narrowing of the spinal canal, nerve root canal, or tunnels of intervertebral foramina.[5] Spinal stenosis can be either congenital or acquired. Acquired stenosis may be due to degenerative conditions (spondylolisthesis, see below), failed medical procedures (postlaminectomy, postfusion, postchemonucleolysis), or posttraumatic injuries, or it may be secondary to disk herniation (see below). Narrowing can occur in one or several locations of the same vertebral segment or it can affect several segments. The canal space can be narrowed by pathological changes in the soft tissues, scar tissue, or bony tissue impingement (bone spurs). Severe stenosis results in nerve compression. Soft tissue encroachment or abnormal bone growth such as osteophyte formation reduces the size of the intervertebral foramen and causes foraminal stenosis.

Twenty percent of patients diagnosed with spinal stenosis show no pain symptoms. The majority of sufferers experience lower back pain and some impairment of sensory or motor function in the leg(s) when walking or standing. Patients with spinal stenosis are more comfortable sleeping in the fetal position but they still experience a stiff back upon awakening. This stiffness is diminished in the course of daily activities but increases with prolonged standing and walking.

Some patients with spinal stenosis experience numbness or a burning sensation in both legs. Narrowing of the spinal canal or nerve root canal causes the painful condition known as a pinched nerve, which also irritates muscles and causes muscle pain. Acupuncture needling can relax the groups of erector spinae muscles from the neck to the sacral regions, thus reducing tension and increasing blood circulation between vertebral joints, which alleviates the pressure on the nerve roots and may help reduce swelling or inflammation of soft tissues in the affected region. Based on this mechanism, acupuncture therapy is helpful in mild cases of spinal stenosis especially when applied in combination with proper physical exercise. For example, one of our patients developed both spinal and foramenal stenosis at age 74 after four lumbar surgeries. Acupuncture therapy was able to reduce the pain to a very tolerable level and this patient now resumes normal life, including home office work and some gardening. Acupuncture therapy is not effective for severe cases of stenosis. When the cause of pain is not physiologically repairable such as in severe stenosis, acupuncture provides limited or no relief.

Radiculopathy

Radiculopathy is a common pain pattern seen in both the neck and the lower back. A spinal nerve leaves the spinal cord through the intervertebral foramen to innervate the skin, muscles, joints, or organs. The spinal nerve root or its membrane (dura) becomes inflamed and painful when the intervertebral foramen becomes reduced in its size due to herniated disks, bone spurs, osteoarthritis, or pathological changes in the soft tissues. The pain from the narrowing nerve root causes pain anywhere along the course of this spinal nerve to its target organs, especially the arm or the leg. This pathological condition is called radiculopathy.

In the case of radiculopathy, pain is manifested along the distribution of the painful nerve trunk. This condition also results in decreased muscle strength or a loss of sensation or reflex. Some radiculopathic pain may be referred pain and may manifest itself in an area distanced from the affected nerve because of cross communication between the nerves. For example:

1. Cervical radiculopathy often manifest itself as neck, shoulder and arm pain
2. Thoracic radiculopathy may cause upper back pain due to muscle shortening
3. Lumbar radiculopathy results in lower back and lower limb pain

Both radiculopathy and spinal stenosis (see above) can reduce blood circulation and cause one or more of the affected limbs to become a little cooler or paler than the healthy one. Some patients with lumbar radiculopathy may experience changes in bowel or bladder habits, with more frequent nighttime urination or leakage of urine when coughing or laughing.

Needling of the HAs and symptomatic acupoints (SAs) in cases of radiculopathy and stenosis reduces pain as a result of:

1. Relaxation of the joints, and paraspinal and limb muscles that are shortened by the pain
2. Increased blood circulation in the affected regions, achieved by reducing peripheral resistance in the blood vessels after the muscles are relaxed
3. Balanced autonomic nervous activity, which increases the diameter of the blood vessels

Spondylosis

Spondylosis refers to an acquired immobility of the joints caused by pathological conditions such as traumatic injury, infection, inflamed joint coverings, or degenerative spinal changes due to osteoarthritis. The majority of spondylosis cases are related to chronic rheumatoid arthritis, when the affected joint tends to assume the least painful position and may become more or less permanently fixed in this position. Pain from the affected joint spreads to the adjacent muscles and can cause extensive soft tissue pain and inflammation.

Application of needling relaxes the muscles and reduces soft tissue pain and inflammation. Relaxation and reduced inflammation of the muscles result in relaxation of the joint. The efficacy of acupuncture therapy in the treatment of spondylosis directly depends on the severity of the condition and the general health of the patient. If the spondylosis is caused by acute soft tissue injuries, needling will provide fast and significant relief due to the localized and restricted nature of the symptoms. If the spondylosis is of a chronic nature, which involves extensive tissue damage and even degenerative destruction, acupuncture can provide only limited, temporary, or no pain relief. In healthier patients a quicker and more complete recovery can be expected, and conversely recovery is slower in patients with greater medical problems.

Spondylolisthesis

Spondylolisthesis is the forward displacement of a vertebra over a lower vertebra. Usually this out-of-alignment condition happens at the fifth lumbar vertebra over the sacrum, or the fourth lumbar over the fifth. The forward slippage of the vertebra can lead to spinal stenosis and radiculopathy, which result in muscles that are tight and painful in response to movement, especially movement in the back and buttocks area.

Usually, acupuncture provides only temporary relief for this condition by reducing the muscle pain. It cannot secure stable pain relief because in this case reducing muscle spasm does not result in realignment of the affected joints.

Sciatica

Sciatica is one of the three main clinical manifestations of lower back pain. The other two are pain caused by spinal stenosis and nonspecific back pain symptoms that are often related to problems with various back muscles.

The term "sciatica" is used to describe a number of disorders directly or indirectly affecting the sciatic nerve. Patients with sciatica often feel pain along the anatomic path of the sciatic nerve and its branches: along the lumbar spine through the gluteal area, down along the back of the leg and calf to the sole of the foot or the big toe. Sciatica pain can have a constant or intermittent character. The sharpness of the pain sensation varies and may increase and decrease over a short period of time. The character of the pain can be described as an unpleasant electric shock, heat, tingling, or a stabbing or almost unbearable pain sensation.

Because of its significant size and length (it is the biggest nerve in our body), the sciatic nerve is subject to many types of injuries and inflammations. For example, sciatic pain can be caused by a herniated disk, arthritis of the spine, and pressure on the nerve from certain types of exertion. The sciatic nerve also can be damaged by toxic substances such as lead or alcohol. Occasionally diseases such as diabetes mellitus, gout, or vitamin deficiency contribute to sciatica pain.

In the majority of sciatica cases, where pain and inflammation are caused by soft tissue injury, a proper combination of HAs and SAs produces the optimum pain relief by reducing the inflammation of nerves and muscle. Nerve inflammation is liable to cause pain in the muscles it innervates. Needling and its resulting lesions activate an anti-inflammatory reaction that reduces nerve sensitization. Needling also relaxes the painful muscles and increases blood circulation. The general effect of the acupuncture needling is to reduce the inflammation of nerves, muscles, and other soft tissues, and this results in relief from the pain of sciatica.

When patients have sciatica of unknown etiology, and do not experience significant relief after sufficient acupuncture sessions (Chapter 6), they should be referred for further medical evaluation.

Piriformis Syndrome

The piriformis muscle arises from the anterior surface of the sacrum, then is distributed through the greater sciatic foramen and is surrounded by neurovascular structures that enter the buttock. The piriformis muscle is attached to the upper border of the greater trochanter of the femur. Functionally, it is a lateral rotator of the thigh at the hip. Its task is to ensure, in concert with other muscles, a lateral rotation of the femur, and this is very demanding. When the piriformis muscle is fatigued, it becomes tight and generates pain when forced to stretch.

Current medical opinion holds that lower back pain with sciatic radiation may be caused by a compression of the sciatic nerve by the piriformis muscle as the nerve emerges from under the muscle in the buttock (Figure 9-8). The piriformis syndrome is characterized by pain along the sciatic nerve. The pain is usually more severe in the sitting position than in the standing position, and it is often more troublesome early in the morning if patients sleep on their backs. Tenderness in the buttock area, especially at the center of the gluteus maximus muscle, can be palpated. This tenderness is located at acupoint H16 inferior gluteal in our INMAS. This acupoint is sensitive in most healthy people but this does not mean they all have piriformis syndrome.

Patients with piriformis syndrome experience pain and a restricted range of motion when trying to cross the affected leg over the healthy leg because this action demands stretching of the piriformis muscle. After a prolonged period in a sitting position, patients may experience numbness, tingling, weakness, loss of reflexes, strange discomfort sensations, and even a temperature difference in the parts of the body served by the sciatic nerve, which starts from the roots of L4, L5, and S1. In a few cases, patients with piriformis syndrome experience a tingling sensation in the testicles or labia majora.

Some in the medical profession believe that the piriformis syndrome cannot trigger such a significant amount of pain because the piriformis muscle is too small to have such a powerful impact on the sciatic nerve. Regardless of whether this opinion is justified, patients with piriformis syndrome can be benefited by acupuncture needling. The practitioner can easily find the tender acupoint H16 inferior gluteal and needle it deeply with a long needle all the way to the piriformis muscle. This needling

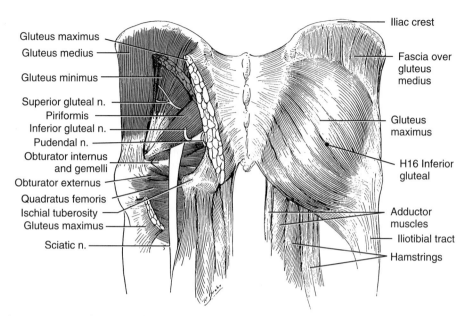

Figure 9-8   Piriformis syndrome: some experts believe that the piriformis muscle compresses the sciatic nerve as it emerges from under the piriformis muscle in the buttock. (Modified from Jenkins D: *Hollinshead's functional anatomy of the limbs and back,* ed 8, Philadelphia, 2002, WB Saunders.)

of the piriformis muscle itself reduces tension and inflammation. If there are other tender points around H16, they should be located by palpation and needled for complete pain relief.

INTERVERTEBRAL DISKS (HERNIATED DISK)

An estimated 5% to 10% of all back pain is nerve pain caused by herniated disks (ruptured disks) that have broken and lost their gelatinous center. Displaced disks, or slipped disks (also called a disk bulge), usually cause less nerve pain than herniated disks but occur more frequently.

Each disk lies between two vertebral bodies, one above and one below. The disk functions as a joint and allows certain movement. The disk performs a double function: it provides flexibility of the vertebrae above and below and ensures stability against excess motion. A disk also absorbs mechanical shock during movement.

Each disk has an inner core called the nucleus pulposus (nucleus) and an outer shell called the annulus fibrosus (annulus). The annulus keeps the nucleus in its proper space. The annulus is made of annular collagen fibers, fat, and water, which give the disk highly hydrodynamic characteristics and allow normal physiologic elongation and recovery.

During daily activities, such as standing or sitting, the water is squeezed out of the disks by our body weight (gravitational pressure), while during sleep the water is restored back to the disks. In young people, the disks contain more water and less fat, so their bodies are an inch higher when they wake up in the morning than when they go to bed at night. As we get older, the water content of the disks diminishes and the disks become thinner, causing our older selves to become shorter than our younger selves. The hydrodynamic nature of the disk permits both a little flexion and a little translational motion in each functional unit of two adjacent vertebrae.

In addition to gravitational pressure, the disks are affected by muscular contraction. Approximately 3% to 10% of disk fluid is lost during 10 hours of daily activity but is recovered after at least 2 hours of rest.[6] Tight or stiff back muscles reduce the flexibility of the spine and impede water recovery of the disks.

Both herniated and displaced disks are often caused by chronically poor posture, weak muscles in the back, damage to ligaments, degeneration of vertebral components, acute injuries, and pregnancy. Disk degeneration starts to appear after midlife because of the continuous process of water loss in the spinal disks. Most cases of herniated disks in people between the age of 35 and 50 are attributed to performing tasks that are too physically challenging. After the age of 50, most people will have some degeneration in about 90% of their disks.

Innervation of the annulus may trigger neck and back pain. In a healthy disk, the outer one-third or the annulus has nerve endings that are sensitive to pressure and possibly to inflammatory chemicals as well. In most individuals, some disk degeneration is part of the inevitable aging process and usually it does not cause pain. However, in some cases the degenerating disks become a cause of chronic neck and back pain, which originates from the stimulation of the nerve endings in the annulus.

Acupuncture treatment will help slow down this degenerative process. Any pain resulting from pathological changes in the spine structure will cause paraspinal muscle pain and sometimes will manifest as referred pain. Pathological changes in the spine cause the paraspinal muscles to become tight, which results in stiff vertebral joints and low blood circulation in the paraspinal area. Acupuncture needling relaxes those muscles that are suffering from chronic lack of nutrients and oxygen due to poor blood circulation. Needling restores or improves the regional blood circulation and induces an antiinflammatory reaction that will help slow down the degenerative process of the disk. Clinically we have helped patients with disk problems to experience a reduction of their back and neck pain and resume normal work and lifestyle for years.

Herniated Disk (Herniated Nucleus Pulposus)

A herniated disk may cause pain because of anatomic abnormality and chemical irritation.

Excessive and nonphysiologic motion of the functional unit of the spine, especially rotation (twisting), damages the annular fibers. The centrally located nucleus is thus allowed to herniate outward through the disrupted annular fibers. This outward bulging, the herniation, may encroach on the posterior longitudinal ligament and the dorsal root ganglion and its dural sheath within the intervertebral foramen, thus creating a radiculopathy or spinal stenosis, affecting multiple nerve roots.

In addition to mechanical encroachment, the injured disk releases nociceptive chemicals of the matrix, leading to inflammation of the dural sheath, ligament, and nerve roots. Inflammatory cells such as macrophages, lymphocytes, and fibroblasts are found in surgically removed disk

material. Recent research shows that cytokines and chemokines also play a role as pain triggers.[7]

In cases of a mild herniated disk, acupuncture needling relaxes the tight back muscles, thereby reducing the pressure applied to the joint by these muscles. The relaxed muscles are enabled to obtain sufficient blood circulation, which causes an increase in nutrition, oxygen supply, and removal of toxins, allowing the self-healing potential to bring under control the biochemical irritation to the nerves. According to some researchers, the body tissues are even able to absorb the herniated materials.[8]

Self healing of a herniated disk is a very important concept as described by the well-known neurosurgeon Dr. Frank T. Vertosick, Fellow of the American College of Surgeons[10]:

> Why does the pain go away? A smashed nerve should be a smashed nerve forever, but the body does find ways to heal itself, a good thing considering that we've been rupturing disks for thousands of years but only operating them recently. In some cases the extruded piece of disk material is absorbed and the nerve becomes slowly decompressed. In effect, the body performs spinal surgery upon itself (and without preapproval from an HMO, I might say).

When our body can absorb the herniated disk in mild cases, acupuncture will accelerate this process.

In cases of a severely herniated disk, the large mass of the herniated material occupies the space and passage of the spinal cord or nerves and constantly irritates the sensory nerves. The irritated nerves cause pain and inflammation in muscles and other soft tissues. In this case acupuncture needling relaxes the tight and painful muscles. In the presence of persisting neuropathologic irritation, pain relief by means of acupuncture is possible but temporary. However, even temporary pain relief is beneficial to patients because it slows down the degenerative or necrotic process as well.

Constant pain causes constant tightness of the muscles, which results in reduced blood circulation and aggravates the process of degeneration. When the tight muscles are relaxed, the blood circulation is increased, which leads to increased supply of nutrients and oxygen to the affected tissues, removing metabolic wastes, and activating tissue regeneration. Thus, needling mechanisms will slow down the tissue degeneration. Unfortunately, because of the herniation, the needle-induced muscle relaxation will not last long, so acupuncture will serve only as a supplementary therapy for this condition.

Several patients with severe lower back pain and MRI-confirmed herniated disks came to our clinic for pain relief before making a decision about whether or not to have surgery. After treatment in our practice some of these patients experienced a reduction in or total relief of pain and decided to delay surgery indefinitely.

TENDONS AND LIGAMENTS (TENDINITIS)

Both tendons and ligaments are made of the same type of tissue called collagen. Tendons connect muscles to bones, which allows the muscles to move the bones. Ligaments connect bones to bones in the area of joints to maintain an anatomically correct distance between bones. Some of the joints are movable, such as shoulder joints; some are less movable, such as the sacroiliac joints.

There is a tendon at each end of every muscle. When a muscle contracts, both tendons pull on the bones to either move them or hold them in place. A tendon contains sensory nerves that will inhibit muscles when the pull on the tendon is too strong. When muscles are injured by overuse, acute trauma, or chronic internal disease, they become shortened and tight. Tight muscles are no longer able to contract or relax. Thus, when forced to move the bones, tight muscles are liable to overstretch or pull the tendons to the point of fraying or breaking. Particularly in the case of athletes, these conditions manifest clinically as swollen Achilles or painful hamstring tendons.

Ligaments hold bones together and maintain an anatomically correct distance between bones. Ligaments produce pain when they are torn or strained and inflamed by excessive motion or injuries.

Tendinitis

Tendinitis means inflammation of tendons and of tendon-muscle attachments. It is frequently associated with a calcium deposit (calcific tendinitis), which may also involve the bursa around the tendon or near the joint, causing bursitis (see below).

Overstretched tendons, whether strained or sprained, will be inflamed. Many professional and amateur athletes have experienced tendinitis, such as pain in the region where the hamstring originates on the ischial tuberosity, or the insertion area on the medial side of the knee, or the upper part of the medial surface of the tibia. In upper limbs, lateral epicondylitis (tennis elbow) and medial epicondylitis (golfer's elbow) are very common tendon injuries. These types of tendinitis are caused by repeated and

excessive extension-flexion motions and, in the upper limbs, by rapid pronation-supination. These repeated motions first make muscles tight and fatigued so they cannot relax fast enough or to a sufficient extent. Then the tight muscles start to exert force on the tendons, which results in tendinitis. Upon examination of the affected muscles, tender points are found in the affected tendons and muscles as well. In most repetitive injuries, tendinitis is clearly caused by tight, shortened, and fatigued muscles (Figure 9-9).

To treat tendinitis, both the affected muscles and the inflamed tendons should be needled simultaneously. Focusing only on inflamed tendons is a common mistake in treating tendinitis. The inflammation of the tendon is the effect, and the cause is the tight and fatigued muscles. We get very good results in treating tendon and ligament inflammation by proper simultaneous needling of both tight muscles and inflamed tendons. Practitioners should carefully palpate the sore muscles and inflamed tendons to detect all the tender points, and all these points should be needled.

Note that in cases of tendon or ligament inflammation caused by overstretching from athletic activities, patients should take complete rest or perform only mild exercise during the course of the first few acupuncture treatments.

JOINTS

There are various types of joints. Facet joints are among the major structures that link the 26 vertebrae together. Each vertebra has four facet joints: two superior and two inferior. The superior joints of the vertebra below connect with the inferior joints of the vertebra above. The sacrum, which is the root of the spine, forms an immovable joint with the two iliac bones. Pathological changes related to either type of joint, superior or inferior, can generate pain.

Facet Syndrome

The majority of joints in the spine have smooth surfaces of cartilage. Each joint is bathed in a slippery lubricating liquid and enclosed in a rough pleated capsule. Facet joints have a rich nerve supply from the medial branch of the dorsal ramus of the spinal nerve.

Facet joints of the spine, like all joints in the body, are mechanically aligned to sustain and secure movement. For example, due to the mechanical design necessary to meet the functional demands of the body, the cervical spine is more

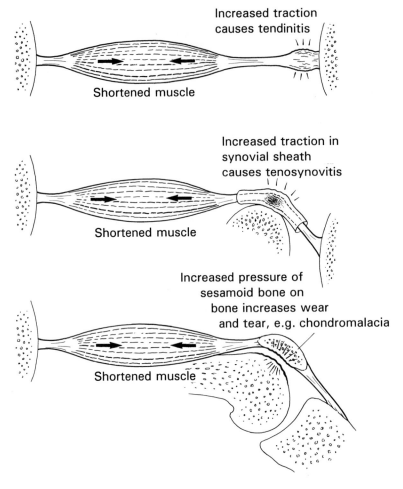

Increased traction
causes tendinitis

Shortened muscle

Increased traction in
synovial sheath
causes tenosynovitis

Shortened muscle

Increased pressure of
sesamoid bone on
bone increases wear
and tear, e.g. chondromalacia

Shortened muscle

Figure 9-9 A fatigued, tight, and shortened muscle can cause tendinitis. (From Filshie J, White A: *Medical acupuncture: a Western scientific approach,* Edinburgh, 1998, Churchill Livingstone.)

mobile but less stable while the lumbar spine is less mobile and more stable. Therefore the facet joints of the cervical spine are designed to allow flexion (bending forward), extension (bending backward), and rotation to the side while the lumbar facet joints resist rotation.

High-tech medical equipment such as X-rays, CAT, and MRI scans often provide the necessary data for identifying the underlying cause of a patient's pain, but medical doctors are aware that the source of pain cannot always be detected by these means. In some cases patients feel pain when their joints appear normal on X-rays, CAT, or MRI scans. Alternatively, the joints can appear damaged while no pain is experienced by the patient. Thus, acupuncture practitioners should keep in mind that high-tech data presented to them by a patient may be valuable, but the underlying cause of the pain can be much more complicated than the data can reveal.

Pathology of facet joints may result in neck and back pain. For instance, in chronic whiplash cases, disturbed facet joints are the single most common cause of neck pain. Once a facet joint is injured in an accident or through excessive motion, a patient experiences pain even when performing tasks within their normal range of motion.

In young people, strong or abrupt movement can cause the lumbar facet joints to slip out of normal alignment. When this happens, the facet joints become locked and extremely painful. With aging many minor traumas are accumulated at the joint surface. The accumulated effect of these injuries gradually produces permanent swellings and deformities on the joint surfaces, which are no longer smooth. When such joints are forced to move or to support weight, the deformities bear the full impact of pressure that is normally evenly distributed over the entire joint surface. This pathological condition chemically and mechanically provokes the nerves to create pain.

Acupuncture needling relaxes tight muscles, increases blood circulation, activates the secretion of endorphins, and stimulates immune reactions, thus reducing the pain and inflammation associated with muscles, nerves, tendons, and ligaments and restoring normal physiology. This process is likely to contribute to a slowing of the degeneration of the facet joints. However, when facet pain is related to degeneration caused purely by aging, acupuncture is helpful in reducing pain but cannot cure the cause of the pain.

Acupuncture is very useful in treating mis-aligned joints because it relaxes the shortened muscles that pull the joints out of alignment or immobilize them. Relaxing the tight muscles and ligaments loosens the joints and thereby allows them to realign. In addition, the effect of needling in promoting blood circulation and stimulating the immune reaction, which reduces swelling and inflammation of soft tissues of the joints, helps to restore the physiologic structure of the affected joint.

This mechanism of needling plays a significant role in preventing the traumas that accumulate on the surface of facet joints as a result of aging. Regular acupuncture maintenance treatments and proper exercise help to develop healthy, strong paraspinal muscles and an enhanced blood supply. With the increased nutrition and oxygen that this brings, aging-related degeneration slows down, and the possibility of trauma in this region is greatly reduced.

Sacroiliac Joint Derangement

The erect position of the human body makes it prone to SI joint derangement. The entire spine and all related structures such as the head, ribs, arms and the weight of the inner organs are resting on the spade-shaped sacrum bone. Both sides of the sacrum form immovable SI joints with the iliac bones. Therefore the entire weight of the body above the waist is supported by these two joints. As noted at the beginning of this chapter, daily movements such as twisting, bending, running, pulling, pushing, and lifting, as well as improperly carrying heavy loads, subject the SI joints to an enormous amount of stress.

The surfaces of the two joints are very rough and irregular, with numerous notches and tabs that must fit exactly into each other. The joints are stabilized by the strongest ligaments of the body. The normal range of motion for this part of the spine is only a few millimeters, which means that the SI joints are practically immovable.

Pain from SI joint derangement can be different on the left and right sides of the body. The pain is increased while performing certain movements, such as lifting the feet when getting in or out of a car, getting out of bed in the morning, or bending down with the knees locked. Usually twisting to one side hurts more than twisting to the other. The pain can be felt in the area of the SI joint and the iliac crest and also along the pathway of the sciatic nerve. Changing position or shifting body weight may help to alleviate the pain for a short time.

There is a difference of opinion in the medical profession as to whether SI joint injuries are a common cause of back pain. Some believe that SI joint injuries account for many cases of lower back pain because the mechanical stress of the spine converges on the SI joints. When a person flexes forward asymmetrically or rotates the body, most of the stress of supporting the motion is borne by one of the two SI joints. In a study on two hundred patients with "workmen's compensation" type of injuries of the lower back, it was found that more than 80% of the patients could localize their pain to one or both SI joints while injuries involving the spinal ligaments, muscles, iliolumbar ligaments, facet joints, ribs, or protruding disks were less common.[4]

Others believe that SI joint injuries are rarely the source of lower back pain except in unusual types of arthritis or pelvic dislocation,[11] and the reasons usually given are that SI joints form a very stable intersection, that SI joints are very well fused in adults, and that the ligaments on either side of the SI joints are among the strongest in the body. It is interesting to note that SI joint derangement does not show up on X-rays, MRIs, or electromyography (EMG).

The theoretical disagreement on SI joint etiology does not affect the good results achieved by acupuncture therapy in most patients diagnosed with SI joint problems. In the case of lower back pain, an acupuncture practitioner should carefully examine and palpate the lumbar, sacral, and iliac crest areas including the surface just on the top of the SI joints. Usually, if the SI joint area is sensitive, the iliac crest area, buttock muscles, and iliotibial band area are also sensitive and tight. In this case the acupoints H14, H15, H16, and H18 are very sensitive or even painful upon palpation because all the peripheral nerves are irritated or inflamed because of the injured SI joints. Desensitizing these nerve points reduces pain, relaxes the affected muscles, and improves regional blood supply, thus helping the recovery of the soft tissues of the SI joints.

Subluxation and Dislocation

Extended joint strain can cause a mild change in the position of the bones. Subluxation is a condition occurring when the articular surfaces of the bones inside a joint are not in perfect spatial relationship with each other. This slight misalignment of one or both bones produces pain in the joint and related soft tissues. Subluxation turns into dislocation when the bone surfaces are so far out of alignment that severe pain results.

Acupuncture needling relaxes the muscles that move the joint. The stimulation activates both the local blood circulation through the vasodilation mechanism of the autonomic nervous system and the neuroendocrine function of the central nervous system. The improved blood circulation eliminates swelling, reduces inflammation, desensitizes the irritated nerves, and alleviates the pain. Orthopedists or neurosurgeons can take care of severe dislocation, and modalities such as chiropractic, osteopathy, or physical therapy will address realignment of the subluxated bones.

Osteoarthritis

Osteoarthritis is a degenerative joint disease that can be caused by both normal and abnormal wear and tear on the joints. Consequently, there more patients who complain of pain from osteoarthritis than of pain caused by herniated disks.

Cartilage smoothly lines the surfaces of all joints and is constantly being worn away and replaced by fresh secretions. When the cartilage-producing cells of the joints are injured by normal wear and tear, their secretions form a slightly irregular surface on the joints. The progressive accumulation of such secretions results in more friction between joint surfaces and consequent damage. In more serious cases, the structural changes invade the bone and are sufficient to narrow the spinal canal (spinal stenosis) or intervertebral foramen (radiculopathy).

Patients with osteoarthritis suffer from painful and reduced motion of the arms, legs, and spine. Such sufferers experience a constant ache, which is usually worse in the morning and in the evening. As the osteoarthritis develops, the affected bones may deform, which changes the normal alignment of the joint, creating pain and tightness in the muscles that move the joint. This condition can compress the nerve roots, and the resulting pain often has a shooting or stabbing character. The neck is more prone to osteoarthritis than the rest of the back because the neck joints have greater mobility combined with weaker structural support.

Osteoarthritic pain irritates muscles and other soft tissues, resulting in tight muscles and swollen soft tissues. This process applies physical pressure on the joints and induces chemicals that irritate other joint tissues, including bone and blood vessels. Joint degeneration progresses with the resulting low blood supply, which causes an energy crisis: low nutrition and low oxygen supply, both of which are detrimental to healing. If the energy crisis persists, the affected tissues undergo constant and finally irreversible degeneration. Acupuncture relaxes tight muscles and restores blood circulation, thus ending the energy crisis. The relaxed muscles reduce the physical pressure applied on the joints and the restored blood circulation brings more nutrition and oxygen, which slows down the process of joint degeneration.

Please note that after the needles are removed, the needle-induced lesions in the muscles remain and continue to prevent the muscles from tightening, thus providing longlasting therapeutic effects. Acupuncture therapy effectively reduces muscle and joint pain as well as reducing tissue inflammation in patients with mild osteoarthritis or in the early stages of the disease.

Rheumatoid Arthritis

Current medical theory describes rheumatoid arthritis as an autoimmune disease that occurs when the body attacks the collagen in its own joint linings. This pain is accompanied by joint stiffness as well as a sporadic sensation of heat. The effectiveness of acupuncture in treating it depends on the degree and duration of the pathological condition in each patient, much as it does with osteoarthritic cases. Please note that the INMAS protocol can be successfully used for pain management regardless of the underlying cause of the pain in many cases. The success of acupuncture treatment will depend on the physiological repairability of the particular symptoms in each case combined with the ability of the body to support the self-healing process.

Acupuncture needling is helpful in treating early stages of rheumatoid arthritis by reducing swelling, inflammation, and pain, and it does so by desensitizing the peripheral nerves and improving the regional blood circulation. As the rheumatoid arthritis progresses, the efficacy of acupuncture becomes less.

GYNECOLOGICALLY RELATED LOWER BACK PAIN

Many teenage girls and adult women experience neck and lower back pain during their premenstrual (PMS) and menstrual period. Women also may experience neck and lower back pain caused by endometriosis, pelvic inflammation, or pregnancy.

PMS may be caused by a combination of psychoemotional and physiologic disturbances such as rapid hormonal changes during puberty or after a pregnancy, the discontinuation of oral contraceptives, and so on. Acupuncture is able to reduce pain related to PMS and regulate the period by affecting the neuroendocrine system. Treatment should start after ovulation and continue at a rate of two treatments per week up to the early days of the menstrual period, over 3 consecutive months. Clinical experience shows that acupuncture treatment alleviates the symptoms of PMS, and since this is a hormone-related symptom, this result is possibly due to interaction between the neural and endocrine systems.

Patients with endometriosis or pelvic inflammation also can be helped by acupuncture treatments, and its effectiveness in these cases depends on the severity of the disease and the healing potential of the body.

Acupuncture is effective in treating lower back pain caused by pregnancy. However, both classic and modern acupuncture literature warns that some acupoints like H12 superficial radial and H6 tibial may induce abortion, especially during the first 3 months of pregnancy. In China, there is a difference of opinion among medical professionals about the safety of administering acupuncture treatment to pregnant women. Experience has shown that some pregnant women are so sensitive that acupuncture stimulation to any acupoints on their bodies can induce abortion. In any event, as the average age of pregnant women increases in modern society, acupuncture practitioners should be aware of the risk of abortion when treating pain during pregnancy. The practitioner should use the least number of needles and apply very mild stimulation with short needle retention; for example, select H14, H15, H16, and H18 and retain the needles for less than 2 minutes. Continue with two treatments a week for as long as needed. Acupuncture should not be used if the patient has a history of abortion or miscarriage.

Gynecological pain can be caused by ovarian or uterine cysts. In such cases acupuncture provides only temporary pain relief and patients should be referred to a gynecologist.

NEUROPATHY, AMYOTROPHIC LATERAL SCLEROSIS, MULTIPLE SCLEROSIS

These three neurological diseases can be the cause of severe back pain.

Neuropathy

Neuropathy means that the peripheral nerve fibers and their myelinated sheaths are damaged and the nerves do not conduct any signals. Thus, patients with neuropathy lose their skin sensation and muscle strength. Neuropathy can be caused by toxic substances, diabetes, an ischemic condition, renal or thyroid diseases, or traumatic injuries. According to research conducted in China and also in our clinical experience, acupuncture can slow down the progress of neuropathy in early and mild cases but is not effective in more advanced cases, especially when the numbness has already invaded the regions above the wrist and ankle.

Amyotrophic Lateral Sclerosis (Lou Gehrig's Disease)

Amyotrophic lateral sclerosis (ALS) is a progressive neurologic disease characterized by degeneration of the cell bodies of the lower motor neurons in the gray matter of the anterior horns of the spinal cord and of the brainstem motor neurons. This condition kills motor neurons but does not affect sensation or mental capacity. Once the motor neurons die, the muscles supplied by those neurons become weak and atrophy. Lower back pain results from weakness of the muscles of the lower extremities, abdomen, and back. Although there may be periods of remission, the disease usually progresses rapidly. Acupuncture can provide different degrees of pain relief by relaxing the painful muscles and improving the blood circulation, but the efficacy is only short-term. After the muscles are deprived of their innervation of motor neurons, they gradually atrophy and the sensory nerves within the muscles become supersensitive.

Multiple Sclerosis

Multiple sclerosis (MS) is a chronic neurological disease in which sclerotic patches form in the myelin sheath of the nerves in the central nervous system (the spine and brain). The course of the disease is usually prolonged, with remissions and relapses over many years. The prevailing medical opinion is that an inherited immune response is probably responsible for the production of autoantibodies that attack the myelin sheath of the central nervous system. Patients with MS often show symptoms in two or three limbs; for example, tingling in one leg and numbness in one arm, trouble controlling bowel and bladder, dimming vision in one eye, and weakness in one leg. Acupuncture is helpful in providing temporary pain relief by relaxing muscles, improving blood circulation, and desensitizing the peripheral nerves but does not have long-term therapeutic results due to the irreversible process of the disease.

PARESTHESIAS AND NUMBNESS

Some patients with back or neck problems also have paresthesias or numbness, for example, neck pain with numbness of the fingers or back pain with paresthesia on the thigh.

Numbness is defined as diminished or absent skin sensitivity. It indicates that the nerves are no longer conducting impulses and that there is damage in the peripheral nervous system or in the central nervous system. Diabetes, a condition of too much sugar in the bloodstream, is toxic to the nerves and can cause numbness. Kidney and thyroid diseases also cause numbness. Other factors that induce numbness include autoimmune diseases and exposure to toxic substances such as heavy metals or drugs. A blow to the head can cause a concussion and result in numbness of the face. Prolonged pressure on the arm or leg will produce temporary numbness because of reduced blood circulation. Emotional tension quickens breathing and may cause numbness because of an increased ratio of oxygen in the blood.

Paresthesias are the strange sensations that some patients feel on their skin when there is no stimulation of any sort. For example, patients experience tingling, burning, tightness, pins and needles, or ants crawling on their skin without any real stimulation. Prevailing medical opinion is that abnormal, erratic firing of impulses by nerves produces paresthesias. Possibly these abnormal nerves are compressed or pinched in the spinal canal at the root level, in the plexus where the spinal nerve roots meet and regroup.

It is not uncommon for neck and/or back pain to be accompanied by numbness and paresthesias, especially among professionals who spend a lot of time in front of the computer, such as programmers. In general, acupuncture is more effective in treating pain than in treating numbness and paresthesias. Acupuncture can eliminate paresthesias and numbness in some cases if the pathological sensation is caused by peripheral conditions like tight muscles or low blood circulation. If nerve degeneration is the underlying cause, acupuncture has no effect.

OTHER UNDERLYING MEDICAL CONDITIONS CAUSING LOWER BACK PAIN

An acupuncture practitioner should understand that a small percentage of back pain is caused by underlying medical conditions such as a bone fracture, spinal tumor, spinal tuberculosis, inflammation of spinal meninges, metastatic prostate cancer, or kidney pain such as kidney stones. Patients suspected of having such complex medical conditions should be directed to a specialist for medical evaluation, although acupuncture may provide short-term pain relief.

UPPER BACK (THORACIC) PAIN

Most upper back pain is derived from pathologic conditions of the paravertebral soft tissues, the paraspinal muscles, and ligaments of the upper thorax. The thoracic paraspinal muscles are long longitudinal muscles in numerous layers. The joint facets are also involved in pain of this region.

Forceful activities such as lifting, repetitive overwork such as playing musical instruments, or prolonged sedentary work will instigate tender points because of the tightening of muscles in the upper back area.

Acupuncture is routinely effective in relaxing the tender acupoints and de-stressing the muscles. However, practitioners should be very cautious while working in this region because deep needling can cause pneumothorax. Needles always should be tilted toward the spinal cord and should not exceed 1 inch in length. To effectively and safely needle a particular tender acupoint, if the lung is below the acupoint, a practitioner can grasp and lift up the muscle while inserting the needle (Figure 9-10). The INMAS protocol for treatment of upper back pain will be provided at the end of this chapter.

SPECIAL CONSIDERATIONS IN TREATING NECK PAIN

The neck serves two basic functions: (1) as a passage for blood, nerves, food, and air; and (2) as a pedestal to support the head. The neck connects the head, trunk, and upper limbs. Many important

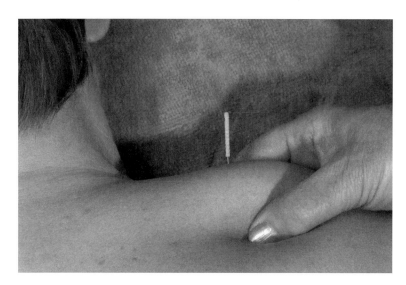

Figure 9-10   To effectively and safely deactivate a particular tender acupoint (for example, if the lung is below the acupoint), a practitioner can grasp and lift up the muscle when inserting the needle. The needle should be removed immediately.

structures are crowded in these areas. Physiological problems with the neck, including the neck pain itself, have a systemic impact on the physiology of the whole body, causing problems in the respiratory system, the cardiovascular system, the endocrine system, and the digestive system, as well as affecting activities of the autonomic and lymphatic systems. Clinical evidence shows that treating neck pain will help to improve many other pathologic conditions of the body.

It is important to note that neck pain and lower back pain symptoms are closely related and are often interconnected because functionally and anatomically the neck and lower back should be understood as a single entity and treated as such if pain occurs in either area.

About two dozen muscles in the neck and upper back support and move the neck and head. In general, the muscles in the back of the neck are responsible for bending the head backward (extension); the muscles on the sides of the neck are responsible for bending to the left or right and rotating the neck and head; and the muscles in the front are responsible for bending the head forward (flexion). The muscles between the shoulder blades (the scapulae) form a platform that supports the neck and head. These muscles have a very stressful task in supporting the weight of the head (about 10 to 15 pounds) and the frequent motion of the head (bending and rotation). Strain, fatigue, low blood circulation, inflammation, or other injuries to any of the muscles and their ligaments can cause pain.

Weakness or tightness in one or more muscle groups causes the disks and joints to support more weight than they should, which in turn may lead to chronic damage to these structures. Muscle problems can spread to the lymph nodes, joints, and disks, and vice versa. For example, an injury to the deeper structures of the neck, such as an inflamed joint or a herniated disk, causes the muscles to work harder to protect these injured structures. As a result, the muscles fatigue quickly and produce pain that is in addition to the pain from the deeper injured structures.

Due to the mobility of the neck, the joints and disks are prone to wear and tear, which may cause inflammation or even deformation of the joints. Adopting a correct neck posture, holding the head up and erect by the neck muscles, keeps the neck muscles from overworking and protects the joints and disks.

When treating neck pain, an acupuncture practitioner should carefully palpate the entire neck to find the location of the pain. Often a practitioner will not be able to identify whether the pain is caused by muscles or other structures. However, regardless of the cause, needling in the precise location will ease all of the inflammation and pain in the muscles and other structures. Manual palpation on the neck is not able to differentiate if the pain or inflammation is on the muscles, other soft tissues, or facet joints. In general, joint problems often create soft tissue inflammation and pain, and vice versa. Needling painful or tender points on the neck will improve soft tissues by relaxing the muscles and increasing blood circulation. This process reduces pressure on the neck joints due to the relaxation of the muscles, which eventually will eliminate swelling and inflammation of the soft tissues.

It is important to note that proper neck exercises following the treatments will help to strengthen the neck muscles and joint structures and to prevent a recurrence of pain.

Onset of Neck Pain

Neck pain can be triggered by whiplash from a car accident; by a sports injury such as a fall from a bicycle or being struck on the head by a football; by hitting the head on an overhang; or by a fall, and so on. The impact from these accidents applies force to the neck and injures disks or joints, which generates muscle spasms. These types of impacts may also cause traumatic close brain injury and bring changes in memory, mental processes, and mood. Mild acute neck pain may come from bad posture during work-related activities or improper sleeping position. Most of the neck pain seen in our clinic is due to cumulative trauma from frequent repetitions of the same activity or from sports or car accidents.

Degenerative diseases such as arthritis or osteoarthritis are some of the major causes of chronic neck pain in people over 40 years old.

Whiplash from car accidents is a common neck injury. Most often neck pain begins hours or days after the accident, with most pain symptoms diminishing within several weeks afterwards. However, the pain may last as long as 4 to 6 months and research studies show that about 10% to 20% of those who experience whiplash are left with some degree of chronic neck pain. Some people who have neck pain soon after an accident recover initially but develop pain symptoms 5 to 10 years later. In these cases, the accident may have caused a minor injury to a disk that appeared to have healed. The injury may cause the affected disk or joint to degenerate much faster than normal and so eventually cause pain many years later.

Some neck pain is usually not a serious medical condition by itself, but it could be a signal of a more significant problem. Since shoulder injuries can refer pain to the neck, neck pain can be indicative of shoulder injuries. Neck pain with fever can indicate an infection. Neck pain that occurs during eating may indicate problems with the esophagus. Neck pain can be caused by problems with the thyroid gland or the lymphatic nodes. A heart problem can cause referred neck pain with or without chest pressure. Neck pain accompanied by weight loss may indicate a tumor. A practitioner should be aware of these possibilities when treating neck pain.

Other symptoms associated with neck problems, especially related to untreated whiplash, include headache, nausea, vomiting, dizziness, blurry vision, pain between the shoulder blades, and numbness in the upper limbs or fingers.

In general, acupuncture needling relaxes the muscles of the neck, shoulder, and lower back. This muscle relaxation also loosens the joints of the spine, increases the blood circulation to the soft tissue and joints, reduces inflammation and swelling, and desensitizes the irritated nerves. All these processes promote self-healing of the needled regions.

Patterns of Neck Pain

The pattern of the pain may serve as a clue to the nature of the pain and helps to predict the result of the treatment. Here we list a few pain patterns from our clinical experience.

Tenderness usually comes from muscles, joints, or both. A disk tear or herniation may compress the nerve root and cause severe neck and/or arm pain. If pain is worse after prolonged periods of reading, writing, or computer work, it is possible that a disk is damaged. Pain that is made worse by looking upward may be originating from an inflamed facet joint. It is common for pain from disks or facet joints to be referred (i.e., experienced in a different region, such as the shoulder blades, the upper arm, the base of the skull, or the head).

The pain pattern and/or level of pain may reveal the location of the injured joints and may help in determining the location of the SAs to be used in addition to the HAs. Pain in the upper neck and the occipital area is usually related to C2-C3. Pain in the upper neck and the levator scapulae muscle may originate from C3-C4. Pain in the lower neck and upper part of the shoulder may radiate from the joints of C4-C5. Pain to the lower neck and the supraspinatus area may originate from the joints of C5-C6. Pain in the sizeable area over the blade of the scapula may be caused by the joints of C6-C7.

In general, pain in the back of the neck is caused by injured disks, joints, muscles, or other soft tissues. Pain in the front of the neck may be due to a medical problem such as an infection in the lymph nodes, thyroid gland, or salivary gland. Persistent pain in the front of the neck, especially if associated with fever, difficulty swallowing, or weight loss, requires consultation with a physician.

A detailed evaluation is required in cases where pain has persisted for more than 3 or 4 months.

Whiplash

The leading source of trauma in developed countries is automotive accidents. Most of these create some degree of whiplash, so it is not surprising that whiplash has become a common cause of neck and lower back pain. The mechanics of whiplash are clearly understood but the extent and type of injuries vary greatly. All whiplash victims should seek early treatment regardless of whether or not they experience pain immediately following the accident because, as discussed above, a whiplash injury that is not painful after the accident may cause pain as much as 5 to 10 years later. If early treatment is provided, acupuncture can effectively reduce most whiplash pain, and it will also activate the recovery of most soft tissue injuries, as well as improving other related symptoms such as arm or lower back pain or numbness, dizziness, and nausea. The efficacy of acupuncture decreases proportionally as the treatment is delayed because in time the tissue damage invades deeper tissues and structures.

Whiplash injuries to the neck, especially after a rear-end collision, are caused by a combination of factors such as the sudden forced neck extension (backward), compression (upward), shearing (forward), recoiling, and possibly some lateral forces. During a rear-end collision, the force of impact pushes the torso forward and upward while throwing the head and neck backward (extension), all within one-tenth of a second. The upward movement of the torso compresses the cervical region from below and the backward movement of the head narrows the space between the cervical vertebrae and compresses the facet joints. Approximately six-hundredths of a second later, the neck begins to move forward, which produces a shearing action and reduces the front intervertebral space, thereby pressing the front edge of the disks. After the initial backward-forward motion, the head recoils backward. These combined movements apply great pressure on the facet joints and disks, resulting in immediate or potential injuries. For example, if the weight of the whiplash victim's head is 10 pounds, the impact force on the neck can be as high as 170 pounds even in a low-speed rear-end collision. Due to the shape of the neck, the region from C5 to C7 suffers most from the strongest impact force and the region from C1 to C3 absorbs the remainder of the impact force.

During a rear-end collision some lateral neck flexion may occur with a slight rotation. This lateral force causes compression of the ipsilateral facet joints and distraction of the contralateral facet joints. Thus, the ipsilateral joints and disk can be damaged, while the joint capsules of contralateral joints sustain strain or enormous stress. In severe cases, possible fracture of the odontoid process and fractures of the laminar and superior process can occur and CT scanning is needed to confirm these injuries.

Most people with whiplash begin to have pain within 24 hours of the accident but often the pain begins later. Immediately following the accident, the body activates the hormonal mechanism that releases endorphins and adrenaline to help the body manage stress. This physiologic process suppresses the sensation of pain from the injury. A few days later, the hormone level drops, the injured structures become gradually inflamed, and the suppressed pain is liberated and increases over time. Acupuncture treatments immediately following the accident effectively reduce pain and inflammation. After the accident, it may take hours or days to develop the symptoms, but if acupuncture treatments are applied before the symptoms become severe or uncontrollable, the recovery will be easier, faster, and more complete. The needling provides better blood circulation to the injured tissues and introduces an antiinflammatory reaction, which prevent more severe or chronic consequence from the injuries.

All whiplash injures involve damage to some or all tissues in the neck and back area such as muscles, nerves, ligaments (soft tissues), facet joints, and disks. Acupuncture is effective in treating most whiplash symptoms. The INMAS protocol provides adequate treatment to both the neck and other parts of the body like the shoulder and lower back. Soft tissue injuries should heal within at most 1 to 4 months. If there is still pain after acupuncture therapy, it is usually due to injuries to facet joints or disks, or both. In these cases, additional evaluation is required.

If whiplash results in injury to cervical soft tissue, the direct consequence is sustained, continuous neck pain. Other complaints that may result from whiplash include headache, neck stiffness, and restriction of movement. The headache is typically at the occipital or temporal region, which is innervated by nerve roots from C1 to C3. A headache also can result from a concussion or from an injury to the lateral atlantoaxial joint. If there are injuries to the upper cervical facet joints of disks, the headache is usually located at the base or the top of the skull, the forehead, or the face and jaw.

Pain caused by whiplash-related injuries may radiate to the shoulders, arms, and the area between the shoulder blades. Pain in the shoulder, between the shoulder blades, or in the arms can be referred from the neck nerves or facet joints. Numbness, tingling, or heaviness in the arm and/or hand, especially in the ring and little fingers, are common symptoms. Lower back pain is also among the common complaints.

Some whiplash patients experience sleep disturbances, fatigue, dizziness, vomiting, ringing in the ears, or visual disturbances. Dizziness may be caused by inner ear disequilibrium or damage to the cervical musculature. About one-third of whiplash patients have shown deficits in concentration or problems with memory. Changes in personality are also observed in some patients who become irritable, depressed, or short-tempered because of neck pain.

If a whiplash patient has a history of neck pain, arthritis in the neck, or headaches prior to the accident, the whiplash may have caused more severe injuries to the neck structure, creating a higher risk that the patient will develop chronic neck pain months or years later.

Acupuncture therapy can effectively improve the majority of the physical symptoms associated with whiplash. In our clinic we have achieved very good results in whiplash patients with severe chronic neck pain, even where some of the patients were involved in several whiplash accidents. With the INMAS protocol, the neck and the whole muscular system receive appropriate treatment and the healing is optimal. However, mental or psychological symptoms associated with whiplash, such as personality changes, require longer treatments and multidisciplinary approaches because one modality will not solve all the complex problems involved.

NECK AND LOWER BACK PAIN CAUSED BY SPORTS AND RECREATIONAL ACTIVITIES

Most pain resulting from sports and recreational activities is associated with musculoskeletal problems. In order to successfully treat and prevent sport-related injuries, it is very important for a practitioner to understand the mechanism of such injuries.

The majority of pain from sports is due to bad body posture (bad mechanics), overused muscles, or insufficient time to warm-up the muscles before exercise. Whenever pain occurs, patients should first check their posture (mechanics). A detailed description of good mechanics is beyond the scope of this book. However, if muscle or tendon pain is felt during an exercise, the exercise should be discontinued or modified. For example, if a runner feels pain during running, he or she should stop running but may resume walking. Immediate treatment should be sought, accompanied by short-term

rest (1 to 3 days, for example). If a person who feels pain continues to exercise, whether with or without pain medication, he or she is taking the risk of permanently damaging the affected muscles or tendons.

There are several mistakes that should be avoided. One common mistake is relying solely on pain medication. Muscle or tendon pain is usually a warning signal of potential or existing damage. The pain sensation can be immediately stopped or suppressed by pain medication but the damage needs time to be repaired and the recovery of muscular functions requires an even longer time. Pain medication can neither repair the damage nor recover the function. Another common mistake seen in our clinic is that when people feel pain during exercise, they continue to stretch the muscles and tendons, trying to help the muscles. The majority of muscle and tendon pain during exercise is caused by overstretching, and so continued stretching will make the injured tissue worse.

Our clinical experience shows that it is important to start acupuncture treatment immediately in cases where pain occurs during exercise, regardless of the cause of pain. Slight or mild pain can be relieved within 1 to 3 days and swelling or inflammation can be drastically reduced within 3 to 7 days. Recovering the function of the muscle or tendon requires a longer time, about 5 to 10 days. Usually we recommend that after the first acupuncture treatment the patient should rest for 2 days and then resume mild exercise if he or she does not feel pain while doing so. Patients should not resume their regular exercise routines until after recovery is complete, otherwise the pain will quickly return.

Prevention is the best strategy. This may include many procedures such as scientific planning of training, nutrition, and warming-up exercises. Regular acupuncture treatment is also an important preventive measure. No matter how carefully the training is planned and how successfully an athlete maintains good biomechanics, repetitive motions always tighten the muscles, which puts stress on the tendons and disturbs the coordination of different muscle groups. The INMAS protocol provides a way of comprehensively examining injured muscles: the 24 HAs are the road map to find the affected areas and tender points in the major muscles. Relaxing the tightened muscles before exercise will reduce the risk of muscle and tendon tear.

Bicycling

Bicyclists may suffer neck and lower back pain; wrist pain; hamstring muscle pain from road vibrations;

strain and fatigue of the muscles in the back of the neck, shoulders, and between the shoulder blades; and strain and fatigue of the lumbar muscles and leg muscles. They also may suffer from the consequences of poor body and/or head position, such as excessive extension or flexion of the neck and flattening of the lower back lordosis. All of the above may also result if the bicycle is not properly adjusted to the height of the user.

Running

The majority of runners have a flexible and relaxed neck but get lower back and leg problems. Their necks are in good condition possibly because they maintain a good neck posture and make little neck motion while running. The leg muscles, however, are subject to repetitive overuse injuries. If some muscles, like hamstring muscles, become tight or are injured, they are able to restrict or change the movement of the pelvis, which creates stress on the lower back muscles. Frequent acupuncture treatment will relax the tight lower back and lower limb muscles and increase blood supply to them. If the muscles are kept healthy, flexible and not tight, well-supplied with nutrition, and strong, there will be fewer problems during and after exercise.

Tennis

Tennis players are prone to several injuries. The forearm flexor muscles of tennis players are frequently stressed, which causes tennis elbow. Also, the need to look up and rotate the head rapidly can cause problems in the facets of the neck spine. A practitioner should carefully check the neck of a tennis player and needle the tender muscles and joints.

Swimming

When in the water, a swimmer's neck does not bear the weight of the head but the head needs to be frequently rotated so the neck is routinely extended or flexed, which may cause neck strain or sprain. A practitioner should regularly check the neck of a swimmer and needle the sore neck muscles.

Golf

Golfers face many physiomechanical problems. A survey published in the June 2003 issue of the *American Journal of Sports Medicine* provides useful data regarding golf-related injuries.

Researchers surveyed 703 golfers (643 amateurs and 60 professionals) from 24 golf courses in Germany during two golfing seasons. They found that more than 80% of reported golf injuries were due to overuse. Golfer's elbow was the most common overuse injury among amateur golfers, followed by back and shoulder pain. Professional golfers had more injuries in the back, wrist, and shoulder. There were also occasional reports of sprained ankles. The research showed that professional golfers suffer an average three injuries a year compared with an average of two injuries per year among amateurs.

The research further showed that players who warmed up for 10 minutes or less had an average of about one injury per player compared with an average of only about 0.4 injuries per player for those who warmed up for more than 10 minutes.

Overall, the golfers surveyed lost about 4 weeks of golfing time per injury, although a significant number had injuries that kept them from playing for up to 6 months. Our clinical experience shows that regular acupuncture treatments can reduce the likelihood of golf-related injuries and that acupuncture treatments that are received immediately after the injury can allow golfers to return back to the green much earlier.

When examining the ball and determining their swing, golfers often adopt a posture where the waist is bent and the neck is flexed, which can strain the neck muscles. The backswing, which requires rotating the shoulders and flexing the neck, also strains the neck and lower back spine.

When treating a golfer, a practitioner should always carefully examine the neck, shoulders, elbows, upper back, and lower back, and identify and needle all the tender points.

LOWER BACK PAIN OCCURRING IN THE WORKPLACE

Most lower back pain occurring in the workplace involves muscular overexertion injuries, with asymmetric bending and twisting motions being the predominant cause. Most of these lower back pains are injuries of the soft tissues, especially the back muscles. Acupuncture needling is very effective in treating soft tissue injuries because needling is able to relax the tight muscles and the vasoconstriction, restoring blood circulation and activating antiinflammatory reactions. Early treatment before the symptoms invade other regions usually provides faster and more complete recovery.

NEEDLING SAFETY IN TREATING NECK AND LOWER BACK PAIN

Needling safety is an important aspect of the clinical procedure to which acupuncture practitioners should always pay attention. When treating neck, upper back, and lower back problems, a practitioner should understand the anatomic configuration at the needle sites. Practitioners should always remember that under no circumstances should they forcefully push the needles into the hardening tissues of the neck, upper back, and lower back ligaments unless they know that it is absolutely safe to do so, as it is, for example, in the case of sacral ligaments.

The Neck

The neck spine has seven vertebrae. Palpation of this part of the spine is very important for finding needling locations. In adults there is often a light hollow posterior to the C1 vertebra (atlas) that does not have a spinous process. When needling this area, a practitioner should stop inserting the needle when resistance is felt.

However, the tip of the transverse process of C1 (atlas) can be felt 1 cm anteroinferior to the tip of the mastoid process (Figure 9-11). A practitioner should first find this point and then ask the patient to rotate the head slowly from side to side, which movement allows the practitioner to feel the transverse process of C1. If a neck injury patient feels a tender sensation during palpation of this region, the transverse process of C1 should be needled all the way to touch the bone.

C2 has a longer spinous process than C3, C4, and C5 and can be palpated with little pressure. The spinous processes of C3-C5 are short, lie deep to the surface, and are difficult to feel. The spinous process of C7 is more prominent than that of C6 (Figure 9-12) but both spinous processes are easily palpable when a patient's neck is flexed as far as possible.

It is important for acupuncture practitioners to understand that the transverse processes of the neck vertebrae divide the neck into anterior and posterior parts. The anterior part of the neck contains many important organs and neurovascular structures, and therefore deep needling should be avoided. If needling is necessary when treating skin problems such as neurodermatitis, fine needles of 1.5 cm in length can be used in this area.

The posterior part of the neck is responsible mostly for extension and side rotation. The back muscles must be sufficiently strong to perform such motions. The back muscles (extensors) sustain more stress than the front muscles when the cervical curve is not properly maintained, such as when working on computers, or overextended, as when looking upward. As the stress accumulates, the back muscles are subject to tightness, spasm, inflammation, strain, or sprain, and these may lead

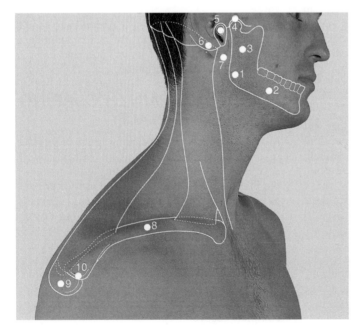

Figure 9-11   Lateral aspect of the neck: bones. *1,* Angle of mandible. *2,* Body of mandible. *3,* Ramus of mandible. *4,* Temporomandibular joint. *5,* External acoustic meatus. *6,* Mastoid process. *7,* Tip of transverse process of atlas. *8,* Clavicle. *9,* Acromion. *10,* Acromioclavicular joint. (From Lumley J: *Surface anatomy: the anatomical basis of clinical examination,* ed 3, Edinburgh, 2002, Churchill Livingstone.)

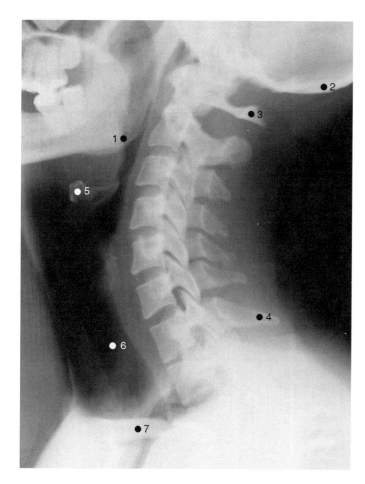

Figure 9-12   Lateral view of the cervical spine. *1*, Angle of mandible. *2*, Occipital bone. *3*, Posterior arch of atlas. *4*, Spine of seventh cervical vertebra. *5*, Hyoid bone. *6*, Tracheal gas shadow. *7*, Clavicle. (From Lumley J: *Surface anatomy: the anatomical basis of clinical examination*, ed 3, Edinburgh, 2002, Churchill Livingstone.)

to reduced blood circulation and hypoxia in the muscles.

The needles are inserted from the back, tilting to the midline or toward the lamina or the transverse process, all the way to the bones. In treating joint problems, needles have to touch the joint coverings. Depending on the patient's body size, the needling depth is from 2.5 cm to 5 cm. As noted above, the needles can be inserted all the way from the skin surface to the bone surface.

The sternocleidomastoid muscle should be mentioned. This broad straplike muscle divides the neck into anterior and posterior triangles and is one of the most used and stressed muscles in the neck. Contrary to expectation, however, this muscle does not often contribute to pain or stiffness in the neck. Superficial to the sternocleidomastoid muscle, the external jugular vein descends obliquely across about half way along the anterior border of this muscle. Deep and close to the anterior border of the muscle there are neurovascular structures, including the vagus nerve, the common carotid artery

(which is divided into the internal and external carotid artery), and the internal jugular vein and its tributaries.

If the sternocleidomustoid muscle needs needling, the upper third can be needled with needles of 2.5 cm in length, whereas fine needles of 1.5 cm in length are suitable for the lower two thirds of the muscle. Be mindful that the apex of the lung is just behind the lowest part of these muscles (see below). Avoid needling the external jugular vein and the apex of the lung. Injury to the external jugular vein, especially in the lower part of the muscle, may cause air to be sucked into the vein during inspiration and leads to venous air embolism, which may result in dyspnea (shortness of breath).

The Back

The importance of understanding the anatomy of the back cannot be overemphasized. *All acupuncture practitioners should have a solid working knowledge of the anatomy of the back.* The back is the most important part of the body in acupuncture medicine. The spinal cord sends its peripheral nerves to all organs through structures related to the back. Sensory nerve roots and autonomic ganglions are located close to the back. Acupoints in the back are used to treat almost all the symptoms that are treated by acupuncture.

Avoiding Puncturing the Lungs (Pneumothorax)

Most accidents occurring from acupuncture needling are related to pneumothorax. If a needle punctures the pleural cavity when needling the anterior, lateral, or posterior surfaces of the thorax, air may be sucked into and accumulate in the pleural cavity after the needle is removed. Special attention should be paid to patients who are long-time smokers, who are extremely thin, or who have scoliosis. These patients have weaker and thinner back muscles or weaker lungs and are more prone to pneumothorax.

Figure 9-13 shows the outline of the pleura and lungs, as viewed from the back during gentle respiration. Viewed from the back, the apices of the lung are close to the transverse processes of T1. However, if observed from the front, the apices of the lung project superiorly through the thoracic inlet into the neck posterior to the sternocleidomastoid muscle. Practitioners should be very careful when working in the area just above the medial part of the clavicle bone and should use fine needles of 1.5 cm in length. Deep needling also should be avoided when needling acupoint H3 spinal accessory on the top of the shoulder because the apices of the lung are close to the base of the neck; a needle of 2.5 cm in length suffices in most cases. When deeper needling is needed such as when a nodule is detected in deep tissue, a practitioner can grasp and lift the trapezius muscle so as not to puncture the apex of the lung below (see Figure 9-10).

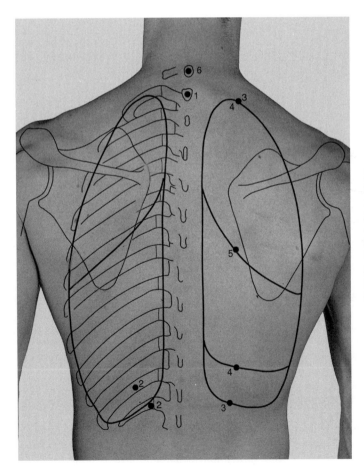

Figure 9-13   Surface markings of the lungs and the pleura: posterior view. *1,* Spine of first thoracic vertebra. *2,* Floating ribs. *3,* Pleural markings. *4,* Lung markings. *5,* Oblique fissure. *6,* Vertebra prominens. (Modified from Lumley J: *Surface anatomy: the anatomical basis of clinical examination,* ed 3, Edinburgh, 2002, Churchill Livingstone.)

Three parameters are critical when using paravertebral acupoints (PAs) in the thoracic area (T1-T12) shown in Figure 9-13: (1) the direction of the needle; (2) a safe distance from the needling point to the midline of the spine; and (3) the depth of needling.

Figure 9-14 shows the transverse section of the lung at the T3 level. To avoid puncturing the pleural cavity, it is safer to tilt the tip of needle toward the body of the vertebra (toward the midline). T3 and the base of the spine of the scapula (medial angle) are at the same level. The safe distance at the T3 level can be determined by first palpating the medial angle of the scapula and then locating the tip of the spinal process of T3. The medial one third of the distance between the medial angle and the spinal process of T3 is the safe distance for needling. Needling at a distance farther from the midline runs the risk of puncturing the pleural cavity. The depth of needling depends on the physical size of a patient's body. For the sake of safety, it is best to needle at a depth of 2.5 to 3.0 cm for an average-sized person. If a patient is suffering from neuralgia or herpes simplex/zoster, fine needles of 1.5 cm in length should be used.

Avoiding Puncturing the Kidneys

Another pair of organs that acupuncture practitioners must take care not to puncture when needling the lower back area are the kidneys. Clear knowledge of surface anatomic markings on the back is necessary to avoid such an accident. The same three parameters are critical when needling in this region: (1) the direction of the needle; (2) a safe distance from the acupoint to the midline of the spine; and (3) the depth of needling.

The kidneys are two bean-shaped organs lying on each side of the vertebral column. The position of the kidneys varies somewhat with posture, body build, and respiration. Each kidney may move vertically about 3 cm when the diaphragm moves during deep breathing. In the prone position, the superior poles of the kidneys are protected by the 11th and 12th ribs (Figure 9-15), while the inferior poles extend to the level of L3 for the right kidney and a little lower than that for the left kidney due to bulky liver lobes. With respect to the midline, the superior poles are in the epigastrium, each 2.5 cm from the midline, while the inferior poles are 7.5 cm from the midline, slightly above the supracristal plane. The right kidney is about a fingerbreadth superior to the crest of the ilium. Based on the above anatomic description and on our clinical experience, the safe needling distance at the L1 level is about 2.5 cm (about 1 inch) from the midline.

The important acupoint H15 is located on the lateral border of the erector spinae at the L2 level. The cross section at this level (Figure 9-16) shows that the distance between the body surface and the posterior surfaces of the kidneys is about one fifth to one sixth of the posterior-anterior body axis at the L2-umbilicus level. It is possible that the usual prone position for needling the low back may shorten this posterior-anterior body axis.

Based on the above information about the topography of the kidneys, it is best to use needles

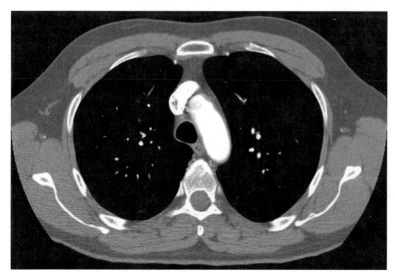

Figure 9-14 Axial CT image at the level of the 3rd thoracic vertebra showing the topography and thickness of the back wall for avoiding needling into the lungs. (From Weir J, Abrahams P: *Imaging atlas of human anatomy*, ed 3, Edinburgh, 2003, Mosby.)

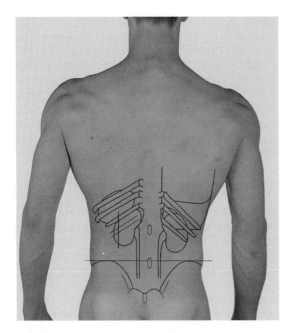

Figure 9-15 Surface anatomical positions of the kidneys. (Modified from Lumley J: *Surface anatomy: the anatomical basis of clinical examination,* ed 3, Edinburgh, 2002, Churchill Livingstone.)

of 4 cm in length for acupoints at L1 levels and to use needles of 5 cm in length for acupoints from the L2 to L5 levels. If the selected acupoints are situated on the ridge of the erector spinae muscles,

the needle should be positioned perpendicular to the muscle surface. If the selected acupoints are located on the lateral border of the erector spinae muscle, the needle is tilted toward the midline.

TREATMENT PROTOCOL OF BACK PAIN (FOR BOTH THE NECK AND LOWER BACK)

When treating the back, a practitioner must first perform a thorough manual examination (palpation) of all the HAs in the neck, upper back, lower back, shoulders, and lower limbs and then identify the SAs to be needled. As noted earlier in this chapter, this is due to the inseparable anatomic and functional relationship between the neck, upper back, and lower back and the referred relationship between the neck and the shoulders and between the lower back and the lower limbs. The procedures for manual examination and acupoint prescription are described below.

Please note that PAs become SAs when treating neck and back problems.

Neck Pain and Upper Back Pain

1. *Examination*

Palpate the following HAs to locate the directly injured area, which will be unique to each patient:

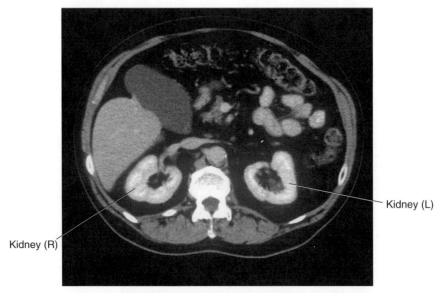

Figure 9-16 Transverse CT image at the level of L2 shows the topography of the kidneys. (From Gosling J, Harris P, Whitmore I, Willan P: *Human anatomy: color atlas and text,* ed 4, Edinburgh, 2002, Mosby.)

Neck: H2 great auricular, H7
                          greater occipital
Shoulder: H3 spinal accessory, H13
                          dorsal scapular
                      H8 suprascapular
Upper back: H20 spinous process of T7, H21
                          posterior cutaneous of T6
Lower back: H14 superior cluneal, H15
                          posterior cutaneous of L2
                      H16 inferior gluteal, H22
                          posterior cutaneous of L5
                      H18 iliotibial

2. *Identify the related SAs.* In the majority of patients with neck pain, the most sensitive HAs are usually H7, H3, and H13. Thus, palpate for SAs around these three HAs. To identify the most sensitive locations, manually examine around these three HAs the skin, muscles, and bones on the back (spinous processes from C2 to C7); the sides of the neck; the upper part of the back; and the shoulders. The most sensitive locations are the SAs. It is very common that the side(s) of the neck is more sensitive than H7 itself.

   Spinous processes from T7 to T1 and the paravertebral area from T7 to T1 also should be manually examined to find possible SAs.

3. *Prescription*
   a. HAs
      H2, H7, H3, H13, H8, H20, H21, H15, H22, H14, H16
   b. SAs
      SAs can be selected on the neck area (Figure 9-17), and around H3.
   c. PAs (paravertebral points)
      Along the cervical spine (C1-C7) and thoracic spine (T1-T7) (Figure 9-18). Some neck pain is caused by upper back pain, so the upper back area should be carefully palpated.

4. *Needling depth*
   a. On the back and sides of the neck (posterior to the transverse processes of the cervical vertebrae), needles can be inserted all the way to the bone. Needles of 4 to 5 cm in length are suitable. The anterior halves of the side of the neck should be avoided or needled only with short needles such as 1.5 cm in length.
   b. On the shoulder area around H3 and paravertebral points from T1 to T7, it is best to use needles of 2.5 cm in length to avoid puncturing the lung. Tilt the

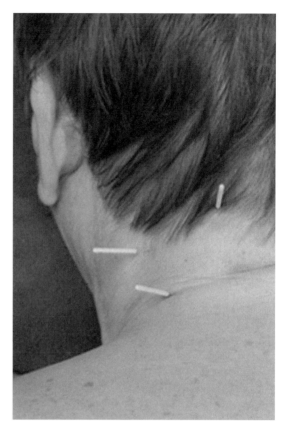

Figure 9-17 Needling the symptomatic acupoints (SAs) on the sides of the neck (posterior to the transverse processes of the cervical vertebrae) for neck pain. Note the right needle is the location of H7 greater occipital. The length of the needles is 4 cm to 5 cm (1½ to 2 inches).

needles toward the spine (midline) when needling the PAs.

Upper Back Pain

1. *Examination*
   To find tender points manually examine: (1) the posterior spinous processes of the spine from C2 to T7 (remember C1 has no spinous process); (2) the paraspinal muscles; and (3) especially the muscles between the thoracic spine and the scapula. Some upper back pain is related to shoulder problems, the treatment protocol for which is discussed in the next chapter.
2. *Prescription*
   a. HAs
      H20, H21, H13, H3, H8

b. SAs

In this case, PAs become SAs. For example, patients with upper back pain, colds, or respiratory problems such as asthma may have tender points along spine T1-T7.

These points serve as both PAs and SAs (Figure 9-18).

3. *Needling depth*

All of the HAs and PAs can be needled safely with needles of 2.5 cm in length. Tender points along the medial margin of the scapula are needled with needles of 1.5 cm in length. When tender points are located deeper along the medial margin of the scapula, a practitioner may grasp and lift the muscle before inserting the needle in order to avoid puncturing the lung and still be able to dissolve deep tender points.

Lower Back Pain

1. *Examination*

Manual examination should be performed from the neck to the leg to understand the location(s) of the pain symptom because lower back pain has very individualized underlying causes.

On the neck and upper back, palpate the area around H7, H3, and H13; and the spinous processes from C2 to T12, including the paravertebral area. On the lower back, we suggest the following procedure:

a. Palpate the spinous processes and the paravertebral area from L1 to the coccyx, paying close attention to L2, L4, L5 and S1-S4.

b. Carefully palpate H15 and the area covered by the latissimus dorsi muscle from the 10th rib to the iliac crest to check for tender points in this area.

c. Palpate H14 and H16 and the area between these two acupoints, including the fascia over the gluteus medius muscle; the gluteus maximus muscle; the tensor fasciae latae muscle on the lateral side of the hip; and the area of the gluteal fold between the gluteus maximus and the hamstring muscles.

d. Examine both lower limbs. Palpate H18 and the iliotibial tract. Palpate the hamstring muscles, especially along the pathway of the sciatic nerve. Palpate H11, both lateral and medial, on the popliteal fossa. Palpate H10, and the two bellies of the gastrocnemius muscle.

The most sensitive or painful area(s) that are identified by carefully performing the examination described above will be the location of the SAs.

2. *Prescription*

a. HAs:

Neck:	H7,
Shoulder:	H3, H13, H8
Upper back:	H20, H21
Low back:	H15, H22, H14, H16
Low limb:	H18, H11, H10

b. SAs:

SAs are located at the most sensitive or painful area(s) found in the above

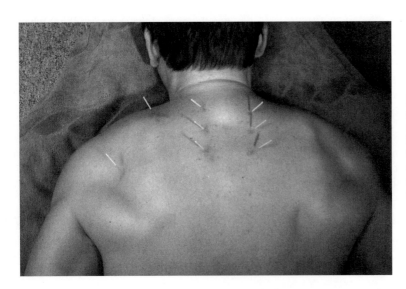

Figure 9-18 Paravertebral acupoints (PAs) from T1 to T4 and shoulder acupoint H8 infraspinatus (at the center of the infrascapular fossa). The other two needles are symptomatic acupoints (SAs) for shoulder pain.

neck-to-leg examination. If the neck is sensitive, one or two SAs can be selected in the neck. In the lower back, usually one of these five areas is sensitive:

1) The area between H15 and H22
2) The area around the sacroiliac (SI) joints
3) The area between H14 and H16
4) The tensor fascia latae muscle and the iliotibial (IT) band
5) The hamstring and the gastrocnemius muscles

   Figure 9-19 shows the standard treatment for lower back pain.

3. *Needling depth*

   Neck: 3-5 cm for H7 and SAs on the back and sides (posterior to the transverse processes of the cervical vertebrae) of the neck

   Shoulder: 2.5 cm for H3 and H13. H8 can be needled all the way to the scapula.

   Upper back: 2.5 cm for H20 and H21.

   Low back: 4 cm for H15. 5 cm for H14 and H22. More than 7 cm for H16.

   Low limb: 2-5 cm, depending on the thickness of the muscle.

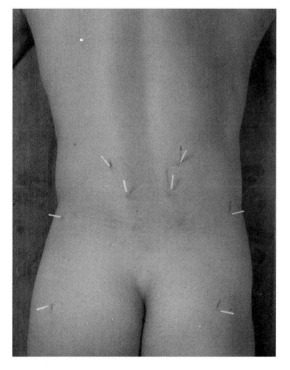

Figure 9-19 Use low back homeostatic acupoints (HAs) H15, H22, H14, and H16 (from lumbar region to buttock).

COCCYGODYNIA (COCCYALGIA, COCCYDYNIA)

Coccygodynia is pain in the coccyx and neighboring regions. Usually this pain is caused by falling down on the back or on the buttocks in the course of playing sports or other routine activities. The effectiveness of acupuncture therapy in reducing the pain depends on the nature of the injury or trauma to the coccyx bone. If there is no bone fracture or only a minor fracture, needling can effectively reduce inflammation, swelling, and pain.

Patients with coccygodynia usually will also have pain in the sacral area. Examination and treatment procedures for coccygodynia are exactly the same as for lower back pain, except that palpation for tender and painful points (in order to locate the SAs) is in the coccygeal area.

INFECTIOUS AND NEOPLASTIC DISEASES THAT CAUSE LOWER BACK PAIN

In a few cases, lower back pain is caused by metastatic conditions, multiple myeloma, and other primary spinal tumors. Some lower back pain is related to infectious diseases such as epidural abscess, vertebral osteomyelitis, or Pott's disease (tuberculosis of the spine, where the vertebral bone is infected by *Mycobacterium tuberculosis*). Depending on the stage of the disease and the patient's condition, acupuncture therapy may be an effective supplementary modality for pain relief.

REFERRED CAUSES OF BACK PAIN

In a few patients lower back pain is caused by diseased internal organs. These pathological conditions include:

Gastrointestinal origin:	Perforated internal organs
Biliary origin:	Obstructed bile duct, distended gallbladder
Pancreatic origin:	Pancreatitis, pancreatic carcinoma
Renal origin:	Kidney stones, urethral stones, pyelonephritis, renal carcinoma, bladder carcinoma
Vascular origin:	Abdominal aortic aneurysm, arterial occlusive diseases

Acupuncture can help patients who suffer lower back pain that is referred from a diseased organ, if it is used as a supplementary therapy.

SUMMARY

Back pain and neck pain are the most common complaints of acupuncture patients. Both classic and modern literature, as well as our clinical experience, show that acupuncture therapy can successfully help more than 90% of these patients, if treatments are properly administered by practitioners.

Pain in the lower back and neck, and sometimes in the upper and lower limbs, are closely related to each other. Therefore, all of these areas should be manually examined and treated together.

Acupuncture practitioners need to know each patient's medical history and the nature of the pain in order to determine whether acupuncture should be used as a primary or a supplementary therapy.

The treatment protocols for back pain, neck pain, and pain referred to or from these regions prescribe largely the same HAs but different local SAs. In patients with neck pain, the SAs are located in the back or sides of the neck and in the upper part of the shoulder. In patients with upper back pain, the SAs are located in the upper back area. In patients with lower back pain, the SAs are located in the low back area, the sacrococcygeal area, the gluteal area, the thigh, or the leg.

Please note that some back pain originates from shortened muscles in the front of the body such as chest or abdominal muscles. These muscles should be examined and treated if needed.

The efficacy of acupuncture therapy will depend on the severity or chronicity of the disease, the self-healing potential of the patient, and the practitioner's skill in administering the treatment.

References

1. Loeser JD, editor: *Bonica's management of pain,* ed 3, Philadelphia, 2001, Lippincott Williams & Wilkins, p 1475.
2. Fishman L, Ardman C: *Back pain: how to relieve low back pain and sciatica,* New York, 1999, WW Norton, p 13.
3. Schofferman J: *What to do for a pain in the neck,* New York, 2001, Fireside, p 15.
4. Ivker RS.: *Backache survival: the holistic medical treatment program for low back pain,* New York, 2003, Jeremy P. Tarcher/Putnam, p 25.
5. Spratt KF, Lehmann TR, Weinstein JW, et al: A new approach to low-back examination: behavioral assessment of mechanical signs, *Spine* 15:96-102, 1990.
6. Gunn CC: *Treating myofascial pain: intramuscular stimulation (IMS) for myofascial syndromes of neuropathic origin,* HSCER, Seattle, 1989, University of Washington.
7. Arnoldi CC, Brodsky AE, Cauchoix J, et al: Lumbar spinal stenosis and nerve root entrapment syndromes: definition and classification, *Clin Orthop* 115:4-5, 1976.
8. Eklund JA, Corlett EN: Shrinkage as a measure of the effect of load on the spine, *Spine* 9:189, 1984.
9. Ahn H, Cho Y-W, Ahn M-W, et al: mRNA expression of cytokines and chemokines in herniated lumbar intervertebral discs, *Spine* 27:9:911-917, 2002.
10. Vertosick FT Jr, *Why we hurt? The natural history of pain,* San Diego, 2000, Harcourt, p 95.
11. Fishman S, Berger L: *The war on pain,* New York, 2001, Quill, p 139.
12. Rosse C, Gaddum-Rosse P: *Hollinshead's textbook of anatomy,* ed 5, Philadelphia, 1997, Lippincott-Raven, p 611.

CHAPTER 10

Upper Limb Pain: Shoulder, Elbow, Wrist, and Hand

INTRODUCTION

Musculoskeletal disorders of the upper limb are among the most common causes of pain and disability. In our clinic, the percentage of patients presenting with shoulder and elbow pain is exceeded only by patients with lower back or neck pain. Acupuncture treatments can achieve very good therapeutic results for pain caused by anything from rotator cuff tears to peritendinitis of the forearm.

As always, the success of acupuncture treatments depends on a practitioner's knowledge of the anatomic structure of the region and on his or her understanding of the pathologic nature of the pain. Thus, this chapter first describes the anatomy, physiology, and biomechanics of the upper limb specifically as these concepts relate to acupuncture therapy, and then we will present the most common disorders of the upper limb. Finally, the chapter introduces a standardized but individually adjustable protocol for treating musculoskeletal upper limb pain.

The upper limb is the organ for manual activity. It consists of the following anatomic parts: the shoulder, junction of the arm and trunk; the arm (brachium) between the shoulder and elbow; the forearm (antebrachium) between the elbow and the wrist; the wrist (carpus) between the forearm and hand; and the hand. In contrast to the lower limb, the upper limb is freely movable and does not bear weight. Since the upper limb is built for mobility, it does not have a bony junction with the vertebral column. Thus, its stability is compromised to gain mobility.

Clinically, pains in the shoulder, elbow, wrist, hand, and even neck are anatomically related and pathologically interrelated. In acupuncture therapy, all of these regions should be examined and treated together even if the patient complains of only local pain.

Most shoulder and elbow pains are caused by soft tissue disorders. In our computer-oriented cul-

ture wrist pain is becoming more prevalent. Common causes of shoulder and elbow pain include degeneration, injuries from sports and daily activities, inflammation, and referred pain from a distant site. Other pathologic conditions such as vascular diseases and tumors may cause shoulder and elbow pain. The reason for the relatively high incidence of shoulder pain is that the stability and smooth motion of the shoulder depend on the integrated function of numerous elements: muscles, ligaments, tendons, and the eight joints involved. The shoulder is not just a single joint but a complex group of articulation, and pain may involve one or more elements of the shoulder complex.

Elbow pain occurs less frequently than shoulder pain, but it is becoming something of an epidemic among computer users and some professional and amateur athletes. Some sports, such as tennis and golf, are likely to cause elbow pain. Like the shoulder, a well-functioning elbow requires stability, strength, and smooth motion. A healthy elbow allows movement of the forearm and enables the hands to be positioned at a desired location. Stiffness, instability, or weakness of the elbow produces pain in use. Common extraarticular problems that cause elbow pain are lateral (tennis elbow), medial (golfer's elbow), epicondylitis, neuropathy of the ulna, and olecranon bursitis. Intraarticular disorders such as arthritis or osteochondritis happen less often.

The wrist and hand are the de facto working units of the upper limb. The shoulder, upper arm, elbow, and forearm form a multijointed lever to place the wrist and hand in an appropriate working position. The hand with its pincer-like thumb serves for grasping and fine manipulation with exquisite sensation and delicate discrimination. The function of the hand is controlled by the brain. The physical activities that the wrist and hand are made to perform render these working units susceptible to accidental injuries and inflammation caused by wear and tear, and most of these injuries may produce pain. The fingers (the digits) are the most mobile parts of the body. The delicate and complex structures of the wrist and hand make recovery of function through acupuncture more difficult than in other parts of the body. However, good results can still be achieved with early treatment.

BASIC ANATOMY OF THE UPPER LIMB AS IT RELATES TO ACUPUNCTURE THERAPY

Anatomic knowledge of bones, nerves, muscles, and major blood vessels is critical to successful acupuncture treatment. However, a detailed anatomic description of the upper limb is beyond the scope of this chapter. This chapter focuses only on the bones, muscles, and nerves that are specifically related to acupuncture practice.

The Bones of the Upper Limb

The bones comprising the upper limb include the clavicle (collar bone) and scapula (shoulder blade) in the pectoral girdle; the humerus in the arm; the radius and ulna in the forearm; the eight carpal bones in the wrist; the five metacarpal bones in the hand; and the 14 phalanges in the fingers (digits) (Figure 10-1).

The Brachial Plexus

The brachial plexus is a complex of nerves serving the upper limb, which provides the following physiologic functions:

1. Sensory information from the skin, the muscles, and deep structures such as the joints
2. Motor control of the muscles

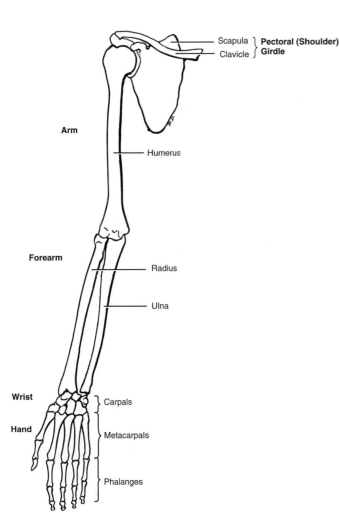

Figure 10-1   The bones of the right upper limb. (From Jenkins D: *Hollinshead's functional anatomy of the limbs and back,* ed 8, Philadelphia, 2002, WB Saunders, p 65.)

3. Influence over the diameter of blood vessels regulated by the sympathetic vasomotor nerves
4. Sympathetic secretomotor supply to the sweat glands

At the root of the neck, the five anterior rami of the spinal nerves from C5 to C8 and T1 unite to form the brachial plexus in the posterior triangle of the neck. (Remember there are seven cervical spinal vertebrae and eight cervical spinal nerves because spinal nerves C1 and C2 originate from the superior and inferior sides of C1, respectively.) The union of the five anterior rami and the rearrangement of the five cervical spinal nerves allow the nerve fibers derived from different segments of the spinal cord to be arranged and distributed efficiently in different nerve trunks to the various parts of the upper limb. The plexus can be divided into roots, trunks, divisions, and cords (Figure 10-2).

The brachial plexus divides its nerves into supraclavicular branches and infraclavicular branches. Supraclavicular branches arise from the rami and trunks of the brachial plexus and are distributed in the posterior triangle of the neck and above the level of the clavicle. Infraclavicular branches arise from the cords of the brachial plexus and are distributed through the axilla (armpit) from where they are distributed to the arm.

Supraclavicular Branches of the Brachial Plexus   Supraclavicular branches include the following nerves and the following major muscles and joints that they innervate:

- Dorsal scapular nerve (C5): scalenus medius, levator scapulae, and rhomboids Acupoint H13 is formed on the levator scapulae muscle
- Long thoracic nerve (C5 to C7): scalenus medius, serratus anterior

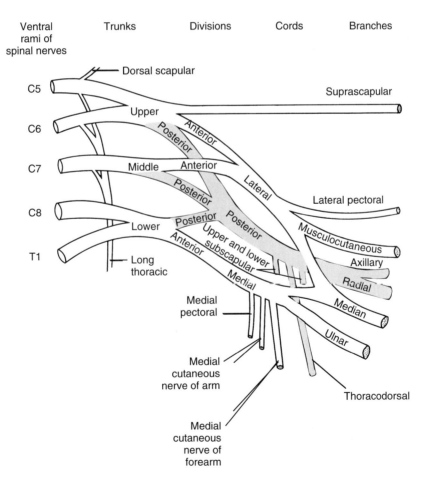

Figure 10-2   Diagram of the brachial plexus. (From Jenkins D: *Hollinshead's functional anatomy of the limbs and back,* ed 8, Philadelphia, 2002, WB Saunders, p 80.)

- Nerve to the subclavius (C5)
- Suprascapular nerve (C5 and C6): supraspinatus, infraspinatus, and the shoulder joint. Acupoint H8 is formed on the infraspinatus muscle.

Infraclavicular Branches of the Brachial Plexus   The lateral cord of the brachial plexus includes three branches:

- Lateral pectoral nerve (C5 to C7): pectoralis major. Acupoint H17 lateral pectoral is formed where the nerve enters the muscle

- Musculocutaneous nerve (C5 to C7): The muscles of the anterior aspects of the arm. This nerve continues in the arm to supply the biceps brachii and the brachialis muscles (Figure 10-3). Just proximal to the elbow joint, this nerve penetrates the deep fascia and becomes a superficial nerve named the lateral antebrachial cutaneous nerve; at this point acupoint H9 lateral antebrachial cutaneous is formed
- Lateral root of the median nerve: This nerve is the continuation of the lateral cord of the brachial plexus. It is joined by the medial root of the median nerve to form the median nerve

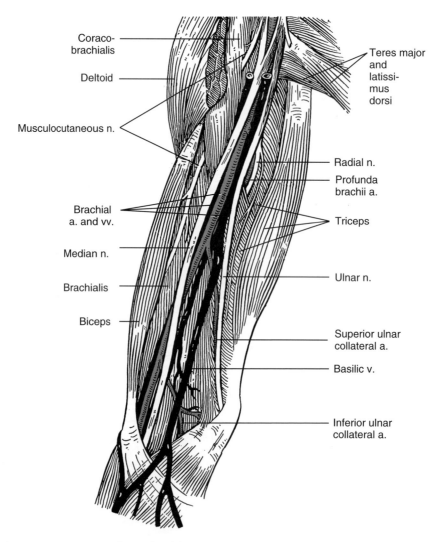

Figure 10-3   Nerves and vessels of the arm. Pay attention to the musculocutaneous nerve. (From Jenkins D: *Hollinshead's functional anatomy of the limbs and back,* ed 8, Philadelphia, 2002, WB Saunders, p 125.)

The medial cord of the brachial plexus includes five branches:

- Medial pectoral nerve (C8 and T1): pectoralis minor and part of pectoralis major
- Medial brachial cutaneous nerve (C8 and T1): the skin over the medial surface of the arm and the proximal part of the forearm
- Medial antebrachial cutaneous nerve (C8 and T1): the skin over the medial surface of the forearm
- Ulnar nerve (C8 and T1): this nerve does not give branches in the axilla and passes through the arm into the forearm and hand. As it enters the forearm from behind the medial epicondyle, it supplies the flexor carpi ulnaris; the medial half of the smallest muscles of the flexor digitorum profundus; and the skin on the ulnar side of the hand. The muscular and cutaneous supply of the ulnar nerve is summarized in Table 10-1
- Medial root of the median nerve: the medial root joins with the lateral root to form the median nerve (Table 10-2), which supplies all the flexor muscles in the forearm (except

the flexor carpi ulnaris) and the skin on the lateral half of the palm. In the palm, the median nerve supplies the muscles of the thenar eminence and the first two lumbricals. The cutaneous branches of the median nerve provide sensory information from the skin on the palmar aspect of the lateral (radial) three fingers and radial half of the ring fingers

The posterior cord of the brachial plexus includes five branches:

- Upper subscapular nerve (C5 and C6): subscapularis
- Thoracodorsal nerve (C6, C7 and C8): latissimus dorsi
- Lower subscapular nerve (C5 and C6): subscapularis and teres major
- Axillary nerve (C5 and C6): this nerve winds around the surgical neck of the humerus to supply the teres minor and deltoid muscles
- Radial nerve (C5 to C8 and T1): this is the major nerve that supplies the extensor muscles of the upper limb and carries sensory information from the skin of the extensor

Table 10-1
A Summary of Main Innervation of the Ulnar Nerve (C8 and T1)

Upper Arm	Forearm	Hand

Elbow joint	Flexor carpi ulnaris
	Flexor digitorum profundus (median half)
	Ulnar artery
	Palmar cutaneous branch
	Posterior cutaneous branch
	Wrist joint
		Muscles of hypothenar eminence
		Adductor pollicis 3rd and 4th lumbricals
		Interossei joints of hand
		Palmaris brevis
		Palmar digital branches to medial
		  1½ fingers
		Skin of medial side of dorsum of hand and
		  medial 1½ fingers

Table 10-2
A Summary of the Main Innervation of the Median Nerves (C5, C6, C7, C8, T1)

Upper Arm	Forearm	Hand
Brachial artery Elbow joint	Pronator teres Flexor carpi radialis Palmaris longus Flexor digitorum superficialis Flexor pollicis longus Flexor digitorum profundus (lateral half) Pronator quadratus	Wrist joint Palmar cutaneous branch Three thenar muscles First two lumbricals Palmar digital branches to lateral 3½ fingers

region, including the hand. After leaving the axilla, the radial nerve runs backward, downward, and laterally between the long and medial heads of the triceps, supplying branches to this muscle. Then it passes through the radial groove in the humerus and enters the forearm where it divides into two branches: the deep and the superficial radial nerves. The radial nerve gives off branches to the anconeus, brachioradialis, and extensor muscles (Table 10-3). An important acupoint H1 deep radial is formed when the deep radial nerve pierces the deep fascia between the brachioradialis and extensor carpi radialis longus. After leaving the radial nerve the superficial nerve runs under the brachioradialis muscle and emerges to the surface at the distal portion of the radius bone. This nerve gives branches as it approaches the web between the thumb and the index finger where an acupoint H12 superficial radial is formed

An understanding of the origin, pathways, and connections of the major nerves is critically necessary for acupuncture practitioners to achieve the desired therapeutic results. This knowledge provides the physiologic and pathologic basis for understanding the nature of a patient's injury and how the pain should be treated.

Sympathetic Supply of the Upper Limb

The brachial plexus supplies the cutaneous and muscular nerves of the upper limb (Table 10-4). The cutaneous nerves are responsible for skin sensations such as touch, pressure, pain, heat, cold, or chemical irritation. The muscular nerves control muscle movement, coordinated muscular contraction, and relaxation.

In addition to the cutaneous and muscular nerves mentioned above, the autonomic nervous system is also important for acupuncture therapy. We have discussed the anatomy of the autonomic nervous system in Chapters 1 and 2. Its purpose is to regulate physiologic functions and it consists of two subdivisions, sympathetic and parasympathetic. The sympathetic system activates emergency or survival-oriented physiologic reactions that include constriction of blood vessels (vasoconstriction) in the skin; sweating; contraction of arrector pili muscles (gooseflesh of the skin); increasing the rate and force of the heart beat (increasing blood supply to the muscles for physical activity); constriction of the sphincters of hollow viscera such as stomach and bladder; and relaxation of the muscles inside the visceral wall, such as bronchi (for more oxygen) and stomach (to reduce digestive activity). All these sympathetic functions are activated when survival appears to be threatened. This process is energy consuming and physiologically stressful, which explains why people are usually exhausted after such emergency or survival reactions.

The parasympathetic nervous system physiologically balances the sympathetic nervous system. The effects of the parasympathetic nervous system include dilation of blood vessels in the skin (vasodilation), reduced rate and force of the heart beat, increased digestive activity (absorption of nutrition), immune reaction (reduction of inflammation), and promotion of tissue healing.

The central autonomic neurons are located in the spinal cord. These neurons send nerve fibers

Table 10-3 A Summary of the Main Innervation of the Radial Nerves (C5, C6, C7, C8, T1)	
Upper Arm	**Forearm**
Lower lateral cutaneous nerve of arm	Posterior cutaneous nerve of forearm
Triceps (three heads)	Extensor carpi radialis brevis
Brachialis (small part)	Supinator
Brachioradialis	Extensor digitorum
Extensor carpi radialis longus	Extensor digiti minimi
Elbow joint	Extensor carpi ulnaris
	Abductor pollicis longus
	Extensor pollicis longus
	Extensor pollicis brevis
	Extensor indicis
	Skin of lateral side of dorsum of hand and lateral 3½ fingers.

Table 10-4 A Summary of the Main Innervation of the Musculocutaneous Nerve (C5, C6, C7)		
Axilla	**Upper Arm**	**Forearm**
Coracobrachialis	Biceps Brachialis (greater part) Elbow joint	Lateral cutaneous nerve of forearm

(preganglionic fibers) to the autonomic ganglia outside the spinal cord. The preganglionic fibers communicate (via synapses) with ganglionic neurons. The ganglionic neurons send their nerve fibers (the postganglionic fibers) to blood vessels, glands, and organs.

The preganglionic fibers for the upper limb originate from the upper segments (T2-T6) of the spinal cord. These preganglionic fibers ascend in the sympathetic chain to join each root of the brachial plexus. Thus, every cutaneous or muscular nerve in the upper limb also contains autonomic postganglionic nerve fibers. The sympathetic nerves innervate blood vessels, sweat glands, and arrector pili muscles in the skin.

When any sensory nerve fibers are needled, the autonomic postganglionic fibers are also stimulated. In general, this stimulation increases the activity of the parasympathetic nervous system, which reduces the activity of the sympathetic nervous system. This explains why needling acupoints in the upper limb can improve pathologic symptoms of the lung, heart, and stomach, such as reducing nausea, vomiting, and the rate of heart beat (even tachycardia), as well as relieving shallow breathing or some allergic symptoms.

ANATOMY OF THE SHOULDER

Anatomically, the shoulder is the junction of the arm and the trunk. Two bones, the clavicle (the collar bone) and the scapula (the shoulder blade), form the structure of the pectoral girdle and connect the humerus and the whole upper limb to the axial skeleton (the bones of the trunk and head) (see Figure 10-1). A number of joints are formed between the girdle bones and the axial skeleton.

This chapter discusses only those shoulder joints or articular interfaces that are significant in the treatment of shoulder pain: glenohumeral, acromioclavicular, claviculosternal, bicipitalhumeral, and scapulocostal.

Glenohumeral Joint

Motion of the arm requires action at all joints of the shoulder complex. The glenohumeral joint has more freedom of motion than any other joint in the body. Therefore this joint is the most important member of the shoulder complex, as well as the most frequent site of pain and impairment. This synovial joint has an incongruous ball-and-socket articulation. The articulation is made up of the large head of the humerus and the small and shallow glenoid fossa. Rather than merely rotating

about a fixed axis, the head of the humerus also slides against the glenoid articulation surface (Figure 10-4). This intrinsic weakness of the joint makes it susceptible to degenerative changes and derangement and also renders the stability of the joint dependent on the supporting soft tissues.

The concave pear-shaped glenoid fossa is located at the lateral tip of the scapula (see Figure 10-4), which allows little close contact of the two articular surfaces. The shallow glenoid fossa is deepened by a lip, the glenoid labrum, surrounding the fossa. The glenohumeral capsule is attached to the lip. The glenohumeral articulation is a multiaxial ball-and-socket joint that allows movement in three axes.

The head of the humerus is larger than the socket of the scapula by approximately a factor of four. When the arm hangs down naturally at the side, the head of the humerus is held in the glenoid fossa against the force of gravity predominantly by the supraspinatus muscle and by the superior aspect of the capsule. The supraspinatus muscle originating within the supraspinatus fossa of the scapula attaches to the greater tuberosity of the humerus. Thus, it is always necessary to manually palpate the supraspinatus muscle and its attachment on the tuberosity of the humerus when treating shoulder pain.

Four scapular muscles—supraspinatus, infraspinatus, teres minor, and subscapularis—form a musculotendinous rotator cuff to protect the glenohumeral joint and provide for its stability (Tables 10-5 and 10-6). All these rotator cuff muscles, except the supraspinatus, rotate the head of the humerus within the glenoid fossa. The tendons of these four muscles join the articular capsule of the glenohumeral joint and form a mass of tendons fused with the lateral part of the capsule. All the rotator cuff and deltoid muscles and their attachments to the head of the humerus should be carefully palpated and needled for any kind of shoulder disorder.

The *capsule* of the joint is thick and strong but lax, especially inferiorly, so as to allow a greater range of motion. Glenohumeral motion will be restricted if pathologic conditions such as inflammation, contracture, or fibrosis occur in the capsule. Acupuncture needling reduces inflammation and relaxes the contracture of the capsule, but is not helpful in cases of fibrosis.

A *bursa* is a flattened sac filled with a lubricant called synovial fluid that enables the two flattened walls of the sac to slide freely over each other. The bursa eliminates the friction that would arise wherever a muscle or tendon could rub against another muscle, tendon, or bone. There are several bursae

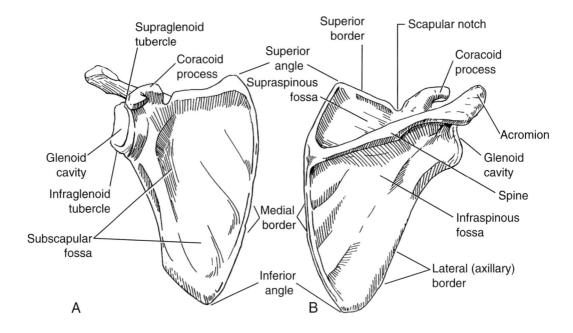

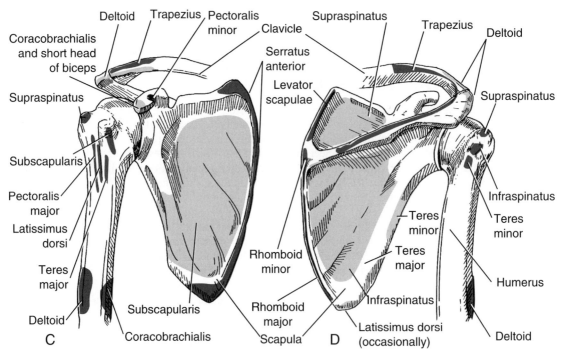

Figure 10-4   The bones of the shoulder joint. Anterior (**A** and **C**) and posterior (**B** and **D**) views of the scapula. Origins of the muscle are gray and insertions are dark. (From Jenkins D: *Hollinshead's functional anatomy of the limbs and back,* ed 8, Philadelphia, 2002, WB Saunders, p 73.)

Table 10-5
Rotator Cuff Muscles

Muscle	Origin	Insertion	Action	Innervation
Supraspinatus	Supraspinous fossa of scapula	Greater tubercle of humerus	Abduction of arm	Suprascapular nerve
Infraspinatus	Infraspinous fossa of scapula	Greater tubercle of humerus below supraspinatus	Lateral rotation of arm	Suprascapular nerve
Teres minor	Upper ⅔ of lateral border of scapula	Greater tubercle of humerus below infraspinatus	Lateral rotation of arm	Axillary nerve
Subscapularis	Subscapular fossa of scapula	Lesser tubercle and crest of humerus	Medial rotation of arm	Upper and lower subscapular nerves

Table 10-6
Prime Movers of the Glenohumeral Joint

Flexion	Deltoid (anterior fibers), pectoralis major (clavicular fibers)
Extension	Deltoid (posterior fibers), latissimus dorsi
Adduction	Pectoralis major, latissimus dorsi, teres major, subscapularis
Abduction	Deltoid, supraspinatus
Internal rotation	Pectoralis major, latissimus dorsi, teres major, subscapularis
External rotation	Deltoid (posterior fibers), infraspinatus, teres minor

specifically associated with the glenohumeral joint (Figure 10-5). The important ones are the subacromial and subdeltoid bursae. These bursae separate the supraspinatus tendon and the head of the humerus from the acromion and the deltoid muscle. Frequently bursitis, the inflammation of the bursae, may occur with shoulder pain. Acupuncture needling is very effective in reducing bursitis. However, needling efficacy is slower if the walls of the bursa adhere to each other (adhesive bursitis).

If a patient is diagnosed with adhesive bursitis, acupuncture needling is still recommended as a noninvasive therapy while the patient is seeking other medical modalities to alleviate the condition.

Acromioclavicular Joint

The acromioclavicular (AC) joint is a plane (flat) synarthrodial joint. It consists of the small convex facet on the lateral end of the clavicle and a small

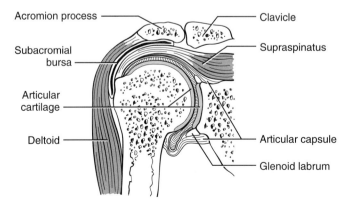

Figure 10-5   Subacromial bursa of the shoulder joint. (From Jenkins D: *Hollinshead's functional anatomy of the limbs and back,* ed 8, Philadelphia, 2002, WB Saunders, p 96.)

concave facet on the acromion of the scapula. This configuration allows rotation. The two bones are joined by fibrous tissue that gradually degenerates and forms a meniscus between them. The AC joint itself is not strong enough to hold the two bones together and is reinforced by the coracoclavicular ligament. This ligament consists of two smaller ligaments: the quadrangular trapezoid ligament and the cone-shaped conoid ligament. These two ligaments prevent separation of the clavicle and scapula. The primary function of the AC joint is to maintain coordination between the clavicle and the scapula during movements of the shoulder (Figure 10-6).

Trauma may tear the fibers of the AC joint, resulting in instability of the joint during shoulder movement. When examining patients with shoulder pain, it is necessary to palpate the area of the AC joint to find local pain or tenderness. Acupuncture needling reduces pain and inflammation, but if dislocation or subluxation is suspected, patients should be referred for further medical evaluation and treatment.

Sternoclavicular Joint

This joint is the only bony articulation between the upper limb and the axial skeleton. The sternoclavicular (SC) joint is formed by the articulation of the sternal end of the clavicle with the flat fossa of the clavicular notch on the superior lateral margin of the sternum and the cartilage of the first rib. A small articular disk is present between these bones with strong ligamentous support (Figure 10-7). The comparatively large sternal end of the clavicle rotates and forms the lateral boundary of the jugular notch. The SC joint allows the clavicle and shoulder to move up and down, forward and backward, or any combination of these movements.

The fibrous capsule of the SC joint is a key structure in supporting the weight of the entire upper limb. The SC joint is well supported and protected by anterior and posterior SC ligaments. The two clavicles are also joined to each other by an interclavicular ligament. Together these ligaments prevent the lateral and upward dislocation of the clavicle. The joint is further strengthened by

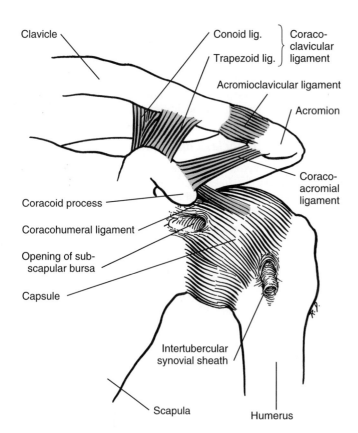

Figure 10-6   The acromioclavicular joint. The joint is covered by the acromioclavicular ligament. (From Jenkins D: *Hollinshead's functional anatomy of the limbs and back,* ed 8, Philadelphia, 2002, WB Saunders, p 75.)

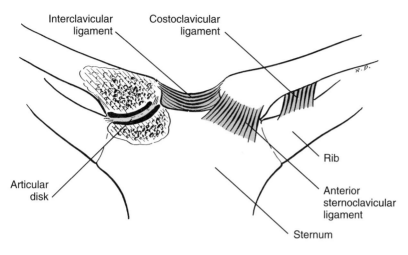

Figure 10-7   The sternoclavicular joint and associated ligaments. The left joint has been sectioned to expose the articular disk. (From Jenkins D: *Hollinshead's functional anatomy of the limbs and back,* ed 8, Philadelphia, 2002, WB Saunders, p 74.)

the costoclavicular ligament that connects the first rib and the inferior surface of the clavicle.

When treating shoulder pain, it is necessary to carefully palpate the SC joint area to find localized pain and tenderness. This area is very close to the lung so practitioners should pay special attention to the direction and depth of needling. It is advisable to use only 1.5 cm needles in this region and to insert needles into the fibrous tissue to reduce pain and inflammation.

Scapulothoracic Joint

The scapulothoracic (ST) joint is not a true anatomic joint but a functional "joint" that maintains a direct relationship between the scapula and the thorax as the scapula slides over the ribs. The movement of the scapula is coordinated with the AC and SC joints.

In a neutral position, the scapula rests on the posterior thorax approximately 5 cm from the midline, between the 2nd through the 7th ribs. From this reference position, the scapula can have movements of elevation-depression (raising or depressing the shoulder), abduction-adduction (away from or toward the midline), and upward-downward rotation (raising the arm over the head or using the hand to touch the lower back). This ST joint is stabilized by the adjacent AC and SC joints and muscles that attach to both the thorax and scapula. Muscle pain associated with scapular movement is a common symptom encountered in most patients.

Acupuncture practitioners should understand the position of the scapula during its movement for three reasons: (1) to identify the painful muscles associated with the scapula, (2) to palpate the acu-

point H8 infrascapularis, which is located at the center of the infrascapular fossa of the scapula, and (3) to ensure safe needling on the thorax when the scapula changes its position.

Many patients complain of pain in the area between the upper spine and the medial border of the scapula. Our clinical experience indicates that about 70% of the patients have pain or tenderness in the levator scapulae, rhomboideus minor and major muscles, especially the parts of these muscles that are close to the medial border of the scapula. When administering acupuncture treatment, we use the following methods to avoid puncturing the lung: (1) use 1.5 cm long needles, (2) grasp and lift up the muscle for deeper needling, or (3) put the patient's forearm on the back to raise the medial border of the scapula and then tilt and insert 4 cm needles to the attachment area of these muscles (see Figure 10-30).

Bicipital-humeral Joint

The bicipital-humeral "joint," like the scapulothoracic joint mentioned above, is also a nonanatomic but functional joint. It is an important area in the treatment of shoulder pain.

The biceps brachii muscle, as its name implies, has two heads, the long and the short (Figure 10-8). Here we focus on the tendon of the long head because it is frequently a source of shoulder pain. The long head has a long tendon that traverses the intertubercular groove on the humerus bone, passes through the glenohumeral jont, and finally attaches to the top of the glenohumeral joint (the supraglenoid tubercle).

Patients with shoulder pain always complain of tenderness or pain at this bicipital-humeral "joint"

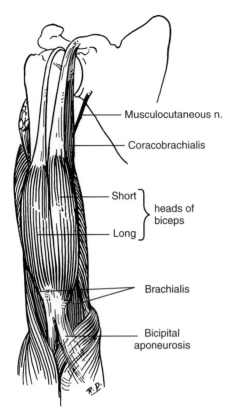

- Musculocutaneous n.

- Coracobrachialis

- Short ⎫
  ⎬ heads of
  ⎭ biceps
- Long ⎭

- Brachialis

- Bicipital aponeurosis

Figure 10-8   The biceps brachii muscle. (From Jenkins D: *Hollinshead's functional anatomy of the limbs and back,* ed 8, Philadelphia, 2002, WB Saunders, p 121.)

upon palpation. Thus, this area contains symptomatic acupoints for treating shoulder pain by acupuncture needling.

MOVEMENTS OF THE SHOULDER

Understanding the movement mechanism of the shoulder joint is necessary for knowing how and where to find symptomatic acupoints to treat shoulder pain. The movements of the shoulder are actually movements between the humerus and the scapula. Muscles, nerves, tendons, bursae, capsules, and articular surfaces of the joints are the elements involved in these highly coordinated movements (Table 10-7), and a disturbance in any of these elements may interrupt their coordination and result in shoulder pain. Knowing how patients move their shoulders greatly helps the practitioner to provide successful treatment.

Here we briefly discuss the major movements of the shoulder and the muscles involved. Shoulder movement involves two components of the glenohumeral joint, the scapula and the humerus. *Scapular movements* consist of elevation, depression, upward rotation, downward rotation, protraction, and retraction (Table 10-8). *Humeral movements* include flexion, extension, abduction, adduction, and internal (medial) and external (lateral) rotation. Any one muscle may perform more than one movement in coordination with other muscles.

Table 10-7 Nerves and Their Innervation to the Shoulder Muscles			
Nerves	**Origin**	**Muscle**	**Main Action**
Accessory	Cranial	Sternocleidomastoid	Lateral flexion and rotation of head
		Trapezius	Elevation of scapula
Nerves to levator scapulae	C3, C4	Levator scapulae	Elevation of scapula
Dorsal scapular	C5	Both rhomboidei	Retraction of scapula
Nerve to subclavius	C5, C6	Subclavius	Depression of clavicle
Axillary	C5, C6	Teres minor	External rotation of arm
		Deltoid	Abduction of arm
Subscapular	C5, C6	Subscapularis	Internal rotation of arm
Suprascapular	C5, C6	Supraspinatus	Abduction of arm
		Infraspinatus	External rotation of arm
Long thoracic	C5, C6, C7	Serratus anterior	Upward rotation of scapula
Lateral pectoral	C5, C6, C7	Upper pectoralis major	Adduction-flexion of arm
Medial pectoral	C8, T1	Lower pectoralis major	Adduction-extension of a flexed arm
		Pectoralis minor	Depression of shoulder
Thoracodorsal	C6, C7, C8	Latissimus dorsi	Extension-adduction of arm

Table 10-8 Prime Movers of the Scapula	
Elevation	Trapezius (upper fibers), rhomboids, levator scapulae
Depression	Latissimus dorsi, pectoralis major (costal fibers), trapezius (lower fibers)
Upward rotation	Trapezius, serratus anterior
Downward rotation	Rhomboids
Protraction	Serratus anterior, pectoralis major and minor
Retraction	Trapezius, rhomboids
Internal rotation	Subscapularis, pectoralis major, latissimus dorsi, teres major deltoid (clavicular fibers)
External rotation	Infraspinatus, teres minor, deltoid (posterior fibers)

Scapular Movements

Elevation of the scapula is produced by four muscles (Figure 10-9). The medial border of the scapula is elevated by three muscles, the levator scapulae and the rhomboideus minor and major. The lateral angle of the scapula is changed by the upper fibers of the trapezius connected to the clavicle, acromion, and spine of the scapula. Often we examine patients with one shoulder higher than the other because of the tightness of these four muscles. The shoulder level returns to normal after proper needling of these muscles.

Muscles involved in *depression* of the scapula include the pectoralis minor and major, subclavius, latissimus dorsi, lower fibers of the trapezius, and serratus anterior (Figure 10-10). In some patients with upper or lower back pain, one shoulder is lower than the other and needling both the lower back muscles and the depressor muscles returns the shoulder to normal level.

When abduction occurs, such as when raising an arm, the scapula rotates upward. Upward rotation is brought about by the combined action of the trapezius and the serratus anterior (Figure 10-11). When reaching down to pick up something from the floor, the scapula rotates downward. Downward rotation is carried out by the combined action of raising the medial border and lowering the lateral angle of the scapula. The levator scapulae and both rhomboids are responsible for raising the medial border, while the pectoralis major and minor and latissimus dorsi, aided by gravity on the free limb, are responsible for lowering the lateral angle of the scapula (Figure 10-12).

The pectoralis major, minor, and serratus anterior bring about protraction (Figure 10-13), while the middle fibers of the trapezius carry out retraction (Figure 10-14).

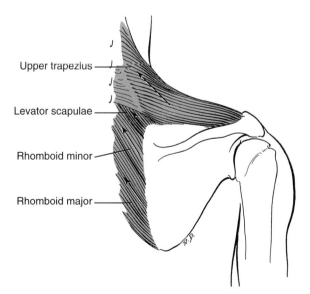

Upper trapezius

Levator scapulae

Rhomboid minor

Rhomboid major

Figure 10-9 Elevators of the scapula. (From Jenkins D: *Hollinshead's functional anatomy of the limbs and back,* ed 8, Philadelphia, 2002, WB Saunders, p 98.)

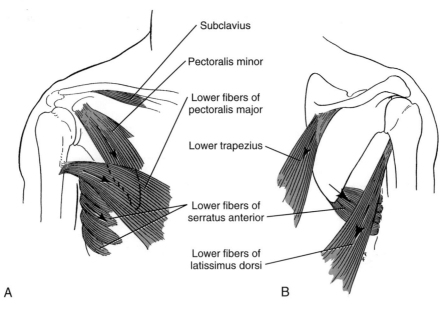

Figure 10-10   Depressors of the scapula. **A,** Anterior view. **B,** Posterior view. (From Jenkins D: *Hollinshead's functional anatomy of the limbs and back,* ed 8, Philadelphia, 2002, WB Saunders, p 99.)

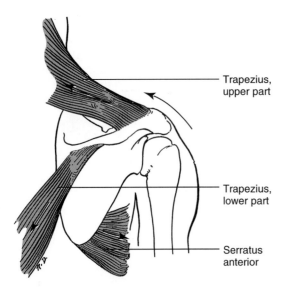

Figure 10-11   Upward rotators of the scapula. (From Jenkins D: *Hollinshead's functional anatomy of the limbs and back,* ed 8, Philadelphia, 2002, WB Saunders, p 99.)

Humeral Movements

Coordinated action of the anterior portion of the deltoid, the clavicular portion of the pectoralis major, the coracobrachialis, and the biceps brachii brings about the flexion of the arm at the shoulder joint. The posterior fibers of the deltoid, the latissimus dorsi, the sternocostal fibers of the pectoralis major, the teres major, and the long head of the biceps brachii are responsible for extension of the arm.

Abduction of the arm is carried out by the deltoid, especially its lateral part and the supraspinatus, while adduction of the arm is carried out by the pectoralis major, teres major, and latissimus dorsi, which are to a small extent assisted by the coracobrachialis and the long head of the triceps brachii.

Internal (medial) rotation is brought about primarily by subscapularis. Other internal rotators include pectoralis major, latissimus dorsi, teres major, and clavicular fibers of the deltoid. External (lateral) rotation is performed by infraspinatus and teres minor, and also by the posterior fibers of the deltoid if extension and lateral rotation are combined. Figure 10-15 explains the topographic relationship between the internal and external rotators of the humerus.

SHOULDER PAINS AND THEIR LOCATIONS

The shoulder is a complex joint and its pathologic conditions are correspondingly complex. The following locations provide very good guidelines for examining and locating symptomatic acupoints when treating different types of shoulder pain.

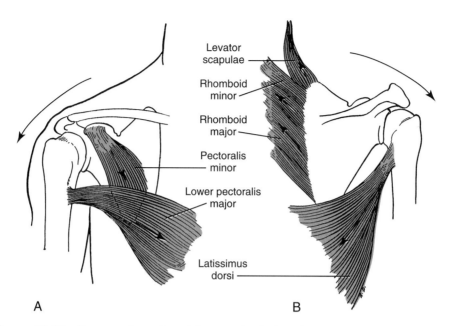

Figure 10-12   Downward rotation of the scapula. **A,** Anterior view. **B,** Posterior view. (From Jenkins D: *Hollinshead's functional anatomy of the limbs and back,* ed 8, Philadelphia, 2002, WB Saunders, p 100.)

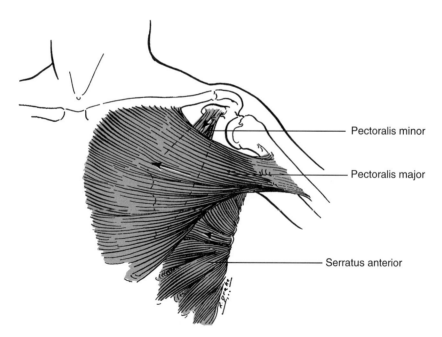

Figure 10-13   Protractors of the scapula. (From Jenkins D: *Hollinshead's functional anatomy of the limbs and back,* ed 8, Philadelphia, 2002, WB Saunders, p 100.)

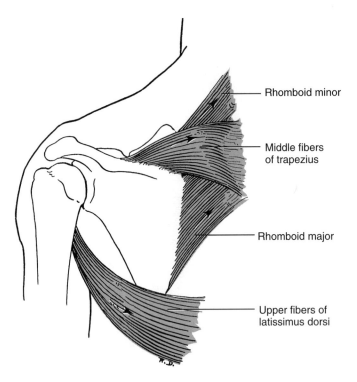

Figure 10-14 Retractors of the scapula. (From Jenkins D: *Hollinshead's functional anatomy of the limbs and back,* ed 8, Philadelphia, 2002, WB Saunders, p 101.)

MEDIAL
ROTATORS

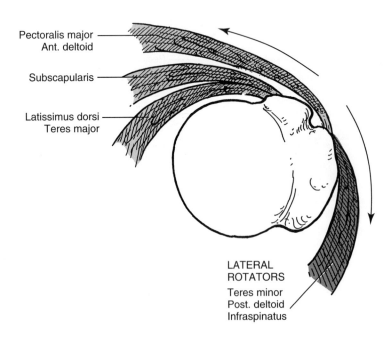

Figure 10-15 Medial rotators and lateral rotators of the humerus. Superior view of the right arm. (From Jenkins D: *Hollinshead's functional anatomy of the limbs and back,* ed 8, Philadelphia, 2002, WB Saunders, p 105.)

Subacromial Space

The subacromial space can be affected with rotator cuff tendinitis, calcific tendinitis, impingement syndrome, and rotator cuff tear.

Bicipital Groove

The bicipital groove can be involved in bicipital tendinitis and biceps tendon subluxation and tear.

Acromioclavicular Joint

Pain in this joint may be caused by degenerative and infectious conditions.

Anterior Glenohumeral Joint

Pain in the anterior glenohumeral join can be caused by glenohumeral arthritis, osteonecrosis, glenoid labial tear, and adhesive capsulitis.

Sternoclavicular Joint

Pain in this joint can be caused by trauma, infection, or degenerative changes.

Posterior Edge of Acromion

Pain found in this region is related to rotator cuff tendinitis, calcific tendinitis, and rotator cuff tear.

Suprascapular Notch

Nerve entrapment may happen at this region, which causes pain.

Quadrilateral Space

Tenderness and pain, which may be caused by axillary nerve entrapment or inflammation, are palpable in most patients with shoulder pain.

Muscle Pain

All of the pain that occurs in any of the above-mentioned locations can cause or refer muscle pain. Carefully palpate this area to examine muscles on the scapula (both infraspinous and supraspinous fossae).

THE MUSCLES AND NERVES OF THE ARM

Muscles

The arm muscles consist of two groups: flexor and extensor (Table 10-9). The flexor muscles are coracobrachialis, biceps brachii, and brachialis. As discussed above, the biceps brachii has two heads, the long head being a common source of pain because of its long tendon, which spans the glenohumeral joint and is attached to the supraglenoid tubercle. Pain from the long head of the biceps brachii is palpable right on the region of the intertubercular groove on the head of the humerus.

The biceps brachii and brachialis muscles are powerful flexors of the elbow. The former also serves as the major supinator of the forearm (for example, allowing us to turn our palms up). The flexor muscles are innervated by the musculocutaneous nerve.

The triceps muscle serves as the prime extensor of the arm. This muscle is a strong extensor of the elbow and a weak extensor of the shoulder. This muscle is innervated by the radial nerve.

Table 10-9 Muscles of the Arm				
Muscle	Origin	Insertion	Action	Innervation
Flexor				
Biceps brachii	*Short head:* tip of coracoid process of scapula	Radial tuberosity and bicipital aponeurosis	Flexion of arm	Musculocutaneous nerve
	Long head: supraglenoid tubercle of scapula		Flexion and supination of forearm	
Brachialis	Lower half anterior surface of humerus	Ulna tuberosity	Flexion of forearm	Musculocutaneous nerve
Coracobrachialis	Coracoid process of scapula	Anteromedial surface of midshaft of humerus	Flexion and adduction of arm	Musculocutaneous nerve

Continued

Table 10-9 Muscles of the Arm—cont'd				
Muscle	**Origin**	**Insertion**	**Action**	**Innervation**
Extensor				
Anconeus	Lateral epicondyle of humerus	Lateral ulna	Extension of forearm	Radial nerve
Triceps brachii	*Long head:* infraglenoid tubercle of scapula *Lateral head:* posterior surface of humerus above groove of radial nerve and lateral intermuscular septum *Medial head:* posterior surface of humerus medial and inferior to groove of radial nerve and both intermuscular septa	Proximal end of olecranon of ulna	Extension of forearm; extension of arm (long head)	Radial nerve

Nerves

Four main nerves traverse the arm: median, ulnar, musculocutaneous, and radial. The median and ulnar nerves do not give off branches to the muscles of the arm (Table 10-10).

The musculocutaneous nerve arises from the lateral cord of the brachial plexus (C5 to C7), passes through the coracobrachialis muscle, and runs between the biceps brachii and brachialis. After sending branches to innervate these three muscles, the musculocutaneous nerve continues as the lateral antebrachial cutaneous nerve, which reaches laterally to the biceps tendon at the cubital fossa. At this location the nerve penetrates the brachial fascia to innervate the skin of the forearm and an acupoint is formed: H9 lateral antebrachial cutaneous.

The radial nerve leaves the axilla and runs posteriorly between the long head of the triceps and the humerus. As it runs deep to the triceps, the radial nerve gives branches to all three heads of this muscle with fibers from C6 to C8.

THE ELBOW JOINTS: HUMERORADIAL, HUMEROULNAR, AND RADIOULNAR

The elbow is a joint complex that mechanically links the arm (the humerus) and the forearm (two bones: the radius and ulna) (see Figure 10-1). The articulating structures of the three bones provide great stability to the joint. The distal end of the humerus has two articular surfaces, the pulley-shaped trochlea and the spherical capitulum (Figure 10-16). The articular surfaces of each forearm bone, radius and ulna, correspond in shape to these two articular surfaces of the humerus. Medially, the trochlear notch of the ulna articulates with the

Table 10-10 Nerves and Their Innervation to the Arm Muscles			
Nerve	**Origin**	**Muscle**	**Chief Action**
Musculocutaneous	C5, C6	Biceps brachii	Flexion-supination of forearm
	C5-C7	Coracobrachialis	Adduction-flexion of arm
	C5, C6	Brachialis	Flexion of forearm
Radial	C5-C8	Triceps	Extension of forearm
	C6-C7	Anconeus	Extension of forearm

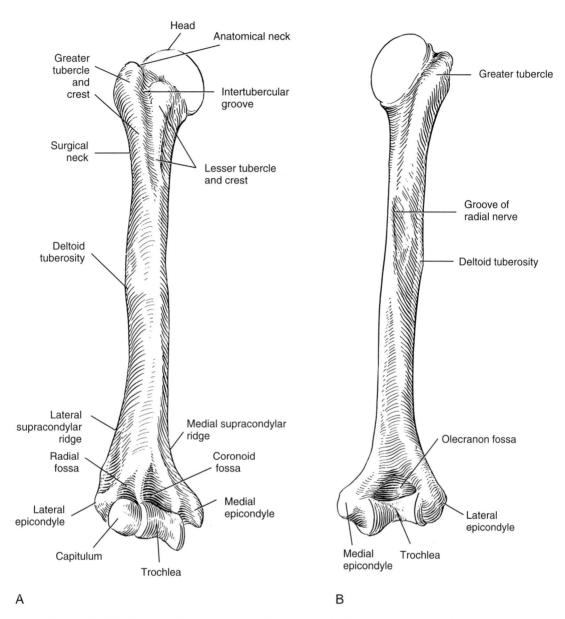

Figure 10-16 Anterior (**A**) and posterior (**B**) views of the humerus. (From Jenkins D: *Hollinshead's functional anatomy of the limbs and back,* ed 8, Philadelphia, 2002, WB Saunders, p 115.)

trochlea, so the ulna bone, and in fact the whole forearm, rotates around the trochlea to perform two-dimensional flexion-extension movement. Laterally the articular surface of the head of the radius is shaped like a cup with a flat concavity that fits into the capitulum. This joint enables the radius bone to rotate along its own axis. The two joints are correspondingly named humeroulnar and humeroradial joints. The third joint, the proximal

radioulnar joint, is formed at the proximal region between the head of the radius and ulna, thus allowing rotation of the head of the radius to produce movements of supination (turning the palms up) and pronation (turning the palms down).

The articular capsule of the joint is relatively thin, but strong collateral ligaments are located on the medial (ulnar) and lateral (radial) sides of the joint and the correspondingly named medial (ulnar) and lateral (radial) collateral ligaments. A ring-like ligament called the annular ligament covers the radioulnar joint (Figure 10-17).

The elbow joint is supplied by four nerves: the musculocutaneous, median, ulnar, and radial.

Elbow tendinitis is one of the most common complaints of patients who seek acupuncture treatment. Our clinical experience indicates that tendinitis is frequently related to muscle injuries. In most patients with elbow tendinitis, more sensitive symptomatic acupoints are found in the related muscles. For example, if a patient complains of lateral epicondylitis, more sensitive points are

palpable in the extensor muscles of the forearm. In our understanding, tight and fatigued muscles are the cause of the inflammation of the tendons. Thus, when treating elbow or any other tendinitis, both muscles and tendons should be needled.

THE FOREARM

The forearm contains 19 muscles, divided into two groups: the 8 flexors (Table 10-11) and the 11 extensors. These muscles act across several joints: the elbow, the wrist, and the small joints of the hand.

Flexors and their Innervation

The eight flexor muscles are arranged into three layers (Figures 10-18 through 10-20). These muscles (Table 10-12) perform the following functions:

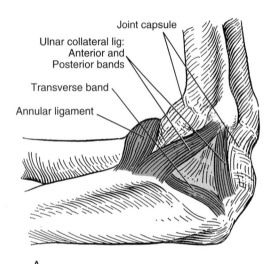

A

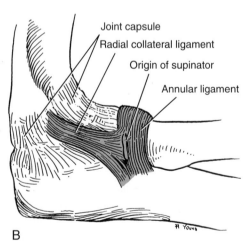

B

Figure 10-17   Medial **(A)** and lateral **(B)** views of the ligaments of the elbow joint. (From Jenkins D: *Hollinshead's functional anatomy of the limbs and back,* ed 8, Philadelphia, 2002, WB Saunders, p 118.)

- Flexion of the wrist: flexor carpi radialis and ulnaris
- Flexion of the fingers: flexor digitorum superficialis and profundus
- Flexion of the hand: flexor palmaris longus
- Flexion of the thumb: flexor pollicis longus
- Pronation of the forearm: pronator teres and quadratus

The superficial layer includes pronator teres, flexor carpi radialis, palmaris longus, and flexor carpi ulnaris. All four muscles form a common tendon that attaches to the medial epicondyle of the humerus. Repetitive wrist flexion or pronation movements occurring in sports (e.g., golf) or other occupations such as the performance of music (e.g., piano, mandolin) may injure these muscles and their common tendon and cause medial epicondylitis.

The flexor digitorum superficialis forms the intermediate layer. It originates from the proximal ulna and the proximal radius. The median nerve passes behind this attachment and may be entrapped. In the distal third of the forearm, the flexor digitorum superficialis muscle gives rise to four tendons: the two superficial tendons go to the middle and ring fingers and the two deep tendons go to the index and little fingers.

The deep layer contains three muscles: flexor digitorum profundus, flexor pollicis longus, and pronator quadratus. The flexor digitorum profundus has an extensive origin from the proximal ulna and the membrane between the ulna and the radius (interosseous membrane). This muscle ends in four tendons that pass the flexor retinaculum and is

Table 10-11
The Flexor Muscles of the Forearm

Muscle	Origin	Insertion	Action	Innervation
Superficial Muscles				
Flexor carpi radialis	Common flexor tendon (medial epicondyle of humerus)	Base of 2nd metacarpal and 3rd metacarpal	Flexion and abduction of hand (radial side)	Median nerve
Flexor carpi ulnaris	Common flexor tendon, proximal two thirds of posterior surface of ulna	Pisiform bone	Flexion and adduction of hand (ulnar side)	Ulnar nerve
Palmaris longus	Common flexor tendon	Palmar aponeurosis	Flexion of hand	Median nerve
Pronator teres	Common flexor tendon; coronoid process of ulna	Lateral surface of shaft of radius	Pronation of forearm and hand	Median nerve
Intermediate Muscle				
Flexor digitorum superficialis	Common tendon, medial aspect of coronoid process of ulna; proximal half of radius distal to radial tuberosity	Middle phalanx of each of four fingers	Flexion of middle phalanx of each of four fingers	Median nerve
Deep Muscles				
Flexor digitorum profundus	Anterior and medial surfaces of proximal two thirds of ulna	Distal phalanx of each of four fingers	Flexion of distal phalanx of each of four fingers	Median and ulnar nerve
Flexor pollicis longus	Anterior surface of middle half of radius	Distal phalanx of thumb	Flexion of distal phalanx of thumb	Median nerve
Pronator quadratus	Distal fourth of ulna	Distal part of radius	Pronation of forearm and hand	Median nerve

inserted on the base of the distal phalanges of each of the four fingers.

The flexor pollicis longus arises from about the middle half of the radius. This muscle forms a tendon that passes through the carpal tunnel and is inserted on the base of the distal phalanx of the thumb.

The pronator quadratus is a flat quadrangular muscle that arises from the distal fourth of the ulna and is inserted on the distal part of the radius. Its action is to pronate the forearm and hand. Therefore this muscle is often subject to repetitive injury. Tenderness can be palpable in this area.

The ulnar nerve runs posterior to the medial epicondyle and enters the forearm (Figure 10-21). In the forearm, it runs along the bone of the ulna, emerges from the lateral side of flexor carpi ulnaris, and continues to the hand. The median nerve runs practically straight down the middle of the forearm (Figure 10-22).

Extensors and their Innervation

The 11 extensor muscles of the forearm (Table 10-13) are arranged into superficial (Figure 10-23) and deep layers (Figure 10-24). The radial nerve innervates all 11 extensor muscles (Figure 10-25) and they perform the following functions:

- Extension of the wrist: extensor carpi ulnaris, radialis, and radialis longus.
- Extension of the fingers: extensor digitorum, indicis, digiti minimi.
- Extension and abduction of the thumb: extensor pollicis longus and brevis, abductor pollicis longus.
- Supination of the forearm: supinator.
- Flexion of the forearm: brachioradialis.

The superficial muscle group arises from the supracondylar ridge and the lateral epicondyle

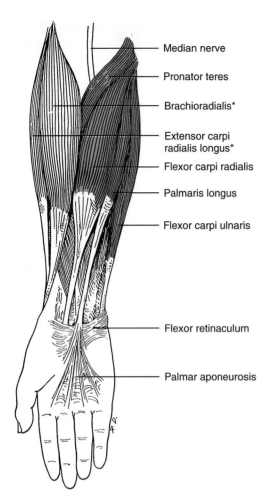

Figure 10-18   The superficial flexor muscles of the right forearm. The starred muscles are extensors. (From Jenkins D: *Hollinshead's functional anatomy of the limbs and back,* ed 8, Philadelphia, 2002, WB Saunders, p 144.)

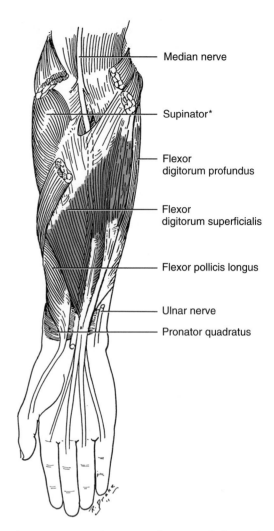

Figure 10-19   The intermediate muscle layer of the right forearm. Supinator is an extensor muscle. (From Jenkins D: *Hollinshead's functional anatomy of the limbs and back,* ed 8, Philadelphia, 2002, WB Saunders, p 145.)

(common extensor tendon) of the humerus. Four muscles attach to this common extensor tendon: extensor carpi radialis brevis, extensor digitorum, extensor digiti minimi, and extensor carpi ulnaris. Repetitive wrist and finger extension such as in some sports and occupations may injure these muscles and cause inflammation of the common extensor tendon (e.g., lateral epicondylitis or tennis elbow).

Tendons crossing the dorsal wrist will be discussed next.

THE WRIST COMPLEX

The wrist (carpus) is the distal joint of the upper limb that relays the tendons of the long flexor and extensor muscles, as well as the major nerves and vessels, from the forearm to the hand. These soft tissues are grouped to cross the narrow tunnel of the wrist. The wrist is structured to allow flexion-extension, adduction-abduction, and circumduction so the hand can assume an optimal position for grasping and manipulation. Movements of the hand occur primarily at the wrist.

Anatomically the wrist is not a single joint, for this region is the junction of the two forearm bones (radius and ulna) and the eight wrist bones (carpal bones). Thus different joints are formed between the radius and ulna, among the eight

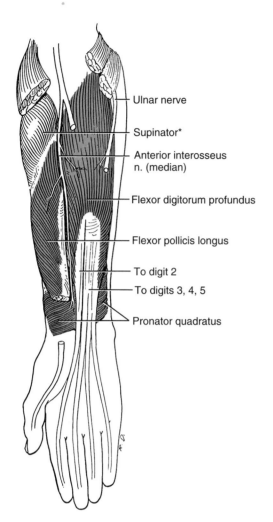

carpal bones, and between the forearm bones and carpal bones. The wrist complex consists of the following joints (Figure 10-26): the distal radioulnar joint, the radiocarpal joint ("the wrist joint"), the intercarpal joints, and the midcarpal joint.

Remember that the proximal radioulnar joint is close to the elbow, so the distal radioulnar joint is close to the wrist. The two radioulnar joints between the radius and ulna make pronation (palm down) and supination (palm up) possible.

The eight carpal bones are arranged in two rows. The three large bones of the proximal row are the scaphoid, lunate, and triquetrum (from the lateral [radial] side to the medial [ulnar] side); the smaller pisiform bone sits on the palm surface of the triquetrum. The proximal row of the carpal bones constitutes the skeleton of the hand. The distal row, also from lateral medial, consists of the trapezium, trapezoid, capitate, and hamate. The eight carpal bones articulate with each other so that, as a whole, the dorsal surface of the wrist is convex and the palmar surface is concave. This concavity, called the carpal groove, contains the median nerve and the long flexor tendons to the hand.

The articular surface of the radius and the distal surface of the ulnar articular disk articulate with the three proximal carpal bones (the scaphoid, lunate, and triquetrum) to form the radiocarpal joint, the "true" wrist joint. The three carpal bones form a convex surface to articulate with the radius so abduction-adduction movement can occur.

The tendons of the long flexor and extensor muscles, together with the nerves and blood vessels, are grouped around the distal ends of the radius and the ulna, the radiocarpal joint, and the carpal bones. To maintain the functional structure, the wrist complex is reinforced by tendons and specialized soft tissues. The forearm fascia (antebrachial fascia) is thickened on the dorsal wrist to

Figure 10-20   The deepest flexor muscles of the right forearm. The supinator (starred) is an extensor muscle of the forearm. (From Jenkins D: *Hollinshead's functional anatomy of the limbs and back,* ed 8, Philadelphia, 2002, WB Saunders, p 145.)

Table 10-12
The Nerves and Their Innervation to the Forearm Flexors

Nerve	Origin	Muscle	Chief Action
Median	C6, C7	Pronator teres	Pronation of forearm
	C7-T1	Pronator quadratus	Pronation of forearm
	C6, C7	Flexor carpi radialis	Flexion at wrist
	C7, C8	Palmaris longus	Flexion at wrist
	C7-T1	Flexor pollicis longus	Flexion of distal phalanx of thumb
	C7-T1	Flexor digitorum superficialis	Flexion of middle phalanges of fingers
	C8, T1	Flexor digitorum profundus (radial part)	Flexion of distal phalanges of digits II and III
Ulna	C8, T1	Flexor digitorum profundus (ulnar part)	Flexion of distal phalanges of digits IV and V
	C8, T1	Flexor carpi ulnaris	Flexion-adduction at wrist

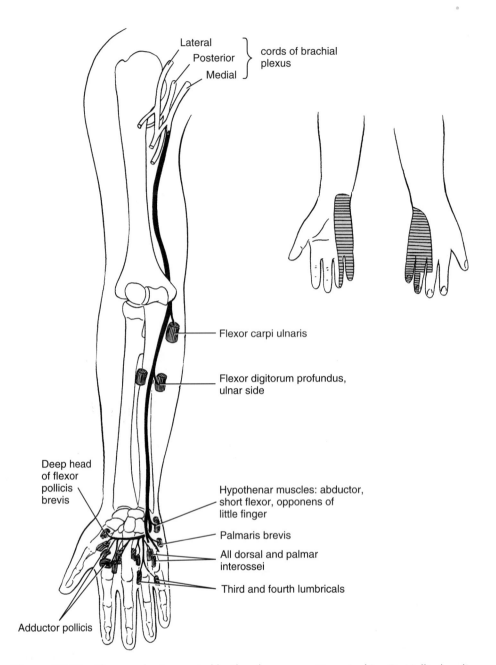

Figure 10-21   The muscles innervated by the ulnar nerve. (From Jenkins D: *Hollinshead's functional anatomy of the limbs and back,* ed 8, Philadelphia, 2002, WB Saunders, p 154.)

form a transverse band called extensor retinaculum, which retains extensor tendons in their position. On the palmar side of the wrist, the deep fascia is also thickened anteriorly to form the flexor retinaculum, which covers the anterior concavity formed by the carpal bones. Thus, the flexor reti-

naculum converts the anterior carpal concavity into a so-called carpal tunnel through which the flexor tendons pass (see below: carpal tunnel syndrome). There are two creases at the wrist. The distal wrist crease indicates the proximal border of the flexor retinaculum. Synovial sheaths surround the long

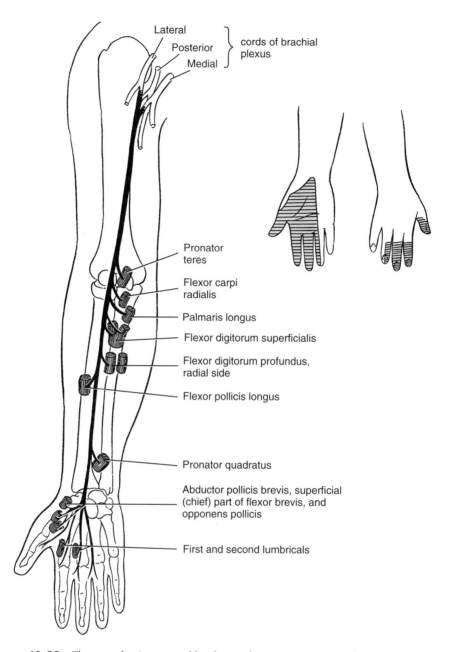

Figure 10-22   The muscles innervated by the median nerve. (From Jenkins D: *Hollinshead's functional anatomy of the limbs and back,* ed 8, Philadelphia, 2002, WB Saunders, p 152.)

flexor tendons and they glide within the fibrous sheath to reduce the friction between the tissues during movement.

The articular nerves of the wrist complex are branches from the median nerve on the palmar aspect, from the radial nerve on the dorsal aspect, and the dorsal and deep branches of the ulnar nerve.

Anatomic relations around the wrist have clinical significance because direct and indirect trauma commonly damages structures around the wrist. Painful irritation of the synovial sheath is common

	Table 10-13			
	The Extensor Muscles of the Forearm: All Are Innervated by the Radial Nerve (C5-C8)			
Muscle	**Origin**	**Insertion**	**Action**	**Segmental Innervation**
Superficial Muscles				
Brachioradialis	Lateral supracondylar ridge of humerus; lateral intermuscular septum of arm	Lateral side of distal end of radius	Flexion of forearm	C5, C6
Extensor carpi radialis brevis	Common extensor tendon (lateral epicondyle of humerus)	Base of 3rd metacarpal	Extension of hand	C6, C7
Extensor carpi radialis longus	Common extensor tendon	Base of 2nd metacarpal	Extension and abduction of hand (radial side)	C6, C7
Extensor carpi ulnaris	Common extensor tendon	Base of 5th metacarpal	Extension and adduction of hand (ulnar side)	C6-C8
Extensor digiti minimi	Common extensor tendon	Middle and distal phalanges of little finger	Extension and adduction of little finger	C6-C8
Extensor digitorum	Common extensor tendon; intermuscular septum; antebrachial fascia	Middle and distal phalanges of each of four fingers	Extension of each of four fingers	C6-C8
Deep Muscles				
Abductor pollicis longus	Posterior surface of ulna and radius	Base of first metacarpal	Abduction and extension of thumb	C7, C8
Extensor indicis	Posterior surface of ulna	Tendon of extensor digitorum	Extension of index finger	C7, C8
Extensor pollicis brevis	Posterior surface of radius	Tendon of extensor proximal phalanx of thumb	Extension of proximal phalanx of thumb	C6, C7
Extensor pollicis longus	Posterior surface of middle third of ulna	Distal phalanx of thumb	Extension of distal phalanx of thumb	C7, C8
Supinator	Posterolateral surface of ulna below radial notch; lateral epicondyle; radial collateral and annular ligaments	Proximal shaft of radius	Supination of forearm and hand	C5, C6

at the point where the tendons of the extensor pollicis brevis and abductor pollicis longus cross over the tendons of the extensors carpi radialis longus and brevis. Inflammation caused by irritation or infection (tenosynovitis) will distend the flexor tendon sheaths. If the pressure of the carpal tunnel is not relieved, the tendons will die due to ischemia. Because of the slow turnover of collagen, tendon rupture may not occur for several weeks, but the median nerve will suffer damage in the carpal tunnel in a very short time.

THE HAND

The remarkable functions of the human hand are achieved by a combination of comprehensive mechanical movement and finely controlled accuracy and tactile sensitivity, which account for a

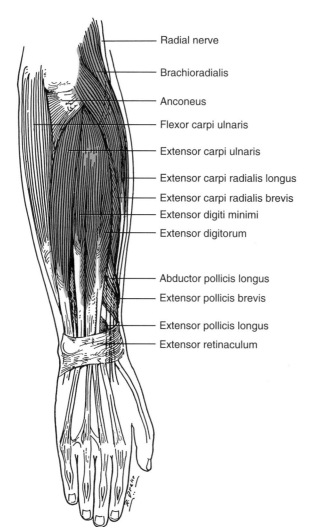

Radial nerve

Brachioradialis

Anconeus

Flexor carpi ulnaris

Extensor carpi ulnaris

Extensor carpi radialis longus

Extensor carpi radialis brevis

Extensor digiti minimi

Extensor digitorum

Abductor pollicis longus

Extensor pollicis brevis

Extensor pollicis longus

Extensor retinaculum

Supinator

Deep branch of radial n.

Extensor pollicis longus

Abductor pollicis longus

Extensor pollicis brevis

Extensor indicis

Ulna

Figure 10-23   The superficial extensor muscles of the right forearm. (From Jenkins D: *Hollinshead's functional anatomy of the limbs and back,* ed 8, Philadelphia, 2002, WB Saunders, p 161.)

Figure 10-24   The deeper extensor muscles of the right forearm. (From Jenkins D: *Hollinshead's functional anatomy of the limbs and back,* ed 8, Philadelphia, 2002, WB Saunders, p 161.)

greater area in the neocortex of the human brain than the functions of any other organ.

The hand is an anatomically complex structure. It consists of 27 named bones with numerous joints between them, the tendons of the extrinsic long muscles, a large number of intrinsic small muscles, and important nerves and vessels.

The base skeleton of the hand is composed of eight carpal bones arranged in two rows, proximal and distal (see the section on the wrist complex). The proximal row of the four carpal bones articulates with the radial to form the radiocarpal joint, the wrist joint. The distal row of carpal bones artic-

ulates with the elongated metacarpal bones (see Figure 10-26). Distal to the metacarpal bones are the 14 phalanges: two for the thumb and three for all the other four digits. Different joints are formed between the bones: intercarpal, carpometacarpal, metacarpophalangeal, and interphalangeal. An important acupoint H12 superficial radial is formed between metacarpals I and II.

The skin of the dorsum is loose and freely mobile with little soft tissue so the dorsal skin and fascia can slide freely over extensor tendons and bones. In contrast, the fibrous bands anchor and stabilize the skin of the palm with the underlying

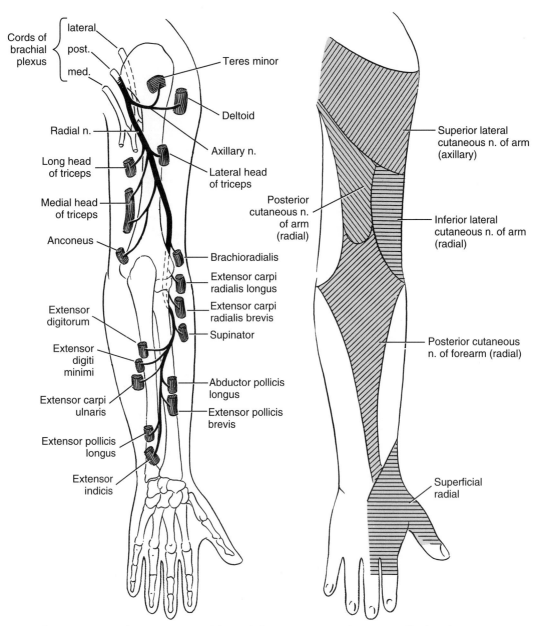

Figure 10-25   The innervation of the radial nerve. (From Jenkins D: *Hollinshead's functional anatomy of the limbs and back,* ed 8, Philadelphia, 2002, WB Saunders, p 168.)

palmar aponeurosis. The soft tissues of the palm are arranged into four layers: just below the palmar aponeurosis is the thenar or lateral compartment containing short muscles of the thumb (thenar), the little finger (hypothenar), nerves, and vessels. The next layer is a central compartment containing vessels, nerves, and the long flexors of the fingers (flexor digitorum superficialis and profundus). The deeper layer contains the adductor muscle of the thumb, nerves, and vessels. The fourth layer includes the four dorsal interosseous muscles lying between the five metacarpal bones.

The tendons of the flexor digitorum superficialis and profundus reach the proximal phalanges and are invested with a synovial sheath. Each tendon of the flexor digitorum superficialis splits

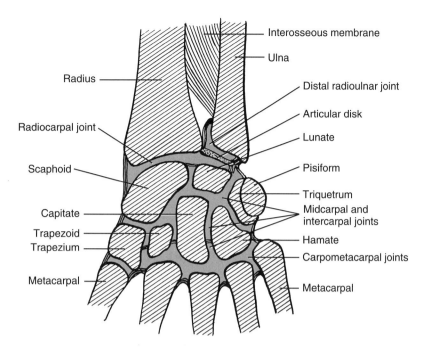

Figure 10-26   The wrist complex: the bones and the joint cavities of the wrist. Note that the radiocarpal and distal radioulnar joint cavities are separate and distinct; that the midcarpal joint is continuous with the intercarpal joints between the proximal and distal rows of the carpals; and that the carpometacarpal joints, except for that of the thumb, are continuous with the intermetacarpal joints and with the distal parts of the intercarpal joints, but have no communication with the midcarpal joint. (From Jenkins D: *Hollinshead's functional anatomy of the limbs and back,* ed 8, Philadelphia, 2002, WB Saunders, p 182.)

into two parts that lie on each side of the tendon of flexor digitorum profundus (Figure 10-27) and finally are inserted into the corresponding phalanx.

In addition to the basic anatomic knowledge of the upper limb from the shoulder to the hand, which is essential for acupuncture treatment, it is also important to know the sensory nerve distribution in the upper limb particularly when treating upper limb pain and numbness. A brief summary of the sensory nerve distribution on the upper limb is shown in Figure 10-28. Please note that in each patient there is a considerable overlap between the sensory territories of different nerves.

UPPER LIMB PAIN COMMONLY ENCOUNTERED IN ACUPUNCTURE CLINICS

Based on our clinical experience, we classify upper limb pain into three groups: (1) soft tissue pain and injuries due to overuse; (2) joint and bone pain; and (3) nerve pain.

Soft Tissue Pain and Injuries due to Overuse (Repetitive Motion Disorders)

Repetitive motion disorders (RMDs)—also referred to as overuse injuries, repetitive stress syndromes, and activity-related musculoskeletal disorders—are often caused by occupations requiring computer use or by sports activities. Many sports participants develop overuse injuries.

The physical processes that cause RMDs can be repetition, sustained loading, and cumulative trauma. RMDs can involve different soft tissues such as muscles, nerves, ligaments, and tendons. Injuries to these tissues show that the accumulated biomechanical stress that has been applied to them is beyond their tolerance. The biomechanical stress is most likely to cause injury at those anatomic locations where tendons change directions, traverse narrow tunnels, pass through a pulley, or are impinged upon by surrounding structures. If the injury is not properly treated, the anatomy and composition of the tendon may change from that of a regularly arranged dense connective tissue to that of fibrocartilage.

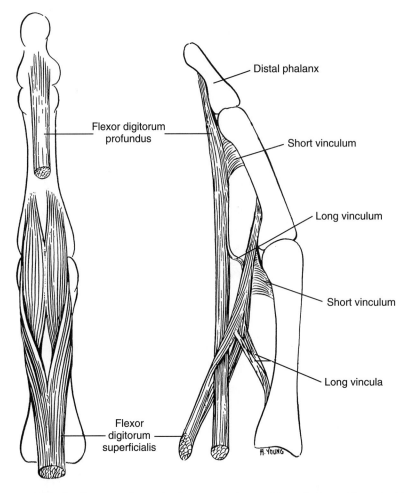

Figure 10-27   The flexor tendons of a finger, anterior and lateral views. (From Jenkins D: *Hollinshead's functional anatomy of the limbs and back,* ed 8, Philadelphia, 2002, WB Saunders, p 188.)

The pathological conditions of irritated tendons may be different. The underlying pathologic entities can be tendinitis (inflammation of the tendon), peritendinitis (inflammation of the tendon and its sheath), or tendinosis (degeneration of the tendon). Our clinical experience shows that most of these tendon problems respond well to acupuncture needling if treated together with their corresponding muscles. Tight muscles always transfer the pulling force to the tendons and cause inflammation of the tendons. The stress on the tendons can only be relieved if the muscles are relaxed and flexible.

Sometimes it is difficult to distinguish a particular pathologic condition because many soft tissues may be involved and different disorders may coexist. For example, shoulder pain in a patient may

represent one or all of these disorders: rotator cuff tendinopathy, subacromial bursitis, acromioclavicular arthritis, or bicipital tendinitis. Acupuncture can achieve faster and better results when the pathologic conditions are simpler and fewer. Slower and less efficient results can be expected when the pathologic conditions are many and complicated.

Rotator Cuff Tendinopathy   Four scapular muscles (supraspinatus, infraspinatus, teres minor, and subscapularis) fuse their tendons with the fibrous capsule of the glenohumeral joint to form a musculotendinous cuff. The rotator cuff protects and stabilizes the shoulder joint by holding the head of the humerus in the glenoid cavity of the scapula (see the section on the glenohumeral

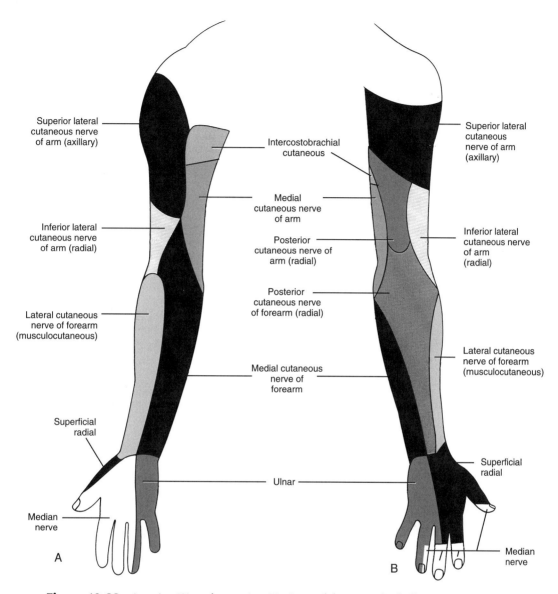

Figure 10-28   Anterior (**A**) and posterior (**B**) views of the upper limb illustrating the sensory innervation to the skin. (From Jenkins D: *Hollinshead's functional anatomy of the limbs and back,* ed 8, Philadelphia, 2002, WB Saunders, p 120.)

joint). The supraspinatus helps abduct the arm and the other three rotator cuff muscles rotate the humerus.

The rotator cuff may be damaged or torn by injury and trauma as a result of prolonged or repetitive use of the upper extremity, particularly in an abducted position. The supraspinatus tendon is the most commonly torn structure of the rotator cuff. Some sports activities, such as baseball pitching, tennis, and bowling, are particularly liable to cause this damage.

Rotator cuff tears are both age-related and activity-related, and create a condition in which neither abduction nor external rotation are possible. During the initial stage, the tear is a relatively minor injury that might not be noted, but if left untreated, the initial tear can develop into a larger tear. Rotator cuff tears can be either incomplete (partial) or complete (total) tears. Pain is often progressive and may radiate to the base of the neck or down the lateral aspect of the arm. Abduction activities become weak and painful.

Degenerative tendinosis of the musculotendinous rotator cuff is a common disease in senior people. Calcium deposits can be formed in the tendon of the supraspinatus and other rotator cuff muscles.

Acupuncture efficacy varies in treating rotator cuff symptoms, depending on the nature of the tendinopathy. Acupuncture alone can achieve good results in patients with early pathologic conditions of the rotator cuff, including minor calcium deposits. The reason for this is unclear, but we speculate that the muscles are relaxed when they obtain better blood circulation and cleansing, so that the minor calcium deposit does not interfere with their movement; or the improved blood circulation may gradually render the minor calcium deposit dissolvable. Acupuncture efficacy decreases as the pathologic condition is more serious. Acupuncture is not effective in cases of severe rotator cuff damage but can be helpful in recovery of the muscles after surgery.

Frozen Shoulder (Adhesive Capsulitis, Adhesive Bursitis)   A normal glenohumeral capsule has a volume of 30 ml of fluid. If the capsular fluid decreases, some parts of the capsule lining will adhere to each other or to the head of the humerus. This pathologic condition reduces the capsular elasticity, resulting in limitation of glenohumeral action. The pain is felt at the end point of any shoulder joint motion. This condition is seen more frequently in patients over 50 years of age. Acupuncture is able to relax the muscles and promote blood circulation, which helps to cleanse wastes, and the needle-induced lesions will reduce inflammation. These functions may help restore the normal structure and function in some patients suffering from frozen shoulder, but in severe cases acupuncture cannot reverse the pathological condition and other medical modalities will be needed.

Subacromial Bursitis (Calcific Bursitis, Scapulohumeral Bursitis)   A bursa is a small fluid-filled sac or saclike cavity situated where friction would otherwise occur. Subacromial bursae lie between the acromion and supraspinatus tendon and extend between the deltoid and greater tubercle. Inflammation of the subacromial bursa can be the underlying cause of acute or chronic shoulder pain (see Figure 10-5). Patients with subacromial bursitis complain of pain and tenderness in the lateral shoulder, with pain that worsens during movement. In chronic cases, the bursa may become thickened and fibrotic, although this pathologic change may not be radiographically detectable.

A calcium deposit can develop in the subdeltoid or subacromial bursa.

Acupuncture treatments are very effective in cases of acute subacromial bursitis and help to reduce pain in mild and moderate cases. Needling the freshly inflamed soft tissues increases blood circulation and reduces the pain, swelling, and inflammation. The tissue reaction to the needling helps to digest the damaged cells and replace them with new cells. However, if the condition becomes chronic, more treatment sessions are needed and the efficacy varies according to the healability of the condition.

Bicipital Tendinitis   The tendon of the long head of the biceps ascends in the intertubercular (bicipital) groove of the humerus and enters the glenohumeral capsule. Within the capsule the tendon crosses the head of the humerus and attaches to the supraglenoid tubercle of the scapula (see Figure 10-8). The long course and angulation of this tendon make it susceptible to tears and degenerative changes. Pain or tenderness is anterior to the shoulder and radiates down the anterior arm.

Acupuncture needling usually helps if only inflammation of the tendon is involved because acupuncture needling induces antiinflammatory reaction and tissue regeneration. The treatment should include needling both the muscles and inflamed tendons. If rupture of the transverse humeral ligament or displacement of the tendon out of the intertubercular groove are suspected, consult an orthopedic surgeon immediately.

Epicondylitis   Medial and lateral epicondylitis is a common cause of pain in the elbow and forearm. The most likely cause of this condition is repetitive overuse or trauma. Age-related degenerative tendinosis may be the underlying cause in some cases. Seemingly the pain is localized over the respective epicondyle with radiation into the forearm. However, tender points can be found by careful palpation of the extensor muscles (lateral epicondylitis) or flexor muscles (medial epicondylitis). These muscle tender points should be needled together with the lateral or medial common tendon.

Epicondylitis, if related to repetitive overuse of the arm, usually results from stressful, tight, or damaged muscles. Needling these muscles is even more important than needling the common tendon. Acupuncture usually provides very good results in most patients with epicondylitis, especially in those with acute onset from sport activities. Self-healable sports injuries such as those caused by repetitive overuse are usually soft tissue injuries with inflammation and swelling. Athletes usually maintain good self-healing potential, so acupuncture needling can achieve satisfactory results. If epicondylitis is caused by age-related necrotic change, less efficacy can be expected and more treatments are needed to reduce the inflammation and pain.

Olecranon Bursitis Symptoms of olecranon bursitis may include pain, tenderness, swelling, and warmth in the posterior elbow. Olecranon bursitis is usually caused by overuse, recurrent trauma, inflammation, or infection. Patients with rheumatic disease may have acute aseptic inflammatory olecranon bursitis.

Because needling can promote immune reaction to reduce inflammation, acupuncture treatments are usually effective in treating olecranon bursitis. Both the inflamed bursa and the muscles of the arm and forearms should be treated together because the inflamed bursa irritates the muscles and makes them tight, resulting in low blood circulation to the inflamed soft tissues. Needling relaxes the muscles and increases the blood circulation, which reduces the inflammation of the bursa and promotes regeneration of the fresh tissues.

Localized Median Nerve Lesion: Carpal Tunnel Syndrome In its course from the neck to the hand, the median nerve can be entrapped in several locations: (1) in the cubital fossa, the median nerve is entrapped by the pronator teres muscle or flexor digitorum superficialis from repetitive strain; (2) in the forearm, the median nerve is injured by direct trauma or forearm fracture, which causes weak thumb activity; (3) the most common median nerve neuropathy is the entrapment of the median nerve in the carpal tunnel at the wrist. We have many patients with carpal tunnel syndrome (CTS) whose professions require substantial use of computers.

The carpal tunnel is a narrow fibro-osseous passage through which 10 structures pass: the median nerve, the flexor pollicis longus tendon, four tendons of the flexor digitorum superficialis, and four tendons of the flexor digitorum profundus (Figure 10-29). All eight flexor tendons in the carpal tunnel share the same common synovial sheath (also called the ulnar bursa) formed by the synovial membrane. Sufficient synovial fluid is contained in the bursa to lubricate and hence facilitate the movement of the tendons beneath the retinaculum.

Any pathologic conditions that significantly increase the pressure inside the carpal tunnel or reduce the size of the carpal tunnel (e.g., edema, inflammation of the flexor retinaculum, anterior dislocation of the lunate bone, rheumatoid thick-

ening of the synovial membrane of the tendon sheaths, and tenosynovitis of the tendon sheaths) may cause compression of the median nerve as well as the tendons. Most patients with CTS are between 40 and 60 years of age and the syndrome is more common in women, possibly because women have less physical training than men. Those workers with jobs that require use of repetitive wrist motion (computer programmers and bank tellers) or forced hand movement are more susceptible to CTS.

CTS is characterized by pain on the palmar-radial aspect of the hand, and the pain often becomes worse at night and may be severe enough to wake the patient. When tapped on the palm side of the wrist, patients experience a tingling or shooting pain into the hand or forearm. The median nerve has two terminal branches (lateral and medial) that supply the skin of the hand. Therefore, there is often tingling (paresthesia), absence of tactile sensation (anesthesia), or diminished sensation (hypoesthesia) in the digits. Often there is a progressive loss of coordination and strength in the thumb, owing to weakness of the abductor pollicis brevis and opponens pollicis muscles. This results in difficulty in performing fine movements of the thumb. As the thenar muscles and the two lateral lumbrical muscles of the other digits are also supplied by the median nerve, the usefulness of the first to third digits may be diminished. In severe CTS cases, wasting or atrophy of the thenar muscles will occur. If the pathologic condition persists, all the tendons will die owing to ischemia.

In most people, a minor tenosynovitis of the tendons within the carpal tunnel can occur without experiencing any CTS symptoms.

Early and proper treatment can relieve pain and numbness and usually can prevent permanent damage to the wrist and hand. Permanent nerve, tendon, and muscle damage will occur if CTS is left untreated.

The efficacy of acupuncture in treating CTS depends on the severity of the condition, the nature of the case, and the general health of the patient. For example, better and faster results are achieved in patients who are suffering from the initial stages of CTS in one hand than in those who are affected in both hands. Acute and recently developed CTS is more responsive to acupuncture needling than chronic CTS in one or both hands. If the CTS is caused by carpal bone dislocation or rheumatoid thickening of the sheath as opposed to inflammation or infection, acupuncture efficacy will be uncertain. Acupuncture may help in reducing some pain, but the major symptoms can be reduced only after the carpal bone dislocation is corrected or the

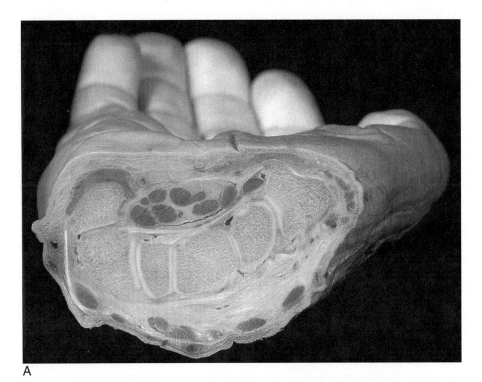

A

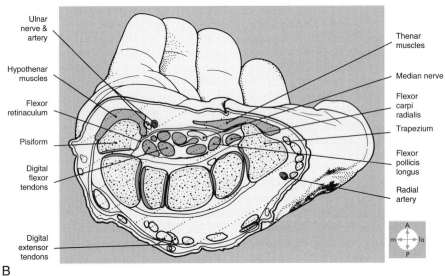

B

Figure 10-29 Transverse section through the carpal tunnel to show its contents. In cases of carpal tunnel syndrome, directly needling into the tunnel helps reduce swelling and pain and promote healing. (From Gosling J, Harris P, Whitmore I, Willan P: *Human anatomy: color atlas and text,* ed 4, Edinburgh, 2002, Mosby, p 119.)

pressure from the rheumatoid thickening of the sheath can be released.

Ulnar Nerve Entrapment: Thoracic Outlet Syndrome

When the lower trunk of the brachial plexus passes over the first rib, the nerve trunks and subclavian blood vessels may be compressed by the scalenus anticus or medius muscles. This nerve compression produces an aching pain in the neck and along the distribution of the ulnar nerve in the forearm and hand, as well as some numbness in the little and ring fingers. Arterial compression may cause severe ischemia of the upper limb, and venous compression results in sudden pain, cyanosis, and swelling of the upper arms. If the condition persists, it results in weakness and wasting of the small muscles of the hand.

Needling scalenus muscles on the side of the neck and the upper limb helps to reduce the compression on the nerve trunks of the brachial plexus and subclavian blood vessels. This helps reduce the pain and restore the blood circulation. Other modalities such as physical therapy are also recommended.

Tenosynovitis

Long tendons run through the hand and into each finger. Each tendon is enclosed within a sheath lined with a membrane called the synovium. This membrane secretes fluid to lubricate the tendon sheaths and the joints, and to nourish the joint cartilage. The tendon sheath keeps the tendon from adhering to other tissue.

Repetitive overuse, forced activity such as in the fingers of a mountain climber, or arthritis may cause the sheath to become inflamed or infected. This condition is called tenosynovitis. Tenosynovitis can occur in the bicipital tendon in the shoulder, wrist, hand, or fingers.

The major symptoms of tenosynovitis are pain and tenderness or pain when moving the affected region, movements accompanied by a crackling sound or feeling, and hot and inflamed joint(s).

Needling of the affected region is very helpful in treating tenosynovitis, especially in the early stage of the condition because the inflammation and other symptoms are localized. The needling improves blood circulation and activates a local immune reaction to reduce the inflammation and promote healing. Once the sheath becomes thickened, needling cannot reverse the condition but may slow down the progress.

Joint and Bone Pain

Upper limb joint and bone pain are common complaints presented by patients who seek acupuncture treatments. Some patients present with acute symptoms but most cases are chronic. The following is a description of the most common conditions seen in an acupuncture clinic.

Acute Joint and Bone Pain

The most common causes of acute joint pain are infectious arthritis and rheumatic fever. Infectious arthritis has been found to be related to several bacterial and nonbacterial agents. Most cases are the result of hematogenous spread, posttraumatic infection, direct infection, or spread from adjacent infected tissue. Rheumatic fever is associated with the presence of hemolytic streptococci in the body and is characterized by fever and joint pain.

Acupuncture is helpful in reducing pain, fever, and infection in younger and healthier patients because they have a better self-healing potential and once it is activated by acupuncture needling, they are able to easily restore their homeostasis. However, exactly the same acupuncture therapy provides reduced or even no efficacy for patients with more severe conditions and lower self-healing capacity. Severe pathological conditions and lower self-healing potentials always accompany each other.

For noninfectious joint pain, direct needling into the joint is an effective method of reducing the pain and inflammation because needling induces local antiinflammation reaction and tissue regeneration.

In cases of infectious arthritis or rheumatic fever, bleeding into a joint can spread and intensify the infection and cause a strong inflammatory reaction, which may result in a rapid form of osteoarthritis. When treating patients with infectious arthritis or rheumatic fever, focus on relieving muscle pain first and avoid deep needling into the joint.

Chronic Joint and Bone Pain

Two common rheumatologic disorders, osteoarthritis (OA) and rheumatoid arthritis (RA), are characterized by chronic pain, stiffness, and loss of function in joints.

OA is also known as a degenerative joint disease. More than 50% of people who are older than 65 years of age have OA in varying degrees of severity. More women are affected than men. The principal feature of OA is wear and tear on cartilage in a joint, affecting the joint's mobility. The major symptoms presented by patients are pain in a joint during or after movement or following periods of inactivity, morning stiffness in one or more joints, and sometimes lumps on finger joints or around knees.

With age, cartilage changes and may lose its elasticity, making the joint more vulnerable to damage from injury or overuse. The breakdown of cartilage causes the synovial membrane of the joint to become inflamed. The inflamed tissue releases enzymes that further destroy cartilage. As a result, the bones become exposed from cartilage loss, thicken, and form bone spurs (osteophytes). Bone rubs against bone and produces pain. People with joint injuries due to automobile accidents, sports, and work-related activity have an increased risk of developing OA.

OA most frequently occurs in the neck or upper back. It breaks down the disks and forms bone spurs on the sides of damaged vertebra. OA may also develop in the knees, hips, hands, or feet. Genetics also play a role in some patients, especially in cases of OA symptoms in the hands.

OA is not curable but acupuncture treatments may provide some temporary relief of symptomatic pain in joints and muscles. OA creates pain and tightness in the muscles as well as in the joints, which reduces blood circulation in the painful area. Acupuncture relaxes the muscles and the joints to which the muscles are attached. This process increases blood circulation, ensuring a fresh supply of nutrients and oxygen to the affected area, thus slowing down the degeneration.

RA is an autoimmune disease in which the body's immune system attacks healthy tissues, specifically the thin synovial membrane of the joint and some internal organs. In affected joints, the inflamed synovium often proliferates, invading and damaging bone and cartilage. Enzymes released from inflammatory cells digest bone and cartilage. Many people with RA have a genetic marker called HLA-DR4. Other genes may also influence the development of RA.

The major complaints presented by these patients include pain and swelling in the joints of the feet, wrist, and hands (especially the small finger joints); redness and warmth over the joints; and diffuse aching and stiffness. In the early course of the disease, joint tenderness, inflammation of the synovium, and soft tissue swelling are observed, accompanied by a decrease in the range of motion, particularly the wrist extension. Later manifestations of RA include pain and deformity resulting from intraarticular and extraarticular tissue injury. Small, usually nonpainful lumps under the skin (rheumatoid nodules) may develop near the elbows, on the fingers, on the feet, along the Achilles tendons, or on the buttocks.

Unlike OA, which affects only the musculoskeletal system, RA is a systemic disease and it may affect several organs such as the heart, lungs, skin, and eyes. It also tends to affect multiple joints. The symptoms tend to appear symmetrically in the body, for example affecting both ankles or both wrists.

Most RA sufferers are between the ages of 20 and 50, although RA may attack any age group. Statistically, about three times as many women as men have RA.

RA is a noncurable disease but acupuncture treatment in the early stages of the disease helps to relax the muscles and desensitize painful nerves so as to reduce pain and stiffness of the joints. As RA symptoms spread to more joints, acupuncture becomes less effective. However, regular acupuncture treatments, for example, two sessions a week, combined with nutrition therapy, seem to slow down the progress of RA.

TREATMENT PROTOCOL

As usual in INMAS, the treatment protocol consists of homeostatic, paravertebral, and symptomatic acupoints.

Homeostatic Acupoints

All homeostatic acupoints accessible in the position the patient uses for treatment (supine, prone, or side) should be needled.

Paravertebral Acupoints

Paravertebral acupoints can be selected from C2 to T7 because all upper limb pain and disorders are related to or derived from either the cervical plexus (C1-C4) or the brachial plexus (C5-T1). The practitioner should carefully palpate the neck and upper back to find the more sensitive region and to select the corresponding segments of the spine from C2 to T7.

Symptomatic Acupoints

Figures 10-30 through 10-33 show some of the typical symptomatic acupoints used for upper limb pain and disorders. Careful palpation should be applied to find these local symptomatic acupoints. Figures 10-30 through 10-33 also show some of the needling methods. With a good understanding of anatomical structure and mechanical function, practitioners can explore more effective needling methods for each particular case.

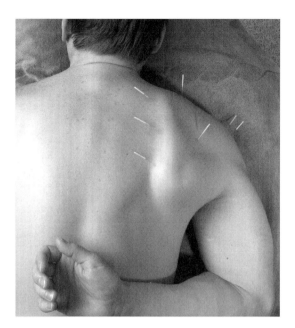

Figure 10-30   Prone position. Left upper limb in cross-back adduction position for shoulder pain.

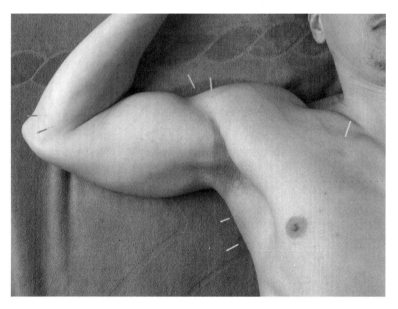

Figure 10-31   Supine position with arm abduction and forearm 90-degree upward flexion. Needles are inserted into the tender points in rotator cuff muscles, latissimus dorsi, pectoralis muscles, and the medial elbow.

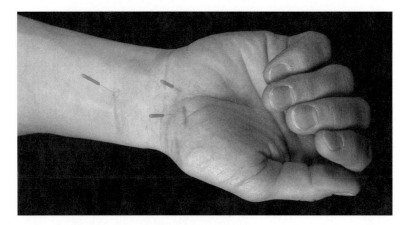

Figure 10-32 Treatment of carpal tunnel syndrome. Needles are inserted into the median nerve point and into the carpal tunnel.

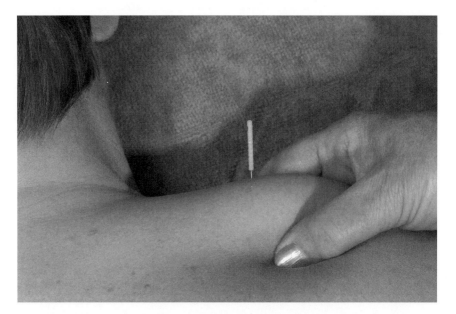

Figure 10-33 Method for needling the acupoints without puncturing the tissues or organs underneath. This photo shows how to needle H3 spinal accessory without inserting needle into the lung tissue below the trapezius muscle.

References

1. Goldstein B: Musculoskeletal upper limb pains. In Loeser J et al, editors: *Bonica's management of pain*, ed 3, Philadelphia, 2001, Lippincott Williams & Wilkins.

2. Kiefhaber TR, Stern PJ: Upper extremity tendinitis and overuse syndromes in the athlete, *Clin Sports Med* 11:39-55, 1992.

CHAPTER 11

Lower Limb Pain: Hip, Thigh, Knee, Leg, Ankle, and Foot

INTRODUCTION

Pain and disorders in the hips and lower limbs are, like lower back pain, among the most challenging conditions in acupuncture pain management. As the baby boomer population ages and more middle-aged people are athletically active, more degenerative and traumatic cases are seen in acupuncture clinics. The task of treating pain and other disorders of these regions is challenging for at least two reasons:

1. Just as shoulder and upper limb pain are often associated with neck problems, pain in the lower limb is often related to lower back disorders, which are among the most common health problems.
2. Unlike the upper limbs, the hips and lower limbs bear weight, which makes them more susceptible to degenerative changes. This also makes the healing of injuries more difficult and prolongs the process of restoring normal physical function.

To overcome this difficult clinical challenge and achieve stable and faster results, it is indispensable to have good knowledge of the anatomic and the biomechanic structure of this region as well as some understanding of the pathologic nature of commonly encountered pain and disorders. This chapter will briefly describe the anatomy, physiology, and biomechanics of the hip and lower limb as it is relevant to acupuncture therapy and then discuss the most common hip and lower limb disorders that are seen in clinical practice. Finally, we will discuss the application of our standardized but individualizable protocol to the pain and disorders presented in this chapter.

The lower limbs are built for locomotion, bearing weight, and maintaining body equilibrium. In contrast with the upper limb, the lower limb has a bony junction with the axial skeleton and, unlike the freely movable and non–weight-bearing upper

limb, the lower limb has more stability at the cost of reduced mobility. For example, the lateral abduction of the lower limb is restricted by the adductor muscles, while the flexion of the thigh is restrained by the hamstring muscles.

The lower limb consists of four major parts:

- *The hip,* which connects the femur (thigh bone) of the lower limb to the vertebral column
- *The thigh*, whose bone, the femur, connects the hip and the knee
- *The leg,* containing two bones, the tibia (shin bone) and the fibula (splint bone, calf bone), which connect the knee and ankle
- *The foot,* consisting of tarsus (bones of posterior and middle foot), metatarsus (bones of anterior foot), and phalanges (bones of toes)

From the perspective of acupuncture treatment, lower back problems and disorders of the hip and lower limb are inseparable. For example, ankle or foot pain will change the gait and shift the center of the gravity of the body, which will put more stress on the contralateral hip. When treating an ankle and foot disorder, both hips and the lower back should be examined and treated, as well as the injured ankle and foot.

Common causes of pain and disorders of the hip and lower limbs include degeneration, neurological origins, injuries from sports and daily activities, and inflammation and referral from a distant site, especially the lower back. Other pathologic conditions such as vascular diseases and tumors may cause lower limb pain for which acupuncture can be used only as supplementary or supportive therapy. This chapter addresses only the common causes of those pathologic conditions that are seen in daily acupuncture practice.

It is important to stress again that acupuncture practitioners must treat the whole body, not only the local symptoms. When treating the lower limb, a practitioner must examine the lower back. If there are tender points in the lower back, a practitioner must examine the upper back and the neck. This is why it is so important for an acupuncture practitioner to understand basic anatomy as it relates to acupuncture therapy and why so many chapters in this book emphasize anatomical descriptions from this standpoint.

BASIC ANATOMY OF THE LOWER LIMB: ITS RELATION TO PAIN AND ACUPUNCTURE THERAPY

The Bones of the Lower Limb

The large, irregular hip bone (os coxae) is composed of three bones: ilium, ischium, and pubis. These bones begin to fuse at 15 to 17 years of age

and the fusion is complete by age 23. Thus, the hip bone is indistinguishably joined in an adult (Figure 11-1). A cup-shaped socket (named acetabulum, after a shallow cup used in ancient Rome for vinegar) is formed where the three bones fuse. The acetabulum and head of the femur form the hip joint.

The femur is the longest, strongest, and heaviest bone in the body (Figure 11-2). A person's height is about four times the length of the femur. The femur consists of a rounded head, neck, and greater and lesser trochanters at the proximal portion of the shaft, and two broadened lateral and medial condyles at the distal portion. The two condyles articulate with the tibia and patella to form the knee joint.

The leg consists of two bones, the tibia (shin bone) and the fibula (splint bone, calf bone). The

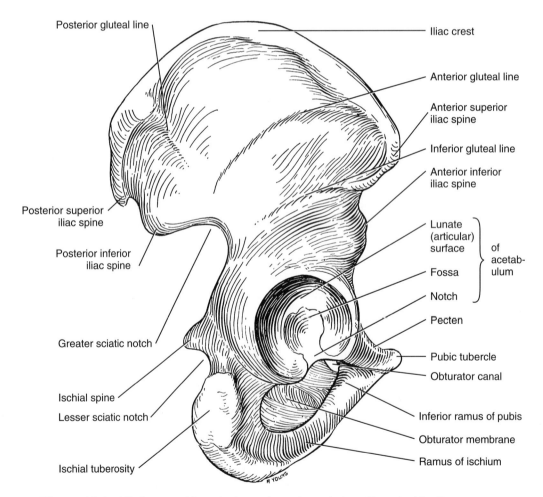

Figure 11-1 Hip bone and its articular surfaces. Lateral view. (From Jenkins D: *Hollinshead's functional anatomy of the limbs and back,* ed 8, Philadelphia, 2002, WB Saunders, p 264.)

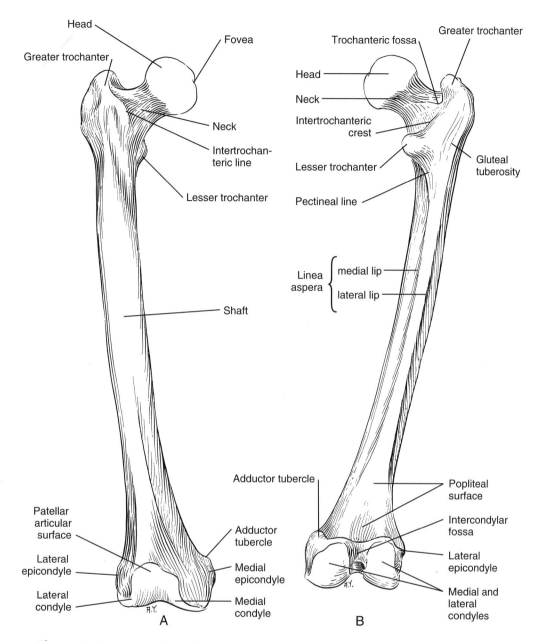

Figure 11-2   Anterior (**A**) and posterior (**B**) views of the femur. (From Jenkins D: *Hollinshead's functional anatomy of the limbs and back,* ed 8, Philadelphia, 2002, WB Saunders, p 269.)

tibia is the second largest bone in the body and is located on the anteromedial side of the leg. The tibia supports most of the body weight. The proximal end of the tibia is large and its lateral and medial condyles articulate with the corresponding condyles of the femur. The patellar ligament from the thigh muscles inserts into the prominent tibial tuberosity. The distal end of the tibia is small and

has articular surfaces for the fibula and talus (Figure 11-3). Here the tibia forms the medial malleolus to stabilize the ankle. The shaft of the tibia is triangular in cross section.

The fibula is a long, pinlike bone (fibula means "pin" in Latin) that articulates with the tibia posterolateral. The fibula serves mainly as an attachment for muscles and gives stability to the ankle

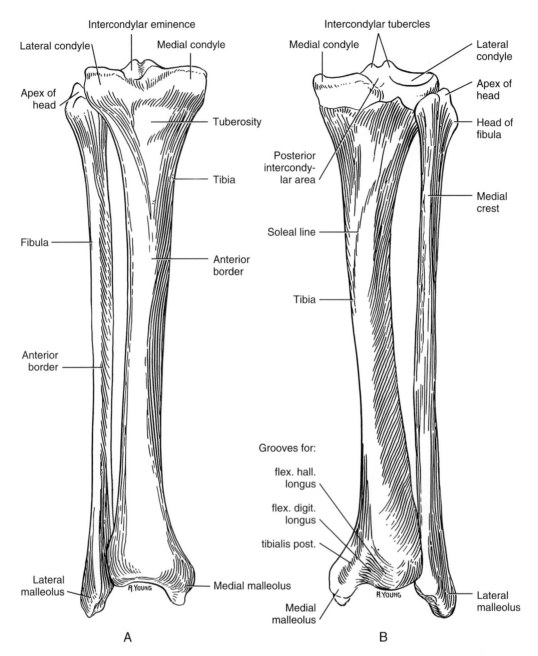

Figure 11-3   Anterior (**A**) and posterior (**B**) views of the right tibia and fibula. (From Jenkins D: *Hollinshead's functional anatomy of the limbs and back,* ed 8, Philadelphia, 2002, WB Saunders, p 329.)

joint. The proximal end of the fibula is its head, which has a facet to articulate with the inferior surface of the lateral tibial condyle. The distal end of the fibula is the lateral malleolus, which helps to hold the talus in its socket (see Figure 11-3).

The foot consists of 7 tarsal bones, 5 metatarsal bones, and 14 phalanges (Figure 11-4). Of the seven

tarsal bones, only the talus articulates with the leg bones. When treating ankle and foot pain, the practitioner needs to understand the anatomy and biomechanics of the foot to know where to find the symptomatic acupoint(s) (SAs). This chapter will focus only on cases that are commonly seen in acupuncture clinics, such as ankle sprain and plantar

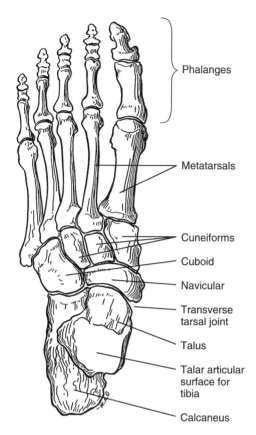

Figure 11-4 The bones of the ankle and foot (dorsal view). (From Jenkins D: *Hollinshead's functional anatomy of the limbs and back,* ed 8, Philadelphia, 2002, WB Saunders, p 330.)

fasciitis, and will therefore not describe the complete anatomy and biomechanics of the foot, although readers may consult the available professional literature for more detailed knowledge.

Muscles

Muscles are the source of most soft-tissue pain. A knowledge of the anatomy, physiology, and pathology of the muscles and peripheral nerves is vital for achieving optimum therapeutic results. The anatomic description of the muscles below shows that they are all supplied by branches of the peripheral nerves of the lumbosacral plexus. When treating pain in the lower back, the gluteal region, and the lower limb, careful manual palpation of the lower back area from T12 to S4 is always necessary because the paravertebral points from T12 to S4 should be selected for needling together with the SAs in the gluteal and lower limb regions.

Thigh muscles are large and the nerve trunks run deeply below these muscles; therefore only one homeostatic acupoint (HA), H18 iliotibial, is formed on the iliotibial band. However, when treating patients with pain or other disorders of the back, gluteal region, hip, knee, or leg, careful palpation can reveal tender points on the adductor muscles, hamstrings, and anterior leg extensor muscles. These tender points should be located by palpation and properly treated by acupuncture needling.

The Gluteal Muscles The gluteal region is important for treating pain in the back, hip, and lower limb. Although there are only two HAs—H14 superior cluneal and H16 inferior gluteal—in this region, additional SAs will appear around these two HAs. Practitioners should be very familiar with the bony landmarks and surface markings of this region.

The iliac crest extends from the anterior superior iliac spine to the posterior superior iliac spine. Between the left and right posterior iliac spines is the posterior aspect of the sacrum. The spinous process of L4 vertebra is at the level of the summit of the posterior iliac crest. The spinous process of S2 is just between the left and right posterior superior iliac spine.

The gluteal muscles include (1) the three large glutei (gluteus maximus, medius, and minimus) and (2) four deeper small muscles (piriformis, obturator internus, gemelli, and quadratus femoris) (Figure 11-5). The three large glutei are extensors and abductors of the thigh at the hip joint and they also stabilize the pelvis. The small muscles are lateral rotators of the thigh at the hip joint and stabilize the femoral head in the acetabulum. Table 11-1 shows a summary of the muscles of the gluteal region.

The Thigh Muscles The large, powerful thigh muscles are organized into three groups: anterior, medial, and posterior. The three groups are separated by fascial intermuscular septa.

The Anterior Thigh Muscles (Flexor Group) The major muscles of the anterior group are iliopsoas, tensor fasciae latae, sartorius, and quadriceps femoris (Figure 11-6). They are accessible to acupuncture needling. Their anatomic function is summarized in Table 11-2.

The Medial Thigh Muscles (Adductor Group) The medial thigh muscles (the pectineus, adductor longus, adductor brevis, adductor magnus, gracilis, and obturator externus) are adductors of the thigh (Figure 11-7). All of these muscles are

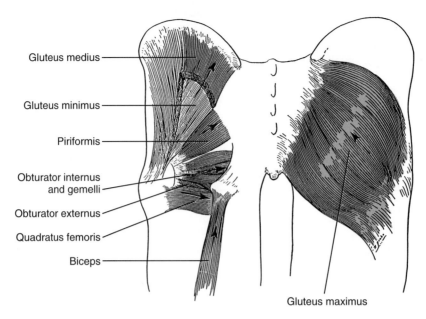

Figure 11-5 The gluteal muscles. (From Jenkins D: *Hollinshead's functional anatomy of the limbs and back,* ed 8, Philadelphia, 2002, WB Saunders, p 316.)

Table 11-1
The Muscles of the Gluteal Region

Muscle	Origin	Insertion	Actions	Innervation
Gluteus maximus	Lateral surface of ilium behind posterior gluteal line; dorsal sacroiliac and sacrotuberous ligament; dorsal surface of sacrum	Iliotibial tract; gluteal tuberosity of femur	Extension, external rotation, abduction (upper fibers), and adduction of thigh (lower fibers)	Inferior gluteal nerve (L5, S1 and S2)
Gluteus medius	Lateral surface of ilium between anterior and posterior gluteus lines	Greater trochanter of femur	Abduction and medial rotation of thigh	Superior gluteal nerve (L5 and S1)
Gluteus minimus	Lateral surface of ilium between anterior and inferior gluteus lines	Greater trochanter of femur	Abduction and medial rotation of thigh	Superior gluteal nerve (L5 and S1)
Piriformis	Anterior surface of sacrum and sacrotuberous ligament	Greater trochanter of femur	Lateral rotation, extension and abduction (when flexed) of thigh	Ventral rami of S1 and S2
Obturator internus	Pelvic surface of obturator membrane and surrounding bones	Medial surface of greater trochanter of femur	Lateral rotation, extension and abduction (when flexed) of thigh	Ventral rami of L5 and S1
Gemelli superior and inferior	*Sup:* ischial spine *Inf:* ischial tuberosity	Medial surface of greater trochanter of femur	Lateral rotation, extension and abduction (when flexed) of thigh	Ventral rami of L5 and S1
Quadratus femoris	Ischial tuberosity	Posterior surface of femur between greater trochanter and lesser trochanter	Lateral rotation	Ventral rami of L5 and S1

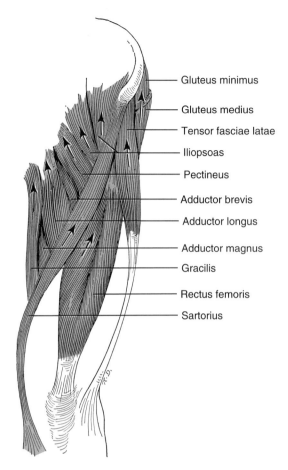

Gluteus minimus

Gluteus medius

Tensor fasciae latae

Iliopsoas

Pectineus

Adductor brevis

Adductor longus

Adductor magnus

Gracilis

Rectus femoris

Sartorius

Figure 11-6   Anterior thigh muscles (flexors). (From Jenkins D: *Hollinshead's functional anatomy of the limbs and back,* ed 8, Philadelphia, 2002, WB Saunders, p 317.)

supplied by the obturator nerve (L2, L3, and L4) except pectineus, which is supplied by the femoral nerve (L2 and L3). The "hamstring" part of the adductor magnus is supplied by the sciatic nerve (L4).

The Posterior Thigh Muscles (The Hamstrings)   Three large muscles (semitendinosus, semimembranosus, and biceps femoris) of the posterior aspect are collectively known as the hamstring muscles (Figure 11-8). These muscles have the same origin on the ischial tuberosity, but the short head of the biceps femoris has an additional origin on the shaft of the femur. These long muscles extend from the hip joint and across the knee joint so they are all extensors of the thigh and flexors of the leg. In addition, they are all supplied by the same sciatic nerve.

Tight hamstring muscles can cause gluteal and back problems because the hamstrings restrict spinal flexion.

The topography of the three groups of thigh muscles is shown in Figure 11-9.

Adductor Muscle Strain   Adductor muscle strain is a common muscle problem that is often overlooked by both healthcare practitioners and patients. Ninety percent of patients with lower back or thigh pain have strained adductor muscles.

When treating patients with lower back disorder or pain of the lower limb, adductor muscles should be palpated and their tender acupoints should be needled.

The Leg Muscles   Anatomically and functionally the leg muscles are divided into three compartments by (1) the tibia, the fibula, and the interosseous membrane between them and (2) the anterior and posterior crural intermuscular septa (Figure 11-10): the anterior, lateral, and posterior. The muscles in the same compartment perform similar functions and share the same nerve and blood supply.

The *anterior* compartment is between the tibia and the anterior crural septum. The muscles of this compartment function as extensors of the toes and effect dorsiflexion of the ankle joint (Figure 11-11).

The *lateral* compartment is surrounded by the lateral aspect of the fibula and anterior and posterior crural intermuscular septa. The two muscles in this compartment are responsible for plantar flexion and eversion of the foot (Figure 11-12).

The *posterior* compartment contains both superficial and deep muscles (Figure 11-13). The three powerful superficial calf muscles affect plantar flexion of the foot. These large muscles support and move the weight of the body. Four smaller deep muscles of the posterior compartment act on the knee joint (popliteus) and ankle and foot joints. These four smaller muscles are not important in acupuncture therapy and therefore are not listed in Table 11-3.

Nerves of Clinical Importance

The Superior Cluneal Nerves   The superior cluneal nerves are branches of the dorsal rami of L1, L2, and L3. They emerge from the deep fascia just superior to the iliac crest and innervate the skin on the superior two thirds of the gluteal region (buttocks). An important homeostatic acupoint, H14 superior cluneal, is formed at the location where the nerves penetrate the deep fascia. Most patients feel tenderness or even pain upon palpation at H14.

■	**Table 11-2** **The Thigh Muscles**			

Muscle	Origin	Insertion	Actions	Innervation
Anterior Muscles				
Iliopsoas				
Psoas major	Body sides of T12 to L5	Lesser trochanter of femur	Flexion of thigh	L1, L2, and L3
Iliacus	Iliac fossa	Lesser trochanter of femur	Flexion of thigh	L2 and L3
Tensor fasciae latae	Anterior superior iliac spine and superior part of external lip of iliac crest	Iliotibial tract that attaches to lateral condyle of tibia	Abduction, mediosuperior rotation, and flexion of the thigh	Gluteal L4 and L5
Sartorius	Anterior superior iliac spine	Superior part of medial surface of tibia	Flexion, abduction, and lateral rotation of thigh at hip joint; flexion of leg	Femoral nerve L2 and L3
Quadriceps femoris		Common insertion of quadriceps femoris	Common action	
Rectus femoris	Anterior inferior iliac spine and groove superior to acetabulum			
Vastus lateralis	Great trochanter and lateral lip of linea aspera of femur	Base of patella and via patella ligament to tibial tuberosity	Extension of leg at knee joint	Femoral nerve L2, L3, and L4
Vastus medialis	Intertrochanteric line and medial lip of linea aspera of femur			
Vastus intermedius	Anterior and lateral surface of body of femur			
Medial Muscles (Adductor Group)				
Pectineus	Pectineal line of pubis	Pectineal line of femur	Adduction and flexion of thigh	Femoral nerve L2 and L3
Adductor longus	Pubic tubercle	Middle third of linea aspera of femur	Adduction of thigh	Obturator nerve L2, L3, and L4
Adductor brevis	Body and inferior ramus of pubis	Pectineal line and proximal part of linea aspera of femur	Adduction of thigh	Obturator nerve L2, L3, and L4
Adductor magnus	Inferior ramus of pubis, ramus of ischium, and ischial tuberosity	Linea aspera (anterior fibers), adductor tubercle of femur posterior fibers	Adduction and flexion of thigh, (hamstring part) extension of thigh	*Adductor part:* obturator nerve: L2 and L3; *hamstring part:* tibial portion of sciatic nerve (L4)
Gracilis	Body and inferior ramus of pubis	Superior part of medial surface of tibia	Adduction of thigh, flexion and medial rotation of leg	Obturator nerve L2 and L3

Table 11-2
The Thigh Muscles—cont'd

Muscle	Origin	Insertion	Actions	Innervation
Obturator externus	Margins of obturator foramen and obturator membrane	Trochanteric fossa of femur	Lateral rotation of thigh	Obturator nerve L3 and L4
Posterior Muscles (The Hamstrings)				
Semitendinosus	Ischial tuberosity	Medial surface of proximal part of tibia	Extension of thigh, flexion and medial rotation of leg, extension of trunk	Tibial division of sciatic nerve L5, S1, and S2
Semimembra-nosus	Same as above	Posterior part of medial condyle of tibia		
Biceps femoris	*Long head:* ischial tuberosity *Short head:* linea aspera and lateral supracondylar line	Lateral side of head of fibula	Flexion of leg, lateral rotation of leg	Sciatic nerve L5, S1, and S2

In patients with chronic lower back or leg pain, the pain may spread over the entire skin area that is supplied by the superior cluneal nerves. In such cases, H14 and adjacent areas should be needled together.

The Inferior Gluteal Nerve

The inferior gluteal nerve branches from the ventral rami of L5, S1, and S2. This nerve leaves the pelvis from the greater sciatic foramen. Accompanying the inferior gluteal artery, the inferior gluteal nerve supplies the gluteus maximus muscle. The motor point, where the inferior gluteal nerve enters the gluteus maximus muscle, is the important HA H16 inferior gluteal. This point is formed deep below the thick gluteus maximus and should be palpated carefully.

The Sciatic Nerve and Its Terminal Branches: the Tibial, Common Fibular (Peroneal), and Sural Nerves   We have discussed this nerve in Chapter 5 and here we emphasize its relation to HAs and pain in the lower limb. The sciatic nerve is the largest nerve in the body. The ventral rami of L4, L5, S1, S2, and S3 converge at the inferior border of the piriformis muscle to form the sciatic nerve (Figure 11-14). Structurally the sciatic nerve consists of two nerves: the tibial and the common fibular (peroneal) nerve. The sciatic nerve leaves the pelvis through the greater sciatic foramen of the hip bone and enters the gluteal region inferior to the piriformis muscle (Figure 11-15). It runs deep below the gluteus maximus muscle, and does not supply any structure there. The sciatic nerve continues down the thigh covered by the hamstring muscles and ends in the lower third of the thigh, at which point the tibial and the common fibular (peroneal) nerves separate from each other.

The tibial nerve, the larger medial branch, descends through the center of the popliteal fossa and sends three articular branches to the knee joint. In the popliteal fossa, acupoint H11 lateral/medial popliteal is palpable. Tender acupoint H11 appears either laterally or medially in different patients. The relationship between H11 and the tibial or fibular nerves is not clear yet.

In the leg region, the tibial nerve supplies the gastrocnemius, plantaris, popliteus, and soleus muscles. In the lower medial aspect of the tibia, the tibial nerve runs very close to the skin, and about 5 to 8 cm above the medial malleolus it forms an important HA, H6 tibial. From this HA, the tibial nerve continues to descend to the plantar aspect of the foot and divides into two branches, the medial and lateral plantar nerve.

The common fibular (peroneal) nerve arises from the sciatic nerve just above the popliteal fossa as a lateral branch. It descends to the lateral aspect of the leg and winds around the lateral surface of the head of the fibula where acupoint H24 common

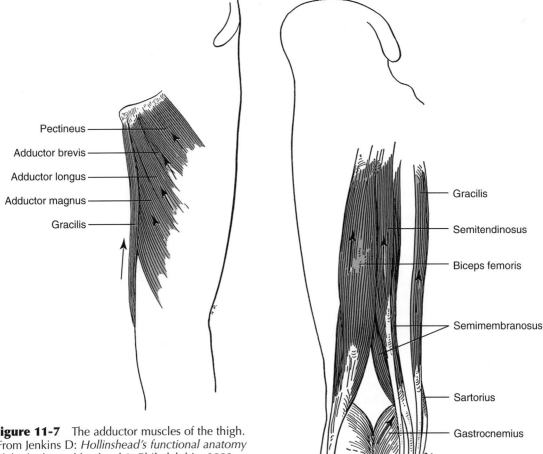

Figure 11-7   The adductor muscles of the thigh. (From Jenkins D: *Hollinshead's functional anatomy of the limbs and back,* ed 8, Philadelphia, 2002, WB Saunders, p 318.)

Figure 11-8   The hamstrings: the flexors of the leg. (From Jenkins D: *Hollinshead's functional anatomy of the limbs and back,* ed 8, Philadelphia, 2002, WB Saunders, p 320.)

fibular (peroneal) is formed. The common fibular (peroneal) nerve enters the lateral compartment of the leg and divides into two cutaneous branches: the superficial and the deep fibular (peroneal) nerves. The superficial fibular (peroneal) nerve innervates the anterior aspect of the skin in the lower leg and ankle area. The deep fibular (peroneal) nerve descends down to the foot and becomes the cutaneous nerve at a point approximately 2 cm proximal to the web between the great and second toes. Here acupoint H5 deep fibular (peroneal) is formed.

In the upper region of the leg, both the tibial and the common peroneal nerve send branches to unite and form the sural nerve, which runs down to the lateral side of the leg through the lateral Achilles tendon all the way to the little toe. Acupoint H10 sural is formed between the two bellies of the gastrocnemius muscle.

Femoral and Saphenous Nerve   The femoral nerve is the largest nerve formed in the abdomen by the branches of the lumbar plexus (L2, L3, and L4) (Figure 11-16). In the thigh area, the femoral nerve gives off muscular branches to supply the anterior thigh muscles. When affected by injury or overuse, these muscles become tender or painful and form SAs.

The cutaneous branch of the femoral nerve, called the saphenous nerve, runs down to the medial aspect of the knee. It passes anteroinferiorly to supply the skin of the anterior and medial aspect of the knee, leg, and foot. As the saphenous nerve pierces the deep fascia on the medial side of the

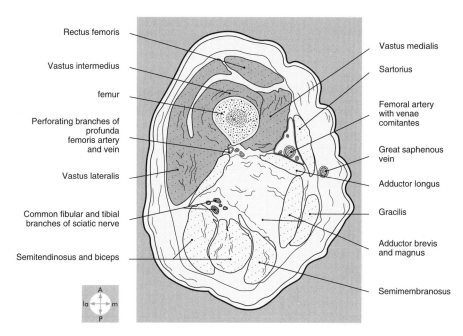

Figure 11-9   Transverse section through the thigh to show the topography of the three groups of thigh muscles. (From Gosling J, Harris P, Whitmore I, Willan P: *Human anatomy: color atlas and text,* ed 4, Edinburgh, 2002, Mosby, p 233.)

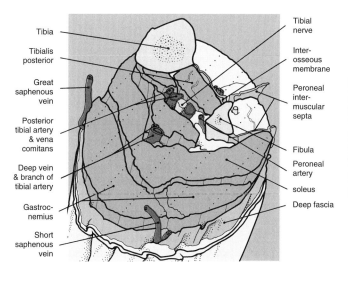

Figure 11-10   Transverse section of the leg to show the three compartments of the leg muscles. Please note that the "small" lateral compartment is surrounded by the fibula and two intermuscular septa. (From Gosling J, Harris P, Whitmore I, Willan P: *Human anatomy: color atlas and text,* ed 4, Edinburgh, 2002, Mosby, p 247.)

knee just below the medial condyle of the tibia, an important HA, H4 saphenous, is formed. You may remember that H4 saphenous and H1 deep radial are used as diagnostic acupoints for quantitative evaluation of acupuncture patients.

Obturator Nerve   The obturator nerve is derived from the same spinal segments as the femoral

nerve (L2, L3, and L4). The obturator nerve leaves the pelvis through the obturator foramen and enters the thigh to supply the adductor muscles (Figure 11-17).

The adductor muscles are involved in many painful conditions of the thigh, especially in athletic persons, but are often ignored by healthcare professionals. Whenever treating patients with leg

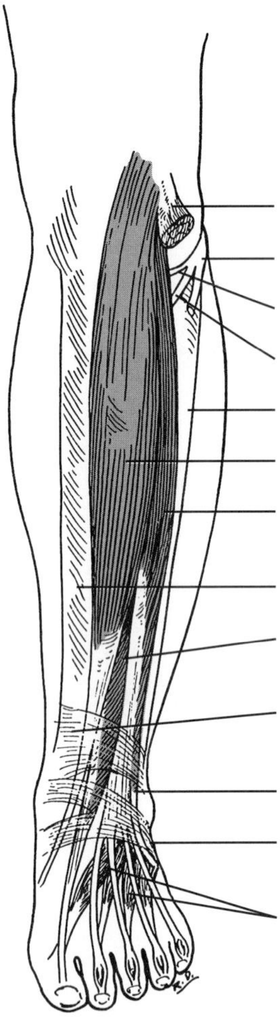
Fibularis longus (cut)
Common fibular n.
Articular branch
Deep fibular n.
Fibula
Tibialis anterior
Extensor digitorum longus
Tibia
Extensor hallucis longus
Superior extensor retinaculum
Fibularis tertius
Inferior extensor retinaculum
Extensor hallucis brevis and extensor digitorum brevis

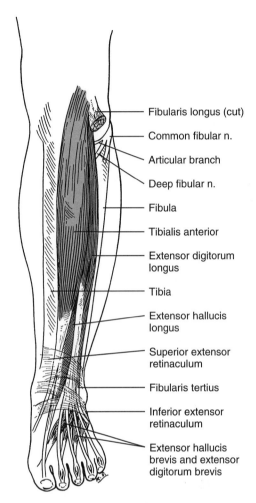

Figure 11-11 The anterior muscles of the leg. (From Jenkins D: *Hollinshead's functional anatomy of the limbs and back,* ed 8, Philadelphia, 2002, WB Saunders, p 339.)

pain, particularly pain in the hamstring muscles, the adductor muscles should be carefully palpated and the tender points in the adductor muscles should be needled.

Joints of the Hip and Lower Limb

The joints of the lower limb include the joints of hip bones, hip joint, knee, and ankle. The discussion of the lower limb joints is limited to how the structure and biomechanics of the joints are relevant to acupuncture therapy.

The Hip Joint The human hip joint is a well-constructed multiaxial joint that has the function of bearing weight, maintaining posture, and facilitating walking. The hip joint is a closely fitting ball-and-socket synovial joint in which the globular head of the femur articulates with the cup-like acetabulum of the hip bone (see Figure 11-1). However, the movement of the femur is limited by the close articular surfaces and strong ligaments of the hip joint. In the case of the shoulder, dislocation of the joints will occur if they are not stabilized by the surrounding muscles. In contrast, the hip joint is able to support the body weight on the head of the femur with little or no muscular energy.

The head of the femur is completely covered by articular cartilage except its small central recess (called fovea). In the acetabulum, only the weight-bearing part of the surface of the ilium, the lunate articular surface, is covered by cartilage.

The joints are enclosed and strengthened by a thick fibrous capsule and ligaments that come from different directions. The ligaments are named according to their anatomic origin: iliofemoral, pubofemoral, and ischiofemoral.

The hip joint permits flexion-extension, abduction-adduction, lateral and medial rotation, and circumduction. Functionally the flexor group and abductor group are the most important muscles in our daily activities. When we walk, for example, the left flexors of the hip raise the thigh as it is swung forward during the gait cycle, while the right abductors stabilize the pelvis during the time that the body is supported only on the right leg.

Understanding the nerve supply to the hip joint helps us to treat the nerve(s) associated with hip pain (Table 11-4). The articular branches of the femoral nerve supply the anterior part of the joint capsule and the iliofemoral ligament. The obturator nerve sends branches to the anteroinferior part of the joint and the medial portion of the capsule. The superolateral aspect of the capsule is innervated by the superior gluteal nerve. The sciatic nerve is believed to supply the posterior portion of the capsule.

General Considerations of Hip Pain Pathology Hip pain and limping are the chief complaints presented by patients in an acupuncture clinic.

Hip joints sustain enormous stress in daily activities such as walking. For example, during walking, when the left limb is lifted, the right hip joint is subjected to compression forces several times greater than the body weight (Figure 11-18). A person does not feel this huge force of compression because there are no nerves in the articular cartilage. When the cartilage is eroded by degenerative disease or aging, the bony head of the

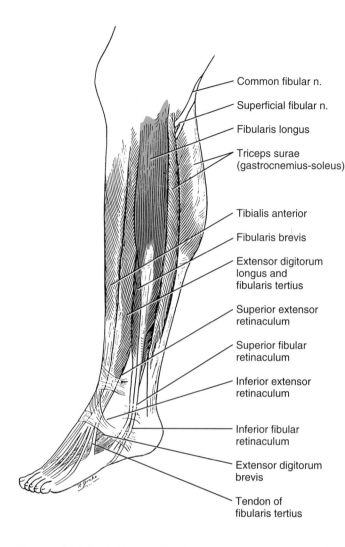

Common fibular n.

Superficial fibular n.

Fibularis longus

Triceps surae
(gastrocnemius-soleus)

Tibialis anterior

Fibularis brevis

Extensor digitorum
longus and
fibularis tertius

Superior extensor
retinaculum

Superior fibular
retinaculum

Inferior extensor
retinaculum

Inferior fibular
retinaculum

Extensor digitorum
brevis

Tendon of
fibularis tertius

Figure 11-12 The lateral muscles of the leg. (From Jenkins D: *Hollinshead's functional anatomy of the limbs and back,* ed 8, Philadelphia, 2002, WB Saunders, p 338.)

femur, which is richly supplied by sensory nerves, produces pain during every step because of this compression force. As a person ages, the articular cartilage becomes thinner and hip pain may gradually develop.

Inflammation of the capsule and/or the ligaments is the major source of hip pain. Soft tissue inflammation of the hip joint is caused by the following conditions:

- Weak or injured muscles put the capsule and ligaments under tension from mechanical forces such as the compression described above
- Trauma or repetitive overuse directly impairs the capsule or ligaments
- Joint diseases such as arthritis or bone infection (osteromyelitis) may develop within the femoral head or neck

Usually hip pain is felt in the groin region, or the pain may be referred to the medial side of the thigh supplied by the obturator nerve. Some hip problems are only felt as knee pain.

If afferent nerves of other organs also originate from lumbar segments of the spinal cord, these organs, if diseased, can refer pain to the hip joint. Such referred pain usually appears in the gluteal region and radiates down the back of the thigh.

Blockage of the internal iliac artery in the pelvis results in ischemia of the gluteal muscles and may cause pain in the buttocks during walking or running (intermittent claudication).

A limp without pain is usually caused by mechanical abnormalities such as a shortened leg, muscle contracture, or muscle paralysis. Careful palpation of the hip, thigh, and leg of the affected limb will reveal that the muscles harbor some tender points. Needling of these tender points relaxes

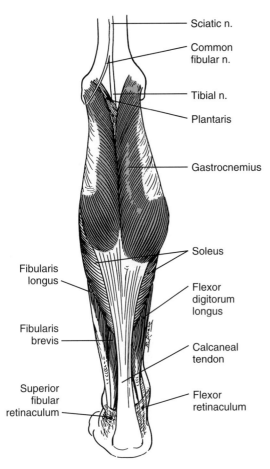

Figure 11-13 The posterior muscles of the leg. (From Jenkins D: *Hollinshead's functional anatomy of the limbs and back,* ed 8, Philadelphia, 2002, WB Saunders, p 333.)

the shortened muscles and helps improve the discrepancy between the two legs.

Trochanteric Bursitis (Iliotibial Band Syndrome) The iliotibial band (IT band) is a sheet of specialized fascia extending from the iliac crest to the lateral plateau of the tibia. In the region just over the greater trochanter the IT band is separated from the bone by a bursa. The hip abductor (tensor fascia lata) and the extensor (gluteus maximus) insert into the fascia. During the gait cycle, both muscles exert a great tensile force on the IT band and the bone below. This tension can cause inflammation of the bursa (bursitis) between the IT band and the greater trochanter.

In some cases, trochanteric bursitis is caused by an imbalance of the muscles. For example, tight abductor muscles of the right thigh may cause the pelvis to tilt to the right and cause the left iliac crest

to be higher than normal. This results in a tightened fascia lata stretching over the left greater trochanter and leads to bursitis.

The pain pattern may vary from patient to patient. The common feature is the tenderness over the bursa. A patient may have such severe pain that he or she is not able to lie on the affected side or sit comfortably. Usually the patient feels pain during activity. The pain can be local, right over the greater trochanter, in the iliac crest, or in the knee region.

Some trochanteric bursitis can be treated very effectively by acupuncture because needling relaxes muscles, activates local antiinflammatory reaction, and encourages tissue regeneration. The muscles and IT bands on both sides of the body should be carefully palpated and the tender points should be needled. In addition, the lower back muscles should be examined and needled to ensure the balanced alignment of the pelvis.

Meralgia Paresthetica (Neuralgia of the Lateral Femoral Cutaneous Nerve) The lateral femoral cutaneous nerve supplies the skin of the lateral thigh. Injury to this nerve causes numbness, hyperesthesia (increased sensitivity to stimuli), and hypoesthesia (decreased sensitivity to stimuli, particularly to touch).

In general, symptoms of numbness are more resistant to acupuncture therapy than symptoms of pain. However, acupuncture helps patients with meralgia paresthetica. We believe that acupuncture needling improves nutrition and oxygen supply to the skin and this may slow down the process of tissue degeneration.

Piriformis Syndrome The symptoms of piriformis syndrome include sciatica and deep pain in the buttocks, especially pain elicited by flexion, adduction, and internal rotation of the thigh.

The exact cause underlying the piriformis syndrome is unknown, but many healthcare professionals believe that the piriformis muscle compresses the sciatic nerve where the nerve passes under or through the belly of the piriformis muscle.[1]

We have successfully treated patients who were diagnosed with piriformis syndrome by medical doctors. The most important acupoint is H16 inferior gluteal because it is just on top of the piriformis muscle. A long needle is needed to reach all the way down to the hip bone. This needling relaxes the piriformis muscle, improves blood supply to the muscle, and reduces inflammation (see Chapter 3).

Degenerative Arthritis Degenerative arthritis is the most common painful and disabling condition of the hip joint. It is generally believed that the pain is caused by (1) degenerative changes in

**Table 11-3
The Leg Muscles**

Muscle	Origin	Insertion	Actions	Innervation
Anterior Muscles (Extensor/Dorsiflexor Group)				
Tibialis anterior	Lateral condyle and superior half of lateral surface of tibia	Medial cuneiform, base of first metatarsal	Inversion and dorsiflexion of foot	Deep fibular (peroneal) nerve (L4 and L5)
Extensor hallucis longus	Middle third of anterior surface of fibula, interosseous membrane	Distal phalanx of great toe (hallux)	Extension of great toe and dorsiflexion of foot	All three muscles are supplied by deep fibular (peroneal) nerve (L5 and S1)
Extensor digitorum longus	Lateral condyle of tibia, superior ³/₄ of anterior surface of fibula, and interosseous membrane	Middle and distal phalanges of lateral four toes	Extension of four lateral toes and dorsiflexion of foot	All three muscles are supplied by deep fibular (peroneal) nerve (L5 and S1)
Fibularis (peroneous) tertius	Inferior ⅓ of anterior surface of fibula and interosseous membrane	Dorsal base of 5th metatarsal bone	Dorsiflexion and eversion of foot	All three muscles are supplied by deep fibular (peroneal) nerve (L5 and S1)
Lateral Muscles				
Fibularis (peroneus) longus	Head and superior ⅔ of lateral surface of fibula	Base of 1st metatarsal and medial cuneiform	Eversion and weak plantar flexion of foot	Both muscles are supplied by superficial fibular (peroneal) nerve (L5, S1, and S2)
Fibularis (peroneus) brevis	Inferior ⅔ of lateral surface of fibula	Dorsal surface of base of 5th metatarsal	Eversion and weak plantar flexion of foot	Both muscles are supplied by superficial fibular (peroneal) nerve (L5, S1, and S2)
Posterior Muscles				
Gastrocnemius	Posterior surface of femur proximal to medial and lateral condyles	All three muscles insert to calcaneus through tendocalcancus	Plantar flexion of foot, flexion of knee joint, heel raising during walking	All three muscles are supplied by tibial nerve (S1 and S2)
Soleus	Proximal ¼ of posterior fibula, posterior head of fibula, soleal line of tibia	All three muscles insert to calcaneus through tendocalcaneus	Plantar flexion of foot	All three muscles are supplied by tibial nerve (S1 and S2)
Plantaris	Lateral epicondyle of femur	All three muscles insert to calcaneus through tendocalcaneus	Weak plantar flexion of foot and weak flexion of knee joint	All three muscles are supplied by tibial nerve (S1 and S2)

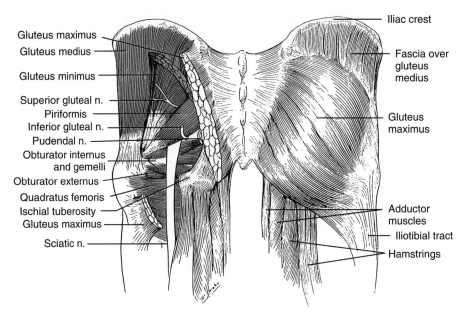

Figure 11-14 Sciatic nerve and the piriformis muscle. (From Jenkins D: *Hollinshead's functional anatomy of the limbs and back,* ed 8, Philadelphia, 2002, WB Saunders, p 300.)

the hip cartilage, causing the bone tissue to directly sustain the huge force of compression and (2) abnormal articular orientation between the head of the femur and the surface of the acetabulum. As noted in the above discussion of hip pathology, the acetabulum is only incompletely covered by cartilage, so the cartilaged surface of the head of the femur must articulate with the cartilaged surface of the acetabulum of the hip bone. During walking, if a person's knees come too close together or too far apart, the orientation of the head of the femur in the joints will change, resulting in hip pain because the heads of the femurs will articulate with the noncartilaged surface of the acetabulum.

Mechanical stress from excessive jogging or running, or repetitive impulsive compression, is believed to be a possible cause of later degenerative changes.

Needling can directly relax the muscles and other soft tissues such as fascia, capsule, or ligaments by breaking the contracture of the muscle fibers and the connective tissues. Thus, acupuncture helps to relax and desensitize the muscles and can reduce pain sensations and thus facilitate posture correction. Since needling is able to improve blood circulation and correct hypoxia, acupuncture also will slow down the degenerative process. However, if the hip pain is caused by damaged cartilage surfaces of the femur and/or acetabulum,

acupuncture needling is not effective in relieving the pain, but is still helpful in slowing down degeneration of the soft tissues such as muscles.

Stress Fracture Strictly speaking, a stress fracture is beyond the field of acupuncture therapy. However, patients with stress fracture, especially athletes, do come to acupuncture clinics for treatment and practitioners should understand the nature of this condition and be able to handle these patients correctly.

A stress fracture is an acute repetitive injury without dramatic trauma history. It is caused by fatigue of the bone during a repetitive activity such as running, or by osteoporosis in elderly patients. A stress fracture may occur in amenorrheic female athletes because of their diminished bone density. Stress fractures may occur in different portions of the lower limb, but the most common site for stress fracture in the hip area is the femoral neck. Stress fractures may be classified as incomplete or complete. Incomplete fractures may not be visible on radiographs and a bone scan or magnetic resonance imaging (MRI) is needed to confirm or rule out the condition.

The possibility of a stress fracture should always be considered if an athlete develops an acute hip problem such as a limp, stiffness in the hip or leg, or pain during weight-bearing or vigorous physical activities.

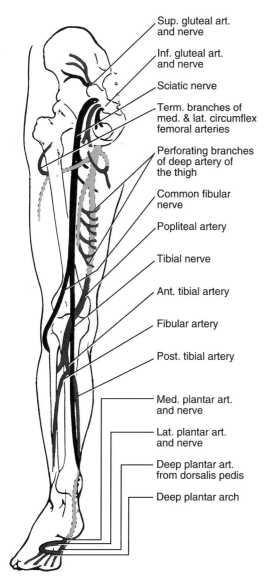

Sup. gluteal art.
and nerve

Inf. gluteal art.
and nerve

Sciatic nerve

Term. branches of
med. & lat. circumflex
femoral arteries

Perforating branches
of deep artery of
the thigh

Common fibular
nerve

Popliteal artery

Tibial nerve

Ant. tibial artery

Fibular artery

Post. tibial artery

Med. plantar art.
and nerve

Lat. plantar art.
and nerve

Deep plantar art.
from dorsalis pedis

Deep plantar arch

Figure 11-15 The distribution of the sciatic
nerve. (From Jenkins D: *Hollinshead's functional
anatomy of the limbs and back,* ed 8, Philadelphia,
2002, WB Saunders, p 259.)

In cases of stress fracture, acupuncture can be
used as a supplementary therapy to reduce muscle
and periosteum pain and to promote bone healing.

The Knee Joint Everyday activities such as
walking, climbing stairs, or rising from a chair, as
well as athletic exercises such as jumping and running, depend on the functional integrity of the muscles of the thigh, as well as on soft tissues such as

the capsules, ligaments, menisci, and articular cartilage of the knee.

Any diseases or trauma to the bone or soft tissues can significantly impair the knee's ability to
perform basic motions.

Knee pain is usually caused by:

- Degenerative changes resulting from musculoskeletal disorders
- Infections, inflammation
- Traumatic injuries from sports, automobile
  accidents, and accidental falls
- Referred pain from hip disorders, spinal
  stenosis, or other lumbosacral spinal disorders. In rare cases, the knee is also affected
  by primary or metastatic neoplasm

**The Two Joints and Three Articulation
Compartments of the Knee** The knee is the
largest joint in the body and consists of three
bones: the femur, tibia, and patella. The knee joint
proper is formed by two joints: the femorotibial
and the patellofemoral within the common cavity
(Figure 11-19). The joint complex consists of three
articulation compartments:

- The intermediate compartment between the
  patella and the femoral trochlea
- The medial compartment between the medial
  femoral condyle and the medial tibial plateau
- The lateral femoral condyle and the lateral
  tibial plateau

The articular surfaces are covered by cartilage.
The medial and lateral compartments are interposed by fibrocartilaginous menisci between the
articular surfaces. Disease processes or injury to
any of the three compartments will cause pain and
deficiency of function in the knee.

The patella is located within the quadriceps
tendon and enhances the extension force of the
quadriceps muscle. The patella and its surrounding
soft tissues, such as the patellar ligament and bursae, are often a source of knee pain. The quadriceps
muscle that is inserted in the patella has five bellies
(Table 11-5). Any injury to one of the five bellies will misalign the five extension forces exerted
on the patellar ligament and will cause knee pain.

All of the structures of the knee, including skin,
capsule, ligaments, muscles, and bursae, are innervated by the femoral and obturator nerves with a
contribution from the sciatic nerve.

The stability of the knee is maintained by ligaments, muscles, tendons, menisci, and the joint
capsule. The bony architecture of the knee depends

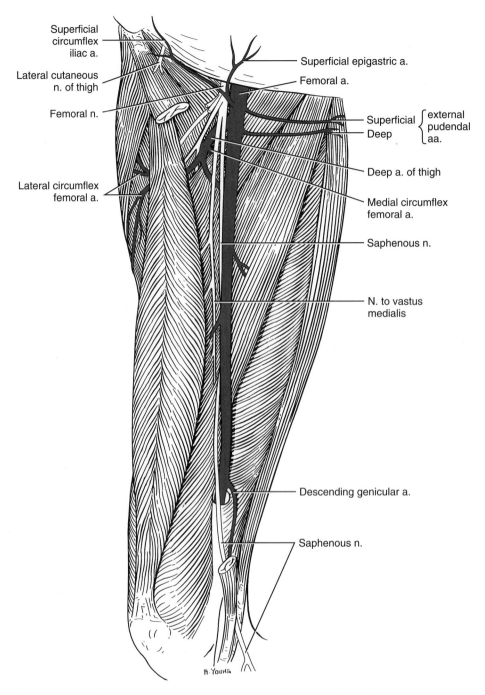

Figure 11-16 The femoral and saphenous nerves of the right thigh. (From Jenkins D: *Hollinshead's functional anatomy of the limbs and back,* ed 8, Philadelphia, 2002, WB Saunders, p 289.)

on the soft tissues for its stability, making the knee the most vulnerable structure in the body to soft tissue injury, and the resulting pain and functional impairment.

From the perspective of acupuncture therapy, this chapter focuses on knee pain caused by or related to soft tissues such as muscles, ligaments, the capsule, and bursae.

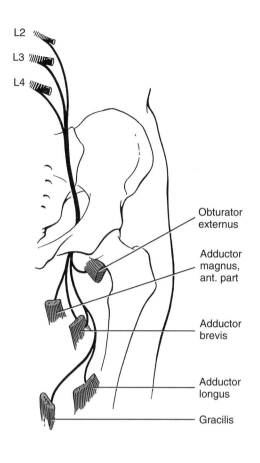

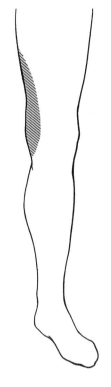

Obturator externus

Adductor magnus, ant. part

Adductor brevis

Adductor longus

Gracilis

Figure 11-17   The obturator nerve. (From Jenkins D: *Hollinshead's functional anatomy of the limbs and back,* ed 8, Philadelphia, 2002, WB Saunders, p 292.)

Table 11-4
Functional Muscle Groups of Hip Motion

Action Roots	Muscles	Innervation	Nerve
Flexors	Rectus femoris, iliopsoas	Femoral nerve	L2-L4
Extensors	Gluteus maximus, hamstrings	Inferior gluteal nerve and sciatic nerve	L5-S1
Abductors	Tensor fasciae latae, gluteus medius and minimus	Superior gluteal nerve	L5-S1
Adductors	Adductor magnus, longus, and brevis	Obturator nerve and sciatic nerve	L2 L4

Muscles Responsible for Knee Movement

The muscles and their functions are summarized in Table 11-5. The extensor quadriceps femoris is composed of four heads. The rectus femoris originates from the anterior iliac spine, and the other three heads come from the shaft of the femur. All of the muscles share the same tendon that attaches to the tibial tubercle.

The flexors of the knee originate from the ischial tuberosity and are all posterior thigh muscles. The semitendinosus muscle descends medially and joins the sartorius and gracilis muscles to

form a common tendon, which is joined by the semimembranosus. This common tendon, the pes anserinus, moves the medial meniscus.

When treating knee pain, these muscles together with the thigh abductor and adductor muscles should be carefully palpated to find the SAs.

The muscles are the most dynamic elements among the possible causes of knee pain. They are the movers of the knee joint and are indispensable components of the knee, and thus they are liable to injuries from repetitive motion or stress due to overuse. Our experience in treating knee pain

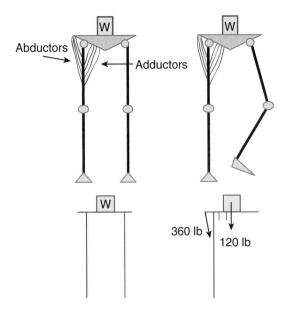

Figure 11-18   The mechanics of the hip abductors. During walking when one leg is lefted, the hip abductors need to exert force at least 3 times more than the body weight to maintain body balance. (Redrawn after Cornelius Rosse: *Hollinshead's textbook of anatomy*, Philadelphia, 1997, Lippincott-Raven.)

shows that most of the pain that is related to soft tissue injuries derives from disorders of the muscle, unless the pain is caused directly by physical trauma to the knee joint. If the muscles are tired or injured, they become tight and resistant to further motion. If they are forced to move under such conditions, it causes overstretching of other soft tissues of the knee such as the ligaments, capsule, bursae, and meniscus, which results in soft tissue inflammation.

If knee problems such as arthritis, infection, or physical trauma are the primary causes of knee pain, they will cause muscle pain because (1) chemical stimuli originate from the diseases and (2) diseased joints and inflamed soft tissues prevent or inhibit the normal coordination of the movement of the muscles, which soon causes fatigue in the muscles.

In acupuncture practice, careful palpation of the muscles and proper needling will help to locate and dissolve muscle tender points by relaxing the muscles, removing the mechanical and chemical stress from the knee structures, and providing a physiologic healing environment with the increased nutrition and supply of oxygen that comes from

improved circulation. Acupuncture treatments will help heal some knee disorders regardless of whether the pain is caused by injury to the knee or by a muscular disorder.

Four ligaments play essential roles in stabilizing the knee joint. The inner layer of the medial collateral ligament (MCL) connects with the medial meniscus and the capsule. The MCL prevents valgus rotation (bending or twisting medially at the joint). The lateral collateral ligament (LCL) passes the lateral epicondyle of the femur to the fibular head. The LCL has no connection with the lateral meniscus but receives fibers from other adjacent ligaments to strengthen the knee laterally.

The two cruciate ligaments are named according to their attachment to the tibia. The anterior cruciate ligament (ACL) originates from the anterior tibial plateau and runs upward and backward to attach to the medial aspect of the lateral femoral condyle. The ACL prevents anterior translation (shear) motion of the tibia on the femur. The stronger posterior cruciate ligament (PCL) runs behind the ACL from the posterior tibial plateau to the anterior part of the lateral surface of the medial condyle of the femur. The PCL restrains posterior translation (shear) motion of the tibia on the femur. The two cruciate ligaments together restrict excessive rotation of the leg.

Of the four ligaments, the MCL is the one most often injured during sports-related activities. The medial meniscus is also vulnerable to mechanical injury as it attaches to the MCL. In the early phases of this type of injury, a patient may feel knee weakness rather than pain. Tender areas can be palpated in the MCL area. Needling this ligament and the painful muscles associated with the injury improves blood circulation and reduces inflammation, thus relieving tenderness and pain, but recovery of function may take longer because the healing of ligament tissue is much slower than that of muscles. The LCL, ACL, PCL, joint cartilage, and joint capsule may also be damaged. Injuries to the LCL are less common but more threatening because they may cause damage to the fibular (peroneal) nerve.

Patients should be referred to specialists for further medical evaluation if severe tearing of the ligaments or meniscus is suspected.

Bursae of the Knee   The knee joint has several bursae to minimize the friction that occurs wherever skin, muscle, or tendon rub against the bone. Inflamed or swollen bursae are frequently the source of knee pain, and acupuncture practitioners should be sure to know the locations of the most important bursae for this reason.

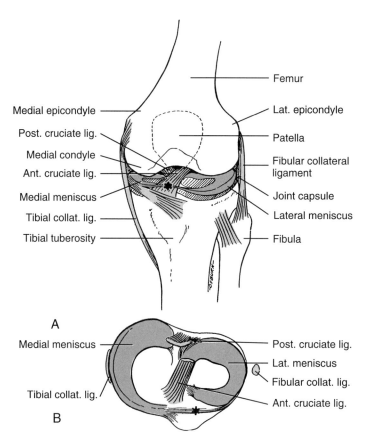

Medial epicondyle
Post. cruciate lig.
Medial condyle
Ant. cruciate lig.
Medial meniscus
Tibial collat. lig.
Tibial tuberosity

Femur
Lat. epicondyle
Patella
Fibular collateral ligament
Joint capsule
Lateral meniscus
Fibula

A

Medial meniscus

Tibial collat. lig.

B

Post. cruciate lig.
Lat. meniscus
Fibular collat. lig.
Ant. cruciate lig.

Figure 11-19   The principal structure of the interior of the knee joint. From front **(A)** and from above **(B)** with the femur removed. Menisci are shown in dark. A transverse ligament (marked with*) may be present, attaching to both the medial and lateral menisci. (From Jenkins D: *Hollinshead's functional anatomy of the limbs and back,* ed 8, Philadelphia, 2002, WB Saunders, p 277.)

Table 11-5
Functional Muscle Groups for Movement of the Knee and Leg

Action Roots	Muscles	Innervation	Nerve
Extensors (five bellies)	Rectus femoris		
	Vastus medialis, intermedius, lateralis, and medialis obliquus sartorius	Femoral nerve	L2, L3, and L4
Leg flexion	Semitendinosus	Sciatic (tibial)	L5, S1, and S2
	Semimembranosus	Sciatic (tibial)	L5 and S1
	Biceps femoris (long head)	Sciatic (tibial)	L5, S1, and S2
	Biceps femoris (short head)	Sciatic (fibular)	S1, S2, and S3
	Gracilis	Obturator	L2 and L3
	Gastrocnemius	Sciatic (tibial)	S1 and S2
Medial rotators	Semitendinosus	Sciatic (tibial)	L5, S1, and S2
	Semimembranosus	Sciatic (tibial)	L5 and S1
	Sartorius	Femoral	L2, L3, and L4
	Gracilis	Obturator	L2-L5
Lateral rotators	Biceps femoris	Tibial	L4, L5, and S1
	Popliteus	Tibial	S2 and S3

There are four bursae anterior to the knee:

- The large subcutaneous *prepatellar* bursa between the skin and the patella
- The *deep infrapatellar* bursa between the patellar ligament and the upper part of the tibia
- The *superficial infrapatellar* bursa between the lower part of the tuberosity of the tibia and the skin
- The huge *suprapatellar* bursa (a hand's breadth in size) sandwiched between the anterior surface of the distal femur and the quadriceps muscle

There are five bursae on the medial aspect between the tendons and the muscles. Four bursae are located on the lateral aspect between the tendons and the muscles. Two posterior bursae are associated with the tendons of the posterior muscles of the posterior knee. All of these bursae may contribute to knee pain if irritated or inflamed.

Acupuncture needling into the bursae relaxes the muscles that sandwich the bursa and improves blood circulation to the muscles and bursa, which helps to reduce inflammation, swelling, and pain. If the patient is suffering from an infectious disease, needling the joint should be avoided to prevent spreading the infection. In such a case, needling the thigh and leg muscles and HAs in other parts of the body should be done to control the immune system and bring the local infection under control.

Anterior Knee Pain   Anterior knee pain, or the pain in the patellofemoral articulation, is one of the most prevalent types of knee pain. Usually it is caused by degeneration of the cartilage of the patella, but it also happens that disorders of the quadriceps muscle can break the coordination among its five bellies during extension and cause misalignment of the patella, producing pain.

Patellar tendinitis is a common symptom of anterior knee pain. It is usually an overuse injury caused by repetitive motions such as running, jumping, and climbing in sports such as basketball, tennis, soccer, and weightlifting.

Acupuncture needling relaxes the muscles, increases blood circulation, and reduces the inflammation and swelling of the muscles, ligament, capsule, and bursae, which help to restore the normal function of patellofemoral articulation. After the stresses of swelling and inflammation are removed, the degeneration process will slow down and partial or even complete recovery of function can be expected, depending on the extent to which the causes of the pain are inherently healable.

The Ankle Joint (Talocrural Joint)   The ankle joint articulates the leg with the foot. The ankle comprises three bones and two articulations. The distal ends of the tibia and fibula form the tibiofibular joint. The inferior ends of the tibia and fibula articulate with the superior part of the talus and form the ankle or talocrural joint (Figure 11-20). The foot itself consists of numerous joints of different types among its 26 bones, the description of which is beyond the scope of this book.

From the perspective of acupuncture therapy, this chapter focuses on pain associated with soft tissues such as collateral ligaments, the calcaneous tendon, and plantar fascia.

The ankle joint is supported by the strong medial and weak lateral collateral ligaments. The MCL is known as the deltoid ligament. Superiorly the ligament attaches to the margin and tip of the medial malleolus. It fans out downward in a delta shape and its broad base attaches from the navicular bone anteriorly to the talus and calcaneus posteriorly. The lateral collateral ligaments consist of three discrete bands that attach the lateral malleolus to the talus and calcaneus: the anterior and posterior talofibular ligaments, and between these two short ligaments—a long, cordlike calcaneofibular ligament (Figure 11-21).

Of the three lateral collateral ligaments, the anterior talofibular ligament is the weakest ligament,

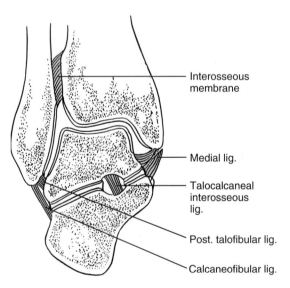

Figure 11-20   Frontal section through the ankle and subtalar joints. Ligaments and interosseous membrane are illustrated. (From Jenkins D: *Hollinshead's functional anatomy of the limbs and back,* ed 8, Philadelphia, 2002, WB Saunders, p 357.)

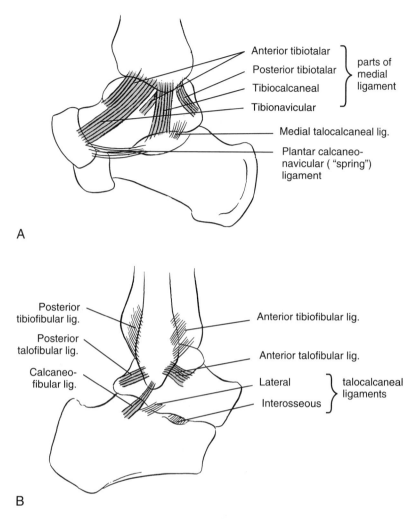

Figure 11-21 Diagram of the ligaments of the ankle and subtalar joints in medial and lateral views. (From Jenkins D: *Hollinshead's functional anatomy of the limbs and back,* ed 8, Philadelphia, 2002, WB Saunders, p 358.)

and the most commonly injured. Ligament injuries are discussed later in this chapter.

Ankle Strains Ankle strains are among the most common injuries to the ankle joint, both from daily activities and from sports like basketball and volleyball. Most ankle strains are caused by excessive inversion and the injury varies from a simple ligament strain (mere elongation of the ligaments with microtrauma) to a major injury with a severe or even complete tear of the ligamentous fibers.

The tibia and fibula are closely joined together by the tibiofibular ligament. The trochlea of the talus is tightly fitted into the space (called the mortise) between the medial malleolus of the tibia and the lateral malleolus of the fibula. During an accident, the excessive force of the inversion created by

the tilted talus will strain or break the tibiofibular ligament and lateral collateral ligaments, especially the anterior talofibular ligament, which is the weakest of the three lateral collateral ligaments. Medially the tilted talus may violently impact the medial malleolus and cause a malleolar fracture.

When an ankle strain occurs, a person feels a sudden sharp pain. This initial pain may soon subside, so that the person may not seek immediate treatment, but if it is possible to apply acupuncture treatment immediately after the injury, the inflammation reaction can be effectively controlled and the healing process is greatly quickened. In the first 6 to 12 hours after injury the ankle gradually becomes swollen and tender points or areas appear on both lateral and medial aspects. Bruising (ecchymosis) also develops in the foot and the lower leg. The patient is then no longer able to perform activities such as running or to bear normal weight on the injured ankle.

When treating ankle sprain, a practitioner should carefully palpate the ankle area, especially the surfaces above the medial and lateral collateral ligaments. Then the practitioner should palpate the entire foot and leg to find the locations of the injured soft tissues. The ankle is a weight-bearing structure, so if the soft tissues of the ankle, such as ligaments or the interosseous membrane, are injured, pain will radiate to the leg muscles and sometimes to the thigh muscles. The swelling and inflammation will spread from the injured ankle to the distal part of the foot and the muscles of the leg.

To reduce pain and heal the injured tissues, the swelling and inflammation should be controlled first. For this purpose, all the injured and affected regions where tender areas are palpable should be needled simultaneously: ankle, foot, leg, and thigh. Usually swelling and inflammation can be brought under control within hours or 1 to 2 days in acute cases.

If severe tears are suspected, a patient should be referred immediately to specialists for further medical examination.

Rupture of the Calcaneal Tendon (Achilles Tendinitis)   Rupture of the calcaneal tendon is often caused by excessive stress on the calf muscles. After overuse caused by repetitive activities such as running or jumping, the calf muscles become fatigued and weak, and tender points develop around acupoint H10 sural. Physiologically the calf muscles start to resist any contraction or relaxation. If the person continues to use the calf muscles, stress is transferred to the calcaneal tendon, finally resulting in tendon rupture.

A patient with a ruptured calcaneal tendon can still walk, but only with a limp. The ruptured site on the calcaneal tendon is usually 4 cm above the point where the tendon is connected, and there will be thickening from edema and effusion of blood. The thickened portion of the tendon is painful or tender upon palpation.

Acupuncture is effective in treating Achilles tendinitis, especially the acute injury. Direct needling into the swollen, painful tendon introduces an antiinflammatory reaction that helps to relieve pain, and the needle-induced lesions activate the process of tissue regeneration. Like an ankle injury, calcaneal tendon injury will radiate pain to the calf muscles. In fact, tight calf muscles are often the cause of calcaneal tendon injury because the tightened muscles subject the tendon to excessive force.

The practitioner should carefully palpate the calcaneal tendon, the whole calf muscle, and both sides of the leg to find the tender points. At the rupture site, a few needles should be inserted deep into the ruptured tissue (Figure 11-22). The tender points on the calf muscles should also be needled. The procedure should be repeated every 3 or 4 days for the first 2 weeks. Pain relief can be achieved almost immediately in acute and fresh cases but recovery of function takes longer. In chronic cases, both pain relief and recovery of function will take longer. During the period of treatment, the patient should use a heel insert to elevate the heel about 2 cm, which will reduce the stretch of the Achilles tendon and the gastrosoleus muscles and thereby facilitate healing.

Plantar Fasciitis   Patients with plantar fasciitis feel moderate to severe pain under the heel, often radiating into the sole of the foot. The pain is worse during the first few steps after getting up in the morning. Weight-bearing activities including normal walking, climbing stairs, or standing on tiptoe increase the pain. Some patients feel more severe pain in the evening, after the day's work. The pain subsides after rest or if the foot resumes stretching exercises. If trauma is not involved, the onset is insidious in most patients.

Plantar fasciitis may occur in one or both feet. Activities such as carrying excessive weight, standing for long periods of time, walking, running, or wearing ill-fitting shoes will increase the risk of plantar fasciitis. We have seen one patient who developed plantar fasciitis after ankle surgery.

Palpation of the foot reveals a deep tender area beneath the anterior portion of the heel, especially at the anteromedial area of the calcaneus, the attachment point of the plantar fascia (see Figure 11-22). In some patients with acute or chronic heel pain, calcium can be deposited at this attachment site to form bone spurs, although most bone spurs will not result in pain. Other conditions causing a similar pain pattern include bursitis under the fascial attachment, atraumatic periostitis, and entrapment of the calcaneal branch of the tibial nerve.

In our clinic we have successfully treated both acute and chronic plantar fasciitis. The practitioner should perform a systemic examination of HAs, especially in the lower back area, posterior thigh, and calf muscles. It is necessary to carefully palpate the sole of the foot and the whole foot, paying attention to the heel bone (calcaneus), to find the most sensitive area. Two or three needles of 4 cm in length should be used to needle this tender area, as well as other tender points on the sole. In addition,

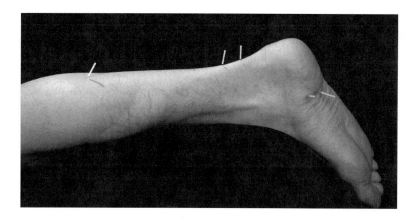

Figure 11-22 Needling method for Achilles tendinitis and plantar fasciitis.

it is advisable to needle HAs on the leg, thigh, buttock, and lower back. After treatments, a patient should resume mild lower limb activities and wear an orthopedic shoe or insert to support the foot arch and to avoid stretching the plantar fascia during walking.

Further medical evaluation is needed in patients with severe foot pain to confirm or rule out a possible stress fracture.

TREATMENT PROTOCOL FOR LOWER LIMB PAIN

Three types of acupoints are used to treat lower limb pain: HAs, paravertebral acupoints (PAs), and SAs.

Homeostatic Acupoints

Practitioners should palpate all 24 HAs to obtain information about which part of the body is most sensitive and to determine the possible origin of referred pain.

Paravertebral Acupoints

For pain and disorders of the lower limb, the area from L1 to S4 should be carefully palpated to see whether specific tender points appear along the lumbar or sacral vertebrae. Based on SAs, practitioners can select lumbar and/or sacral PAs.

Symptomatic Acupoints

Practitioners should carefully palpate the local painful or injured area to find the SAs. An understanding of the local anatomy and the extent and nature of the individual patient's pain or injury will help to find these points and achieve the optimum therapeutic effects. The following are some examples of how to find these SAs.

Hip Pain Palpate the gluteal area around H18, the area around the greater trochanter, the hamstring muscles and the iliotibial band on the thigh.

Thigh Pain Carefully palpate the hamstring, the iliotibial band, and the quadriceps and adductor muscles including their attachments to the hip bone and the knee. Figure 11-23 shows the treatment of adductor muscle strains.

Knee Pain Knee pain is always related to the muscles attached to the knee. First examine the knee area to understand the location of the pain and the possible tendons, ligaments, and bursae involved in this condition. Then carefully examine the muscles. For example, if pain is felt at the area of the MCL and the attachment of semitendinosis, the adductor muscles and semitendinosis should be palpated. The tender and painful points in the knee area and related muscles should be needled (Figure 11-24).

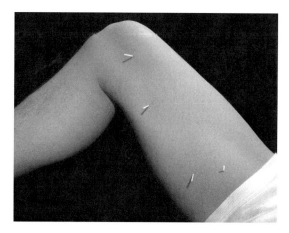

Figure 11-23 Needling method for adductor muscle strains.

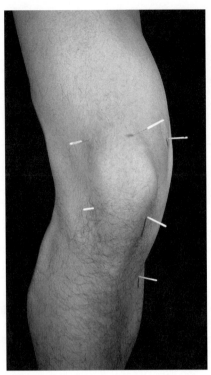

Figure 11-24   Needling method for knee pain. SAs in the thigh should always be needled.

Leg Pain   Examine the leg muscles, thigh muscles, ankle, and foot. The entire lower limb should be treated as one entity. In cases of severe pain where the patient does not experience relief after two to four treatments, the patient should be referred for further medical evaluation to confirm or rule out other causes of underlying pain such as a stress fracture.

Ankle and Foot Pain   Examine the ankle, foot, and leg. The three parts should always be treated together.

Reference

1. Parziale JR, Hudgins TH, Fishman LM: The piriformis syndrome, *Am J Orthop* 25:819-823, 1996.

CHAPTER 12

Systemic Pain–Related Disorders

This chapter discusses a variety of pain symptoms that are encountered in an acupuncture clinic but have not been addressed in previous chapters. The treatment protocol is presented at the end of the chapter.

HEADACHE

General Pathology

Headaches are among the most common complaints presented by patients seeking acupuncture treatments. Some cases respond well to acupuncture treatments, whereas others are rather challenging.

Although brain tissue does not ache, certain structures in the head and outside the skull are sensitive to pain. These include skin, muscles, arteries, the membrane that coats the skull, the eyes, the ears, and the nasal sinus cavities. Pain may result from tension or inflammation of the muscles or arteries of the scalp, or inflammation in the sinuses, ears, or gums.

Pain-sensitive structures inside the skull include arteries, venous sinuses and their tributary veins, parts of the outer membrane at the base of the brain, and cranial and cervical (sensory) nerves. Headache pain may result from dilation or contraction of the arteries, inflammation of brain membranes, or pressure from a tumor or hemorrhage.

The exact nature of headache pain is still unclear. It is believed that headaches occur as the result of an imbalance or changes in brain chemicals called neurotransmitters, such as serotonin and noradrenaline. The unbalanced levels of these brain chemicals cause inflammation of scalp arteries and irritation of the pain-sensitive structures mentioned above. The inflammation or irritation of these structures stimulates the trigeminal nerve, which sends pain impulses to the pain centers of the brain. The pain may be dull, sharp, or throbbing (pulsatile).

A headache is considered chronic if it cannot be relieved or improved after 6 months.

Medical professionals differentiate headaches into four types: migraine, tension, cluster, and organic. Each type of headache has its own pain pattern.

Of the four types of headache, the tension headache is the most common. This headache is characterized by a dull, squeezing knot or pressure pain that involves the forehead, scalp, temples, or back of the head and neck. The cause of this headache is muscle tension, especially the muscles on the neck and shoulder. When physical and/or physiologic tension or stress accumulates in the body, skeletal muscles and smooth muscles (muscles lining the internal organs and blood vessels) become contracted without spontaneous relaxation. This causes low oxygen supply and results in pain in both skeletal and smooth muscles. In such cases some people also feel pain in the stomach; some complain also of pain in the neck or shoulders; and others feel pain only in the head, possibly accompanied by raised blood pressure.

The tension headache responds very well to acupuncture treatments, and the Integrative Neuromuscular Acupoint System (INMAS) protocol proves to be very effective. As discussed in Chapter 3, muscle tension usually changes the homeostatic acupoints (HAs) from the latent phase to the passive phase, making them tender, and INMAS helps to locate these tender points. Locally, the process of needling tender points and the resulting needle-induced lesions effectively relax both superficial and deep muscles all over the body and restore their normal blood and oxygen supply. Systemically, needle-induced neurochemical substances such as endorphins are secreted into the blood stream and cause the relaxation of skeletal and smooth muscles as well as of other systems such as the cardiovascular system, thus normalizing the blood pressure. This combination of local and systemic effects brings about relief of tension headaches.

The underlying cause of migraine headaches is believed to be neurotransmitters, the communicating chemicals within the nervous system. Migraine headaches usually occur as moderate or severe pain on one side of the head, often accompanied by nausea or transient visual disturbance, intolerance to light or sound, or rainbow-like colors called *aura* in the field of vision. The incidence of migraine headaches is higher in females than in males. One of the reasons for the gender difference is that many female patients experience migraine just before or during their menstrual period, possibly due to fluctuation in the level of female hormones. Patients with a migraine headache may feel tightened scalp muscles just as do patients with a tension headache.

The medical history of patients with migraine headaches often shows that they have suffered for many years, and it may also show accompanying problems such as habitual constipation, insomnia, fatigue, or a food allergy. The chronicity of migraine headaches makes treatment challenging. In addition, physiologic problems, such as constipation, that often accompany migraines render the body resistant to any medical intervention. For example, if a migraine patient is also suffering from constipation, the toxins retained in the body as a result of the constipation may be supplementary triggers for the migraine.

A comprehensive approach is needed when treating patients with migraine pain. For example, during the course of acupuncture treatments the practitioner and the patient should work together to find solutions for contributing problems such as constipation, poor diet, fatigue, and lifestyle factors (e.g., lack of proper physical exercise). Acupuncture will not provide longlasting relief from migraine if these conditions are ignored or persist.

Cluster headaches are more common in male patients. The cluster headache is characterized by a steady stabbing pain around one eye or on one side of the head, sometimes with watering and redness of the eye and nasal stuffiness on the same side of the face. The pain episodes may recur at the same time of day or night.

The cluster headache is believed to be caused by a disorder in the hypothalamus, the part of the brain responsible for regulating hormones and physiologic rhythms such as the sleep-wake cycle. A specific chemical present in the brain and some cranial nerves may cause similar symptoms. This brain chemical binds to special receptors in the neck arteries to control the ratio of oxygen to carbon dioxide in the blood supply of the brain. Smoking, alcohol, or certain foods may trigger a cluster headache, especially in patients whose family history shows a similar pattern.

Acupuncture helps to relieve cluster headaches by similar means to those discussed in treating tension headaches. In addition to the local and systemic effects of acupuncture needling as discussed above, the needling stimulates peripheral nerves, which send impulses directly to the hypothalamus. Thus acupuncture stimulation helps the hypothalamus to restore its normal regulatory function and reduces the symptoms of cluster headache.

Organic headaches account for less than 1% of headache cases. These headaches are caused by problems such as inflammation around the brain, elevated blood pressure, brain edema (swelling), or a brain tumor. The underlying causes of organic headaches are life-threatening, and these patients should be examined by specialists. However, clinical evidence shows that acupuncture can be useful as a supplement to conventional approaches in treating such patients. Acupuncture induces the secretion of endorphins, which relaxes blood vessels, promotes blood circulation, and reduces peripheral resistance to blood circulation. By using INMAS and properly selecting symptomatic acupoints (SAs), an acupuncture practitioner can help to reduce tissue swelling and high blood pressure and to control inflammation.

Treatment Protocol

All types of headache, no matter whether acute or chronic, should be treated as systemic problems. This means that the whole INMAS should be used. Treatment should be administered in either prone or supine positions, depending on the patient's health. In general, younger or healthier persons can tolerate more needling than weaker or elderly patients.

Prone Position

Homeostatic Acupoints   Use all of the HAs accessible in this position. Pay special attention to the H2 greater auricular, H3 spinal accessory, and H7 greater occipital acupoints because the degree of their sensitivity and the size of the sensitive area may indicate the duration and severity of the condition. The more sensitive or bigger the acupoint, the more treatments will be needed.

Symptomatic Acupoints   Carefully palpate the neck and shoulder region around H2, H3, H7, and H13 to find the tender SAs and needle them. Usually select four to six SAs in the neck for each treatment. If more than six SAs in the neck are needled, some patients will feel soreness in the neck for a few days.

Paravertebral Acupoints   If there are already four to six needles (SAs) in the neck, then select paravertebral acupoints (PAs) along T1-T7. Five needles on each side are enough. If only two needles are used in the neck, two more needles can be used on each side along C1-C7.

Supine Position
Homeostatic Acupoints Use all of the HAs that are accessible in this position. Pay special attention to the HAs listed below because the degree of their sensitivity and size of the sensitive area may indicate the duration and severity of the condition. The more sensitive or bigger the acupoint, the more treatments are needed. These HAs are H19 infraorbital and H23 supraorbital.

To avoid bruising on the face, smaller needles are suggested for facial needling (1.5 cm in length and 0.2 mm in diameter).

Symptomatic Acupoints Carefully palpate the facial area on the forehead, cheek, and lower jaw and scalp. The tender SAs should be carefully needled in these areas. Do not needle the area around the ocular orbit to avoid bruising.

TRIGEMINAL NEURALGIA (TIC DOULOUREUX)

Trigeminal neuralgia is a recurring pain on one side of the face. The pain is characterized by brief flashes of excruciating pain in the lips, gums, cheek, chin, or rarely, forehead. The patient may describe the pain attack as ripping, darting, or sharply cutting. An attack may last for seconds or a few minutes, accompanied by contraction of facial muscles. The attack can be spontaneous or provoked by mild stimulation such as shaving or applying cosmetics.

The pain is caused by a disturbance in the function of the trigeminal nerve, which is the major nerve that carries the sensation from the face to the brain, but the cause of trigeminal neuralgia is still not clearly identified. A blood vessel that compresses the trigeminal nerve has been blamed for causing trigeminal pain in some cases.

Trigeminal neuralgia is most often seen in patients over the age of fifty and is more common in women than in men.

Treatment Protocol

The treatment procedure is the same as that used in treating a headache. Practitioners should keep in mind that, in general, fewer needles should be used in elderly or weak patients. In such cases it is better to use fewer needles and offer more treatments (for example, twice a week).

The efficacy of acupuncture in treating trigeminal neuralgia depends on the severity of the condition and the patient's health. The quantitative evaluation described in Chapter 6 provides a reliable method to predict the result of the treatment. Acupuncture therapy is effective or helpful for patients in groups A, B, and C. Little or no success can be expected with group D patients.

SHINGLES (HERPES ZOSTER) AND PAIN AFTER SHINGLES (POSTHERPETIC NEURALGIA)

Shingles or herpes zoster is an acute viral disease caused by a herpes virus, the same virus that causes chickenpox. Shingles is caused by a re-emergence of the virus, which has been lying dormant for years within the nerve cells. The virus causes inflammation of the spinal ganglion and a vesicular eruption along the area of distribution of the affected spinal nerves. Patients feel excruciating, burning pain or tingling in the affected area.

If pain persists after the eruption or blisters have healed, the condition is called postherpetic neuralgia. This chronic pain results from damage to the nerve fibers caused by the shingles infection.

Shingles appears in persons who have been exposed to chickenpox. The reactivation of the virus may be triggered by trauma, diseases like pneumonia or tuberculosis, injection of certain drugs, or stress, which suppresses immune functions.

Acupuncture therapy accelerates the healing process through several mechanisms. Needle-induced endorphins systemically relax the whole body, which reduces the stress level. This process restores the function of the immune system, which in turn deactivates the virus and brings it under control. Local needling along the infected nerve stimulates an antiinflammatory reaction and helps recovery or regeneration of the damaged nerve fibers.

Treatment Protocol

Select the proper position, prone, supine, or on the side, to expose the affected area for treatment.

Please note that the infection is limited to the dermatome area of the infected spinal nerve(s), so practitioners need to be familiar with the segmental dermatome distribution of the spinal nerves. For example, the breast and nipple area is the dermatome of T4 and the umbilicus is in dermatome T10. The affected area is usually limited to one side of the body and occupies two neighboring dermatomes. For instance, if the infected skin is just below the nipple, it is the dermatome T5 or T6 or both.

Homeostatic Acupoints   Needle all of the HAs in the body accessible in that position.

Symptomatic Acupoints   Use small needles (1.5 cm in length and 0.2 mm in diameter) and insert them all over the affected skin around the infected nerve. As many as 30 or more tiny needles should be used for each treatment according to the size of the affected skin area. Avoid breaking the blisters to prevent spreading the virus. If the blisters do break, use a cotton cuticle to dry the liquid and apply Betadine to the affected area.

Paravertebral Acupoints   Select the paravertebral points corresponding to the infected spinal nerves. For example, if the affected skin is on dermatomes T5-T6, select the PAs from T3-T8.

TEMPOROMANDIBULAR JOINT DISORDERS AND OTHER SYMPTOMS RESULTING FROM DENTAL WORK

The temporomandibular joints (TMJ) are the hinge-like joints that connect the mandible (lower jaw) to the temporal bone of the skull. As in other joints in the body, the bony surfaces of these joints are covered with cartilage and both articular surfaces are separated by a small disk that prevents the bones from rubbing each other. The muscles that move the joints (open or close the mouth) also stabilize the joints.

As with other joints, any disorder or dysfunction of the TMJs will produce pain. The TMJ is susceptible to various disorders such as inflammation, osteoarthritis, or rheumatoid arthritis. Pain also may result from mechanical damage such as wear and tear on the joints, injury, tightened joint muscles, stress, an improperly aligned bite, and poorly fitting braces or other dental appliances.

Patients may complain of a dull aching pain in front of the ear, a clicking sound or grating sensation when opening the mouth or chewing, or difficulty in opening or closing the mouth. Chronic tension and anxiety may cause a patient to habitually clench the jaw or grind the teeth while sleeping. This unconscious overuse of the TMJs also causes pain and dysfunction of the joints, ligaments, and muscles. Some patients also feel tinnitus, headache, nausea, or even vertigo.

Needling into the TMJs and the muscles that operate them reduces muscle tension and the inflammation of muscle and soft tissues that is associated with the joints. Needling improves local blood circulation and increases oxygen supply, which accelerates tissue healing. Acupuncture is able to repair injured soft tissues and restore joint function. Acupuncture needling also slows down the degenerative process in cases of arthritis. TMJ dislocation or misalignment resulting from dental problems should be treated by the appropriate specialists but acupuncture can be used as a supplementary treatment in such cases.

Similarly to patients with other postoperative problems, patients who have had dental surgery can also be benefited by acupuncture. After dental surgery, patients feel numbness in gums, lips, jaw, and facial skin with edema of soft tissues. Dental surgery, by nature, is an acute trauma to the body. The administration of needling immediately after surgery will greatly reduce edema and swelling. Also needling dilates the blood vessels to reduce peripheral resistance to cardiovascular circulation, which helps to reduce water retention in soft tissues. The accelerated water metabolism increases the metabolism of the anesthetics that were used for the surgery, and so the needling immediately or shortly after dental surgery helps to reduce swelling and to eliminate remnant anesthetics in the oral tissues.

Treatment Protocol

Select the proper position, supine or on one side. If the TMJ problem is chronic, all of the HAs accessible in the selected position should be needled because the patient may have other symptoms like headache, fatigue, tinnitus, or nausea. If the TMJ problem is acute and the patient is healthy (group A or B), only local symptomatic points need to be needled.

To find the local symptomatic points, carefully palpate the area around the TMJ, the temporalis and masseter muscles, the neck muscles including the sternocleidomastoid, and the muscles of the back of the neck.

Use needles 2.5 cm in length (0.2 mm in diameter) for the joints proper and for the thicker muscles like the masseter and the sternocleidomastoid. Use smaller needles 1.5 cm long (0.18 or 0.2 mm in diameter) for areas in the face and thinner muscles like the temporalis and scalp muscles or sutures. Needles 3 to 5 cm long can be used for the muscles on the back of the neck.

COMPLEX REGIONAL PAIN SYNDROME

Complex regional pain syndrome (CRPS) has puzzled clinicians and pain scientists more than any other pain condition. The name itself reflects our incomplete understanding of this disorder. It was first described by Civil War surgeons Mitchell, Morehouse, and Kane in 1864.[1] Currently, medical professionals believe that CRPS is caused by some kind of nerve injuries.

CRPS is classified into two types: reflex sympathetic dystrophy syndrome (RSD, type I) and causalgia (type II). The symptoms of both types are similar, and the difference between them is that causalgia can be associated with an identifiable nerve injury.

In Box 12-1, Dr. Sanjay Gupta suggests the diagnostic criteria for CRPS.[1]

The signs and symptoms presented by CRPS patients may include:

1. Pain and tenderness in the hand or foot
2. Tender, thin, swelling, cool, or shining skin in the affected area, accompanied by increased sweating and hair growth
3. Cold, blue, sweaty limb with "burning" or "stabbing" pain
4. Excessive painful response to cold stimuli or light touch
5. The pain becomes worse at night
6. Emotional stress, depression, or lack of sleep increase the feeling of pain. In some cases, the patient may have had an injury, heart attack, or stroke weeks or months earlier. In other cases the preceding injury may have been very minor and the patient may not even remember it

CRPS usually develops in three stages but any one patient may not necessarily follow the same pattern. Stage I, which is also called the dysfunction stage, is characterized by redness, swelling, and pain in the affected area. This stage usually lasts for 3 to 6 months. CRPS symptoms can be completely reversed by acupuncture treatment if treated at this stage. Some of our young patients were completely cured in about 3 months, after receiving acupuncture treatment twice a week for 1 month and once a week afterwards.

Stage II is also known as the dystrophy stage. Patients exhibit cold and blue skin with sweating and severe pain in the affected area. X-rays may reveal signs of osteoporosis or degenerative changes in the bone. This stage lasts for about 6 months. CRPS is still susceptible to medical treatment at this stage.

Stage III, the final stage, is characterized by pain and signs of atrophy such as muscle and bone wasting. The pain may gradually subside but the atrophy continues to progress. According to current medical opinion, this stage is not reversible.

CRPS commonly results from a fracture in the hand or leg, or nerve and soft tissue damage. It also can be caused by repetitive motion such as typing or operating machines. CRPS is also linked to major or minor body injury or trauma such as sprains, dislocation, laceration, contusions, crushing injuries, amputations, gunshots, or diseases such as stroke.

Acupuncture therapy can provide very effective relief to CRPS patients at stages I and II. Acupuncture needling relaxes the painful and tight muscles, which helps remove mechanical pressure on peripheral blood vessels. It also calms the sympathetic tone and increases parasympathetic activities, which help to improve peripheral blood circulation. This increased circulation provides

---

Box 12-1

Complex Regional Pain Syndrome

Type I: RSD

Continuous pain, with a hypersensitivity to cold stimuli and nonpainful stimuli eliciting a pain response

Evidence of swelling and skin changes with a decrease in blood flow to the affected area

Absence of a condition that otherwise explains the above symptoms

An inciting event or cause may or may not be present

Type II: Causalgia

Continuous pain, with a hypersensitivity to cold stimuli and nonpainful stimuli eliciting a pain response after a nerve injury, but not necessarily following the nerve distribution

Evidence of swelling and skin changes with a decrease in blood flow to the affected area

Absence of a condition that otherwise explains the above symptoms

All three of the above must be present for this diagnosis

more nutrition and oxygen and accelerates the evacuation of metabolic toxins that are retained in soft tissues. Needle-induced endorphins not only reduce pain but also relax the entire body and remove mental tension.

Treatment Protocol

Warning! The affected area should *not* be needled. The area is very sensitive and even a very light touch may trigger excruciating pain (allodynia). Any needling in the affected soft tissues will increase the pain. Remember, do NOT insert acupuncture needles into the affected area.

Homeostatic Acupoints The patient can be placed in a supine, prone, or side position according to the area affected. It is very important to needle all of the HAs accessible in the selected position.

Paravertebral Acupoints Paravertebral acupoints are probably the most important points in treating CRPS.

Follow the dermatome distribution. For example, if the affected area is on the hand, then use PAs along C4-T2. If the affected area is on the foot, use PAs along L2-S4.

Symptomatic Acupoints Do not needle the affected area, according to the above warning, but the neighboring, nonsensitive areas should be examined and needled. For example, if the dorsum of the hand is affected, needle the elbow and shoulder area around the HAs.

To increase the effectiveness of acupuncture treatments, two or three treatments weekly are recommended.

Reference

1. Gupta S: Complex regional pain syndrome (CRPS) or reflex sympathetic dystrophy. In Simon WH, Ehrlich GE, Sadwin A, editors: *Conquering chronic pain after injury: an integrative approach to treating post-traumatic pain,* New York, 2002, Avery, pp 62-64.

CHAPTER 13

Acupuncture Therapy for Non-pain Symptoms

INTRODUCTION

Acupuncture can be used for treating both pain and non-pain symptoms. However, there is a basic difference in treatment between these two types of symptom. When using the Integrative Neuromuscular Acupoint System (INMAS) to treat pain, it is possible to predict the progress and determine the outcome of the treatment: for example: Are the symptoms presented by the patient treatable? If treatable, how many sessions will be needed? How long will the relief last? When treating non-pain symptoms, it is not possible to make such predictions. Thus, the progress and prognosis of treating non-pain symptoms with acupuncture are not so straightforward.

Why is acupuncture effective for such a variety of different disorders? Unlike pharmaceutical therapy, acupuncture employs the *same* principles to treat *different* symptoms and disorders. In other words, it does not correct or target the underlying cause of a *particular* symptom or disease, but activates a series of *general physiologic mechanisms* to accelerate self-healing of healable symptoms or diseases. These physiologic mechanisms ensure that acupuncture therapy can be used to treat any completely or partially self-healable pathophysiologic condition, and consequently this includes conditions that do not manifest symptoms of pain.

Nevertheless, as each symptom has its particular features and each patient presents his or her own personal expression of the symptom or disease, a practitioner needs to pay close attention to the individual features exhibited in each case. The general healing mechanism of acupuncture has to be invoked for the specific symptoms, and although this general healing process can be triggered at most locations of the body, it is by needling a specific acupoint that we purposefully inoculate the healing mechanism into specific tissues or at a specific location. This is the essence of what acupuncture practitioners do in treating pain symptoms: needling the painful soft tissues to bring the self-healing mechanism to particular injured locations. The same strategy, however, is used to treat non-pain symptoms, and the INMAS system of homeostatic acupoints (HAs), symptomatic acupoints (SAs), and paravertebral acupoints (PAs) is equally efficacious.

As we have described in Chapters 1, 2, 3, 5, and 6, the HAs gradually become tender in a predictable pattern as the body's homeostasis decreases, and our body manifests these acupoints to reflect its own pathophysiologic decline. The SAs pinpoint the particular nerves, muscles, and other soft tissues directly affected by the injury, and PAs are selected to assist the SAs. The PAs and SAs belong to the same spinal segment, and needling PAs relaxes the muscles and soft tissues and improves blood circulation at the location of the nerve root; this process helps to desensitize the sensitized nerve endings. Also, PAs are located closer to the autonomic ganglionic chain; clinical evidence has shown that needling PAs balances the mutual interaction between sympathetic and parasympathetic nerves.

In treating pain symptoms, it is very important to find the most effective SAs, and this is equally true when treating non-pain symptoms. The practitioner must locate the tender SAs generated by the diseased organ because of the viscerocutaneous reflex whereby the diseased organ is able to sensitize some of the peripheral nerve endings. When there is no pain, however, it is more difficult to find the SAs because some tender points are innervated by the spinal nerves from the same spinal segment as the diseased organ and other tender points may appear on the spinal nerves from other segments because of intersegmental communication inside the spinal cord.

Some diseases or diseased organs may not produce detectable tender acupoints on the body surface, especially at an early stage of the disease. In these cases, selecting proper PAs provides sound therapeutic results. For instance, PAs along vertebrae T1 to T7 should be selected for respiratory problems such as asthma and PAs along vertebrae

T5 to T12 should be selected for stomach problems such as a gastric ulcer. Knowledge of segmental innervation of internal organs helps the practitioner to select the proper PAs (see Chapter 5).

In general, treating non-pain symptoms, including numbness or tingling, is more difficult than treating pain symptoms. For instance, when we treat a patient with infertility, we will either succeed or fail; partial success is not possible. Although when using INMAS for non-pain symptoms it is not possible to have the same degree of accuracy in prediction, the INMAS quantitative evaluation nonetheless provides useful guidance because it evaluates the healing potential of each patient. This chapter presents several non-pain disorders as examples of using INMAS for treating non-pain symptoms. The symptoms presented are a few samples selected by way of illustration. There is no doubt that INMAS will also be effective in evaluating and treating many more non-pain symptoms than we have described here.

ASTHMA

Asthma is a condition that causes recurrent attacks of dyspnea (shortness of breath or breathlessness), with airway inflammation and wheezing due to spasmodic constriction of the smooth muscles of the bronchi.

Acupuncture needling can relax the spasmodic constriction of the bronchi, accelerate the absorption of mucus by the lining of the bronchi, and reduce the inflammation.

Treatment Protocol

The patient lies in the prone position. Use the following acupoints:

1. HAs: all those accessible in the prone position.
2. PAs: along T1-T8. When treating asthma, PAs along T1-T8 are the most critical points because they provide immediate relief of asthma symptoms.
3. SAs: there are no special SAs for asthma. However, the practitioner should carefully palpate the neck area and may select one or two points on each side of the neck for needling. These neck points may stimulate the vagus nerve to help further relax the bronchi and absorb the mucus.

Treatments may be administered once a day or even twice a day at the beginning. After a few days, the symptoms are usually much improved and the patient may have to continue with two treatments a week to stabilize the condition.

SINUSITIS

Sinusitis is an inflammation of one or more of the paranasal sinuses. The inflamed and swollen mucous membrane of the paranasal sinuses partially or completely blocks the opening between the sinuses and the nasal passage. The mucus that accumulates in the blocked sinus causes pressure on the sinus walls resulting in discomfort, fever, pain and difficult breathing.

Sinusitis can be caused by air pollution, allergies, nose infection, tooth infection, infectious diseases such as pneumonia and measles, physical injury, etc.

Treatment Protocol

The patient takes the supine position. Use the following acupoints:

1. HAs: all those accessible in the supine position. Please note that H19 infraorbital and H23 supraorbital are tender. Their sensitivity and the size of the sensitive area indicate the severity of the symptoms.
2. SAs: carefully palpate the area around H19 and H23. To improve nasal congestion, the nostrils should also be needled as shown in Figure 13-1.

To avoid bruising the patient's face, use needles 1.5 cm in length and 0.18 or 0.20 mm in diameter.

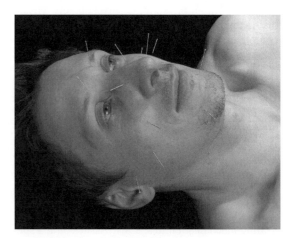

Figure 13-1 Needling method for sinusitis and Bell's palsy. In the case of Bell's palsy, all the affected facial muscles should be needled.

NAUSEA

Nausea is an unpleasant sensation of the epigastrium and abdomen associated with a tendency to vomit. It can be a symptom of minor or serious disorders such as food irritation, chemical toxins, or an imbalance of the autonomic nervous system.

Nausea is usually felt when nerves in the stomach or other parts of the body are irritated. The irritated nerves send signals to the brain center(s) that controls the vomiting reflex. Vomiting results when the signals are intensified.

In addition to stomach disorders, intense pain in almost any part of the body can produce nausea, and strong emotional changes also trigger it.

Acupuncture is very effective in treating nausea due to the following mechanisms:

1. Needling balances the interaction between the sympathetic and parasympathetic nervous systems. Clinical observation suggests that needling calms down sympathetic activities and reduces the muscular tension of the internal organs.
2. Needling desensitizes the sensitized (irritated) nerves through antiinflammatory reactions.
3. Needle-induced endorphins help to reduce physiologic stress throughout the entire body, especially in the cardiovascular system, which causes an increase in blood circulation to the stomach and other parts of the body.
4. Needling relaxes the tight muscles and reduces the sensation of pain.
5. Needling may also help by accelerating the metabolism of toxins if they are the cause of the nausea.

Additional mechanisms may also be involved, and all of these factors work together to reduce nausea and vomiting.

Treatment Protocol

Use both prone and supine positions. Each treatment may use one or two positions. Use the following acupoints:

1. HAs: all those accessible in the position used.
2. PAs: along T5-T12.
3. SAs: palpate the front epigastric region to find tender points. Use needles 2.5 cm in length and insert the needles diagonally and caudally.

4. Empirical point: on the ventral side of the forearm, a point approximately 5 cm above the wrist between the tendons of palmaris longus and flexor carpi radialis (Figure 13-2). Use a needle that is 2.5 cm long and 2 cm deep.

DIGESTIVE DISORDERS, STOMACH ACHE, AND GASTRIC ULCERS

All stomach, duodenum, and intestine disorders, including ulcers, can be treated or helped by acupuncture needling. The treatment protocol for this group of disorders is the same as for nausea.

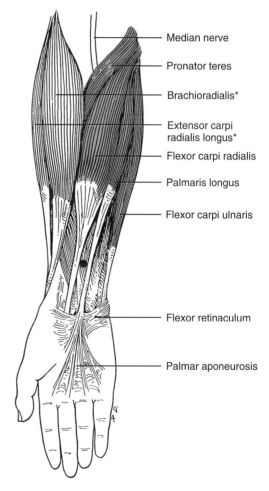

Median nerve
Pronator teres
Brachioradialis*
Extensor carpi radialis longus*
Flexor carpi radialis
Palmaris longus
Flexor carpi ulnaris
Flexor retinaculum
Palmar aponeurosis

Figure 13-2 Empirical acupoint on the forearm for nausea. (From Jenkins D: *Hollinshead's functional anatomy of the limbs and back,* ed 8, Philadelphia, 2002, WB Saunders, p 144.)

Treatment Protocol

For intestinal disorders, palpate the abdominal region and needle it if tender points are felt, with needles 2.5 cm in length. For disorders of the large intestine such as diarrhea, PAs along L5-S4 should be used. In cases of stomach or duodenal disorders, PAs along T8-T12 are usually tender and should be used.

SKIN DISORDERS

Urticaria (hives) is a vascular reaction of the skin characterized by the appearance of slightly elevated red or pale patches (wheals) with severe itching. It may be caused by food, infection, emotional stress, or an allergic reaction to an insect bite or plant contact.

Neurodermatitis is an extremely variable eczematous dermatosis (skin thickening). It is a response to prolonged scratching, rubbing, or pinching to relieve intense itching.

Other general symptoms of skin reaction to insect bites or poisonous plants may include swelling, pain, or itching.

All of these skin symptoms respond very well to acupuncture needling. Itching is mostly a response to chemical stimulation that irritates the nerve endings; this is the underlying cause of allergic reactions of the skin. In addition, itching may originate with inflammation or infection, which can irritate soft tissues of the skin, including nerve endings.

Psychogenic factors can cause noninflammatory irritation of the cutaneous nerves, which produces itching.

Acupuncture needling improves blood circulation, which accelerates the deactivation of the allergen or the metabolism of the toxins. Needling and needle-induced lesions also desensitize the nerve endings. All of these physiologic processes reduce itching and promote tissue repair and regeneration.

Treatment Protocol

The treatment procedure is exactly the same as for other skin symptoms such as herpes zoster. Arrange the patient in the proper position to expose the affected area. Use the following acupoints:

1. HAs: all those accessible in the selected position. Usually skin itching stops immediately after needling the HAs, but recurs after the needles are removed. In subsequent treatments, the relief lasts for an increasing length of time. It is important to densely needle the affected skin as described in the following paragraph.
2. SAs: Insert small needles (1.5 cm or 2.0 cm in length) into the rash or affected area; 10 to 50 needles may be used according to the size of the affected area. This dense needling is the most important procedure for relieving itching, especially during the first few treatments. As itching subsides, fewer needles may be used.
3. PAs: These are not necessary in most cases of skin disorders because usually the itching is distributed all over the body, such as on the neck, elbow, knee, or other areas.
4. Dermal needles, such as Seven-star or Plum needles, can be used by the patients themselves. These hammerlike tools with seven or five needles are very helpful in treating skin itching. The patient should tap the itching area with the dermal needles whenever itching occurs. This will sometimes produce tiny skin bleeding, but this in fact speeds up cell regeneration.

Even chronic neurodermatitis with thickened skin can be treated successfully with dense needling and self-administered dermal needle tapping. Dermal needles can be reused but should be well rinsed and soaked in rubbing alcohol after each use.

GYNECOLOGICAL DISORDERS

Premenstrual syndrome (PMS), or premenstrual tension, consists of symptoms that arise during the period before menstruation or in the early days of the menstrual period. The symptoms may begin at the time of ovulation and become worse or fluctuate until menses. PMS can affect virtually every system of the body and produce behavioral changes. Physical symptoms may include headache, vertigo, common colds, rhinitis, asthma, sinusitis, sore throat, abdominal bloating, nausea, food cravings, breast tenderness, back pain, joint pain, edema, cramps, and other discomforts. The emotional and psychological symptoms may include irritability, fatigue, sleeping disturbances, mood swings, depression, and altered libido.

Menopause normally takes place between the ages of 40 and 58. About 75% of American women reach their menopause by the age of 52. The most recognizable sign of the beginning of menopause is menstrual irregularity, with a gradual decrease in both the amount and duration of flow. In some cases, there may be more frequent and heavier bleeding or bleeding between periods. When menses have ceased for 6 to 12 months, menopause has taken place.

Hormone changes, especially an increased production of follicle-stimulating hormone (FSH), luteinizing hormone (LH), and testosterone, are responsible for physical and psychological symptoms. The most commonly reported symptoms include hot flashes of the face, neck, and upper body; excessive perspiration at night; vaginal dryness; joint pain and back pain; sleeping disturbances; and other physiologic changes.

Infertility is considered a pathological disorder after 1 year of engaging with the same sexual partner without conception. About 35% of infertility cases are due to female factors, the same percent to male factors, and the remaining 30% to a combination of both female and male factors. There is a possibility that acupuncture may help infertile female patients if the patient is confirmed by medical evaluation to have no other physical pathology such as infection, obstruction in the ovarian tube, tumor, and so forth.

Treatment Protocol

The patient alternates between the supine and prone positions, changing for each session.

1. HAs: All those accessible in the selected position.
2. PAs: Select C1-C7, T1-T12, or L1-S4, according to the segmental distribution of the symptoms. For example, if hot flashes appear on the neck, use C1-C7. In case of female infertility, use L1-S4.
3. SAs: If the gynecological problems are accompanied by pain, palpate the area where the patient complains of pain/discomfort.

Patients can be treated regularly (e.g., once a week), for an extended period of time, or only during the occurrence of the symptoms. For example, patients with PMS can be treated twice a week for 2 weeks immediately after ovulation.

BELL'S PALSY

Bell's palsy (facial palsy), a neuropathy of the facial nerve, is characterized by weak or paralyzed muscles of facial expression on one side of the face, inability to wrinkle the forehead and close one eye, and a drooping corner of the mouth on the affected side. The chewing muscles are also weakened or paralyzed so food and saliva dribble out the affected side of the mouth. The onset of Bell's palsy

is often fairly abrupt. Pain behind the ear can precede the palsy by a day or two (the facial nerve exits the skull through the stylomastoid foramen behind the ear lobe). Some patients also complain of pain in the jaw or on the entire side of the face.

The weak and paralyzed muscles of facial expression result from the condition of the facial nerve, but the cause of this neuropathy is unknown. Some cases may be caused by exposure to cold, infection of the face, inflammation or physical injury of the facial nerve, or inflammation of other associated soft tissues along the path of the facial nerve from the skull to the muscles, such as middle ear infection or inflammation of the parotid gland. These swollen tissues apply pressure on the facial nerve and disable its motor function, leading to paralysis of the facial muscles. Bone fracture or tumors may also affect the facial nerve with a similar result.

Bell's palsy is usually a short-term problem, but individual recovery is variable. About 80% of patients with this disorder will show improvement within 2 to 3 weeks and complete recovery within a few months. However, some patients recover so slowly that there is no noticeable improvement even after 6 months or more. We have seen a musician, a trumpet player, who showed no sign of recovery after 2 years. If the recovery is delayed for a long time, part of the facial nerve may degenerate or die as a result of the interruption in the supply of nutrition and oxygen and lack of stimulation from the muscles.

There are other types of facial paralysis with a different etiology. A stroke also can cause one-sided facial paralysis, and if both sides of the face are simultaneously affected, it may be due to Lyme disease (a recurrent multisystemic disease caused by a viral infection from tick bites) or other causes.

Sufferers from Bell's palsy can benefit substantially from acupuncture therapy because it promotes self-healing by reducing inflammation and swelling, and by increasing blood circulation and therefore the supply of nutrition and oxygen. Although most cases of Bell's palsy will heal slowly without intervention, acupuncture can accelerate the process, reducing the suffering associated with speaking, chewing, swallowing, drinking, eye-closing, and sleeping.

Treatment Protocol

The supine position may be used for all treatments because some patients with these symptoms feel uncomfortable in the prone position. Treatment can be administered once every 3 days.

1. HAs: Use all those accessible in the supine position.
2. SAs: Use small needles (1.5 cm in length and 0.18 or 0.20 cm in diameter) for needling the affected facial muscles, including chewing muscles such as masseter and temporalis.

SIDE EFFECTS OF CHEMOTHERAPY

All the side effects of chemotherapy can be reduced partially or completely by acupuncture therapy. These include digestive disorders (stomach upset, constipation, and diarrhea), skin irritation (rash, itching), headache, and ringing in the ears.

Chemotherapy imposes a physiologic stress on the body that interferes with the normal mutual interaction between the sympathetic and parasympathetic nervous systems. The side-effects vary according to the nature of the drug and the body of the patient, but usually the weakest part of the body shows the side-effects first.

The central mechanism of the relief of these side effects is probably the secretion of endorphins at spinal and brain levels under the stimulation of acupuncture, either manual or electrical. These endorphins circulate in the blood stream to the entire body.

The consensus development statement of the National Institutes of Health also indicates that "There is clear evidence that needle acupuncture is efficacious for adult post-operative and chemotherapy nausea and vomiting and probably for the nausea of pregnancy."

Treatment Protocol

Position the patient supine or prone. Use the following acupoints:

1. HAs: all those accessible in either supine or prone position.
2. SAs: palpate the local area to find the tender points and needle them.
3. PAs: select the PAs according to segmental distributions including dermatome, myotome, and viscerotome (see Chapter 5).

UNUSUAL SYMPTOMS WITH UNKNOWN UNDERLYING CAUSE

Here we refer to unusual symptoms that would be classified as "origin unknown" by conventional medical professionals. Consider the example below.

A healthy 28-year-old man presented for treatment. Since the age of 15, every few weeks he experienced headaches lasting for a few hours, red skin rash all over the body, a sensation of discomfort in the testicles, strange changes in taste, and blisters on the lips. He has visited doctors in Germany and the United States, but no one could make a certain diagnosis. We did not see the symptoms when the patient came to our clinic, but we were fairly sure that we would be able to help him because he was a healthy, athletic young man. We used supine and prone positions for each treatment, needling all HAs. The patient received one treatment every week continuously for 4 months. He has not experienced any of these symptoms since the first treatment 2 years ago.

This example shows that health problems with unknown underlying causes can be helped by acupuncture therapy as long as the symptoms are pathophysiologically healable and the patient is reasonably healthy.

Treatment Protocol

For systemic problems as described above, use the HAs accessible to each position (supine, prone, and side). If the patient also presents other symptoms, use SAs and the corresponding PAs.

GENERAL HEALTH MAINTENANCE

Many patients come to an acupuncture clinic for health maintenance, and their experience is that the treatment helps them to feel more relaxed, physically fit, youthful, and mentally alert. These patients show more coordination in their physical movements and their bodies are practically pain free. In some cases, there may be remnant pain, but they are much more able to live comfortably with it.

No healthcare providers can give their patients health. Patients have to make a conscientious effort to regain their health, and after regaining it, the same effort is needed to maintain it.

Acupuncture is a very beneficial modality for health maintenance. Our clinical experience indicates that for people with chronic problems, such as high blood pressure, or even Alzheimer's disease or cancer, regular acupuncture therapy—although it does not remove the problems—will keep the body more functionally stable, with less accumulation of stress. Just as acupuncture helps sick persons to regain their homeostasis without pharmaceutical intervention, it is even more effective in general health maintenance.

Treatment Protocol

For each treatment session, use prone or supine positions, or both, and needle all the HAs accessible in the selected position(s). If a particular symptom is found, palpate to find the local SAs and their corresponding PAs.

SUMMARY

Acupuncture therapy, in principle, is a nonspecific means of promoting physiological balance and thus stimulating the process of self healing (see Chapters 3 and 4). There is enormous potential in using acupuncture for both pain and non-pain symptoms; however, in the case of conditions that are not painful, it is more difficult to predict reliable prognoses.

14

Acupuncture Therapy in Sports Medicine

INTRODUCTION

Acupuncture has been a part of sports medicine since the dawn of Chinese civilization. The concept of *Qi* is the essence of Chinese martial arts as well as of acupuncture, and historically the masters of Chinese martial arts were also experts in traditional Chinese medicine (TCM). They used acupuncture to treat acute and chronic martial arts injuries, and also to "tonify Qi," meaning to activate the healing mechanism of the body to prevent injuries and improve performance.

Today the use of acupuncture in sports medicine is becoming more and more recognized. The continuing growth in popularity of recreational sports and fitness activities creates more injuries like strains, sprains, and broken bones. Now that we better understand the benefits of acupuncture we know that it can be very effective not only for martial arts injuries but also for preventing and treating all kinds of sports injuries for both professional and amateur athletes.

The most common sports injuries are musculoskeletal disorders such as damage to muscles, bursae, ligaments, capsules, and bones. In this chapter we focus on injuries caused by repetitive overuse of muscles, joints, and bones.

Any movement of the human body is a complicated biomechanical process that requires the coordination of many muscles and different parts of the body. When a muscle is weak or injured, it becomes tight, fatigued, inflamed, undernourished, or hypoxic. This injured muscle will disturb the normally synchronous and harmonious coordination between it and other muscles and the result will be pain or injury. This is why muscle injury can spread easily if not treated early. For example, if a group of injured muscles are left untreated, it can result in a stress fracture of the bone. Acupuncture can accelerate the healing of injured muscles and/or injured soft tissues, thus preventing the injury from spreading further. Treating injured muscles also indirectly helps to accelerate the recovery of

injured bones because the healed muscles and the soft tissues allow for an increased blood supply, which is needed for regeneration of bone tissue.

When sport accidents cause severe injuries that affect the bones, orthopedic specialists should be consulted immediately. In these cases, acupuncture can still be used to promote rehabilitation and accelerate recovery after surgery.

Most sports injury pain is of an acute nature resulting from strain and/or sprain. If the acute pain symptoms are neglected (e.g., when some athletes try to perform while ignoring their pain), the acute pain may became chronic and lead to changes in the histological structure of the tissues. The chronic problem will eventually permanently deprive the soft tissues of their functional ability, such as, for example, the full range of contraction of the muscle.

THE DIFFERENCE BETWEEN TREATING PROFESSIONAL AND AMATEUR ATHLETES

There are two basic differences between patients who are professional athletes and those who are amateur athletes. First, professional athletes have a greater risk that a minor injury will become a severe or even disabling condition because their tight schedules do not give them sufficient time to recover. Amateur athletes usually have enough time to adequately treat their acute injuries. Second, the purpose of treating a sports injury in a professional athlete is not pain relief but *functional recovery*, whereas for nonprofessional athletes, pain relief is the primary purpose.

When a professional athlete is injured, the tight schedules of training and competition usually prevent the dedication of sufficient time to achieve proper healing, even in the case of a minor injury. Because of this some professional athletes start to perform again before they are fully recovered. The athletes and their coaches try to find a quick fix such as painkillers or steroid injections. *But there is no such quick fix.* As a result, minor injuries become chronic, and the damage can spread to other tissues. Consequently, many professional athletes have to live with chronic pain or, in some cases, they become disabled, threatening their entire athletic career.

Athletes and coaches should understand that in most cases pain does not appear suddenly but develops as a result of cumulative stress or injury in neuromusculoskeletal tissues, often accompanied by inflammation and swelling. This pathological process, if not completely reversed, gradually reduces the function and structure of the injured tissue to a critical level where the body starts to "cry" for help and protection. Pain means that the injured tissue has been deprived of a sufficient supply of blood, nutrition, and oxygen for some period of time. Acupuncture needling relaxes the stressed tissue and revives the normal supply of nutrients and oxygen. After treatment, the pain will disappear but the process of proper recovery of affected tissues—the replacement of damaged cells by healthy ones and the recovery of normal function and strength—still needs time.

WHAT TO DO WHEN A SPORTS INJURY OCCURS

When pain or injury occurs during sport activities, the athlete should stop and immediately seek a medical evaluation. Acupuncture treatments will be effective to reduce pain, swelling, and inflammation, and the athlete should avoid deep massage or stretching, which may further damage the tissues. An ice pack can be used for the first day or two, to reduce inflammation, and a heat pack should be used to promote blood circulation after the inflammation has been reduced. A few days away from training are essential. Although mild exercise is beneficial for recovery, no physical stress should be placed on the damaged tissues. After recovery is achieved, the athlete still needs to be careful to monitor the amount and intensity of the training, to keep it within a level that is acceptable for the injured tissue, gradually increasing back to a normal level. This may result in a few extra days before the athlete is able to resume training or competition but it will protect the body from permanent injury and minimize the threat to the athlete's professional career.

There is a general agreement among pain specialists that 3 months are needed for natural healing of soft tissues. If pain from a sports injury continues after 3 months, it is regarded as chronic pain. Our clinical experience shows that in cases of minor and moderate acute pain from a sports

injury, proper acupuncture treatment can relieve pain in less than 2 weeks. Without proper treatment, the initially treatable acute pain may become a chronic disorder.

Generally, athletes are healthy and physically active, with a high healing potential. Thus, most of their acute pain symptoms can be treated effectively by acupuncture within a range of a few hours to a few days. The painful tissue is usually physically damaged, energetically starving, physiologically abnormal, functionally disabled, and affected by an abnormal accumulation of metabolic toxins. Acupuncture needling can relieve pain in a very short period of time by desensitizing the nerve endings and reducing swelling and inflammation.

Pain pills, which block the perception of pain in the athlete's brain, also work very well because a healthy body responds better to pain medication than does an unhealthy one.

It is clear that both acupuncture needling and pain pills can stop sports-injury pain in a very short time, but repairing the damaged tissue and restoring function take much more time. Athletes have to be aware that pain relief does not equal functional relief, and to achieve the latter, the normally intense schedule has to be relaxed. It is important to note the difference between acupuncture therapy and pharmaceutical therapy. Acupuncture works on the peripheral level (the local injured tissue), the spinal cord level (gate control in the spinal cord to block pain signals), and the brain level (pain modulation in brain centers). It starts by fixing the damage first, and as the damaged tissue starts to heal, the pain subsides. In contrast, pain medication blocks the pain signal at the spinal cord level or in brain centers and quickly takes away the sensation of pain, but the tissue damage is still waiting for the supply of nutrition and oxygen that is needed for healing. When athletes use pain medication or steroid injections to suppress pain and immediately resume training and competition, the tissue damage becomes more severe.

NO QUICK FIX FOR SPORTS INJURIES

It is understandable that patients want to be healed quickly. Our experience of working with athletes, both professional and amateur, shows that even with the high level of health that they enjoy, healing of injury and pain cannot be accelerated beyond the body's natural rate without the risk of aggravating the injury and leading to disability in the future.

Muscle has an important physiologic character: it has a *memory of its injury.* After an injured or sick muscle is properly treated and recovers, the pain disappears and the flexibility of the muscle fibers is restored, but the memory of the injury will stay for a much longer time, depending on the severity of the injury. As long as the healed muscle retains the memory of its injury, it becomes fatigued and weaker faster and is liable to produce pain and injury again if exposed to the same repetitive overuse. It takes time and a conscious effort toward restraint to erase a muscle's memory of its injury. Athletes with acute muscle pain should not ignore the memory factor, which is an important part of muscle rehabilitation.

PAIN PILLS SHOULD BE USED WITH CAUTION FOR ACUTE SPORTS PAIN

In sports activities, pain appears as a result of cumulative stress or damage to the tissues. The pain is a warning signal intended to protect the damaged or exhausted tissues and to demand additional nutrition, oxygen, relief from the stressful activity, and time to repair and regenerate the tissues. If the demand is ignored, as when pain is numbed by pills or steroid injections, which suppress pain but retard the process of healing, it can result in a future disaster for the injured athlete.

In the context of athletic activity by healthy people, pain is a warning signal, part of the protective wisdom of the body. Chronic pain, however, is a disease in and of itself. For athletes, this difference is important, and different strategies should be used to treat different kinds of pain.

Pain pills are not a solution for restoring the function of injured soft tissue. Athletes should focus on functional restoration as being more important than suppression of acute pain.

INTEGRATIVE NEUROMUSCULAR ACUPOINT SYSTEM FOR SPORTS TRAUMA

The 24 homeostatic acupoints (HAs) of the Integrative Neuromuscular Acupoint System (INMAS) are a map of the most important points for restoring the physiologic function of muscles. Most of the INMAS acupoints are situated in the major muscles that ensure the body's movement and coordination, and all HAs are supplied with major peripheral nerves. Needling INMAS acupoints improves the function and coordination of major muscles and joints. A local injury is always associated with one or more HAs, and stimulation of the local HAs improves the blood circulation and energy metabolism of the injured area.

When pain or injury occurs, the local HAs and SAs should be needled first, and then the distant HAs should be needled to treat possible referred pain, to reduce stress, and to activate homeostatic restoration.

MECHANISMS OF ACUPUNCTURE THERAPY USED IN SPORTS MEDICINE

Acupuncture is effective in sports medicine because, through the healing mechanisms discussed above, it can accelerate the healing of existing trauma, prevent future athletic injuries, and improve athletic performance.

USING ACUPUNCTURE FOR INJURY PREVENTION AND IMPROVEMENT OF PHYSICAL PERFORMANCE

All repetitive strain or overuse injuries from sports activities are caused by physiologically sick muscles. The muscles become injured gradually, without initial warning signals, and the majority of athletes are not aware when a muscle starts to become sick. They may feel some pain or some tightness in the muscle during or after sports activities, but since the pain is not evident during less stressful activities such as walking they believe that there is nothing wrong with the muscle; they believe that massage or a hot bath will take care of the situation. When palpating such affected muscles, however, tender, sore, and even painful spots are felt, and these are symptoms of the sick muscles.

Most of these sensitive spots will not disappear on their own, because, in fact, they are signs of structural abnormality. After repetitive strain or overuse, some muscle cells (fibers) shrink and form contracture spots or bands. Most sensitive spots or bands, if not properly dissolved, can become permanent structures in the muscle. If a muscle harbors these sensitive spots, physiologically the muscle becomes more easily and quickly fatigued; functionally it becomes less flexible and resistant to whole-range stretching and more slow to recover after exercise.

These injured muscles are the weakest muscles in an athlete's body. They disturb the coordination of synchronous muscle movements and cause misalignment of the joints. If the injured muscles are continuously forced to move, they will share the injury with neighboring muscles and tendons in order to protect themselves. As a result, muscle activities are handicapped and even a minor activity can then create a physical injury.

Acupuncture needling is the most effective modality for tight muscles because it physically breaks and dissolves the contracture in a precise way without side effects and thereby accelerates the healing and recovery of the dysfunctional muscles. A healthy, pain- and contracture-free muscle is more flexible and less prone to injury. It works better and longer, and recovers faster from contraction, so it can sustain and adapt to the most vigorous training. This is why acupuncture needling can prevent muscle and soft tissue injury and improve an athlete's physical performance.

TENDINITIS FROM REPETITIVE STRAIN OR OVERUSE IN SPORTS

Tendinitis is a common repetitive strain/overuse disorder in sports medicine. It usually occurs in the tendons of the major muscles associated with the shoulder, elbow, wrist, and knee joints, and in some muscle attachments such as the calcaneal (Achilles') tendon or that between the hamstring muscle and the ischium.

We have seen both professional and amateur athletes with various kinds of tendinitis who came to us because they failed to obtain relief or suffered worse pain after undergoing conventional treatment including surgery, steroid injections, pain medication, physical therapy, and massage. We found that most of these conventional modalities focused on pain and inflammation of the injured tendons but ignored the root of the tendinitis problem: the sick muscle(s).

The muscles are built for contraction and consist of the most dynamic, flexible, and contractible muscle cells (fibers) in the body. The tendons consist of connective tissues that connect the muscles to the bones, and are functionally much less contractible so that they can effectively transfer the muscle's contraction to the motions of the joints and bones. So in the muscle-tendon-tendon attachment structure (tendons attach to the bones, to other tendons, or to dense connective tissues), the muscle creates a contraction, the tendon transfers the contraction to the bones or other tendons, and the bone moves. This is normal functioning.

After repetitive strain or overuse, the mechanism of self-protection is activated and the muscle becomes sick. It is then less contractible (tight) or

may even produce tender contracture inside it that resists further contraction. When the sick, noncontractible muscle is still forced to contract, it tries to force the noncontractible tendon to stretch, which leads to inflammation or physical rupture of the tendon. Similar to the process that occurs inside the muscle, a contracture of the connective tissues is also formed inside the tendon to resist any forced stretch(ing). This type of physical force and physiologic stress is the cause of most of the tendinitis injuries that are found in sports.

Thus tendinitis is usually a secondary injury that is caused by the primary injury—muscle sickness. In some cases, the tendons are damaged first, but very soon the injured tendons cause the muscle to become tight or to manifest tender or painful areas in order to protect themselves. It is clear that all tendinitis is associated with sick muscles, regardless of whether the muscles are the primary or the secondary cause.

Therefore, tendinitis should be treated together with the muscles because a sick muscle always places mechanical stress on the tendon. Fortunately, acupuncture can easily handle both muscles and tendons simultaneously. When treating tendinitis a practitioner should carefully examine both the tendon and the muscle to locate the tender spots in both regions, and needle all of these spots. After the treatments, patients should rest or do only very mild exercise so that the healing process can run its course in both the tendon and the muscle.

We have achieved very good results treating tendinitis, especially when patients come to us immediately after it is suspected. We also have helped patients who had previously tried unsuccessfully to obtain healing from other modalities such as medication, steroid injections, or physical therapy, although more treatments and a longer rehabilitation period were needed because these patients have usually suffered more damage if these other modalities were not beneficial.

It is more difficult to treat tendinitis after unsuccessful surgery because (1) surgery, if not well done, may shorten the muscle and create permanent stress in the muscle and tendon, and (2) surgery usually changes some natural structure, and acupuncture works best with natural pathways.

TREATING SOFT TISSUE DISORDERS IN SPORTS MEDICINE

There are many patients who are suffering from the side effects of drugs (such as long-term use of steroid medication) or the consequences of unnecessary surgery, who could have benefited from acupuncture. Many of the side effects of conventional medical intervention can be avoided or reduced when acupuncture is used alone or in combination with other procedures.

Dr. Alec Meleger of the Harvard Medical School Physical Medicine and Rehabilitation program and Dr. Joanne Borg-Stein of the Tufts Medical School Physical Medicine and Rehabilitation department conducted an in-depth review of published studies on using acupuncture in sports medicine. The review paper by Drs. Meleger and Borg-Stein[1] provided objective data to support the clinical value of using acupuncture for soft tissue disorders in sports medicine.

Acupuncture needling (dry needles) and steroid injections (wet needles) have similar therapeutic efficacy as suggested by Dr. David G. Simons.[2] "Dry needling is as effective as injection of an anesthetic for relief of trigger point symptoms" as long as the dry needling can precisely target the trigger point.

In other research, Dr. Chilton[3] reported a higher success rate with acupuncture and steroids versus steroid-only treatment. We believe, too, that a combination of acupuncture needling and steroid injections provides better results than injections alone because acupuncture can be used for breaking all the tender points detected during a treatment whereas one can make only a limited number of steroid injections in any one treatment. Acupuncture stimulates the natural antiinflammatory process in the body and can be used repeatedly to deactivate muscle and fascia contracture. Thus, acupuncture needling can continue to be used during follow-up treatments without any side effects.

These research conclusions about the use of acupuncture for sports-related injuries completely match the understanding and interpretation of the acupuncture mechanism and its clinical features that are presented in INMAS, which among its other merits helps to explain the nonpharmaceutical self-healing mechanism of acupuncture and the different approaches for treating athletic and nonathletic patients.

We should mention one general misconception about acupuncture, which is to treat it like pharmaceutical therapy and thus try to figure out which problems acupuncture can and cannot effectively treat. However, the efficacy of acupuncture depends on how much healing potential is maintained in the body (which is predictable) and the healability of the injury. The same injury may be effectively healable at the acute stage but unhealable in an advanced chronic stage.

SUMMARY

Scientific studies, clinical evidence, and the history of using acupuncture to treat martial arts injuries all indicate that acupuncture has a special value in treating most soft tissue injuries from sports activities, as well as preventing these injuries and improving physical performance.

When pain or soft tissue injury occurs, immediate acupuncture needling will reduce pain and swelling, limit the extent of the inflamed tissues, and accelerate healing. Acupuncture needling can effectively remove muscle and tendon stress and increase the flexibility of the muscles and tendons by dissolving the contracture that reduces blood circulation and causes muscle pain. INMAS provides an indispensable tool for practitioners to locate the most important acupoints for effectively treating sports-related injuries, preventing future injuries, and improving athletic performance by improving local muscle function and bodily coordination.

References

1. Meleger A, Borg-Stein J: Acupuncture and sports medicine: a review of published studies, *Medical acupuncture*, vol 11, No 2, Fall, 1999/Winter, 2000.
2. Simons DG, Travell JG, Simons LS: *Travell & Simons' myofascial pain and dysfunction: the trigger point manual,* vol 1, Philadelphia, 1999, Lippincott Williams & Wilkins, p 151.
3. Chilton SA: Tennis elbow: a combined approach using acupuncture and local corticosteroid injection, *Acupuncture Med* 15(2):77-78, 1997.

CHAPTER 15

Electroacupuncture Analgesia

INTRODUCTION

Electroacupuncture is not unanimously defined. Professor Ji-sheng Han of Beijing University states that when electrodes are placed on the surface of the skin, and when "the point of stimulation is selected according to traditional acupuncture, the process is usually called electroacupuncture (EA)." The same process, if the points used are not traditional acupoints, is regarded as transcutaneous electrical nerve stimulation (TENS).[1]

Neurophysiologically, there is no difference between the two concepts of EA and TENS. The same author also indicated that, "they operate through very similar, if not identical, mechanisms."[1] Different acupoints may have a different anatomic configuration (see Chapter 1), but sensory nerve fibers are the universal component of any acupoint. Because these fibers are distributed all over the body except nails and hair (which is why we can cut them without pain), acupoints can be found anywhere on the body.

If surface electrodes are placed on a sensitized (tender) point, whether it is a traditional acupoint or not, peripheral stimulation will be provided to the spinal cord through the sensitized nerve endings, which helps to desensitize and calm down the irritated nerve. If the surface electrodes are placed on nonsensitive points, the electrophysiologic process resulting from this peripheral stimulation is exactly the same as with the stimulation of tender acupoints, but with less therapeutic results in terms of desensitizing the painful sensory nerves. As we have already mentioned, the number of traditional and extra-meridian "new" acupoints has reached more than 2500 (see Chapter 1), which means that documented acupoints can be found almost everywhere in the body.

Another method also described as electroacupuncture is the use of needles as electrodes, inserted into the tissue, which is called percutaneous electrical nerve stimulation (PENS). Physiologically PENS is different from both EA and TENS because with PENS *needles are used to create both tissue lesion and electrical stimulation.* Even though EA, TENS, and PENS all stimulate the release of the natural neurochemicals, including endorphins, produced by the central nervous system, PENS with its induced lesions involves other healing mechanisms that are similar to manual needling (see Chapter 3).

Despite the different ways of defining and using peripheral electrical stimulation, all these modalities do the same thing: activating the self-healing mechanisms of the body by balancing physiologic processes. For example, the release of the central nervous system (CNS) opioid peptides known as endorphins is a shared physiologic basis for these modalities, and these substances are physiologic de-stressors whose release can be triggered not only by electrical stimulation or needling, but also by exercise, physical manipulation, and massage.

The therapeutic use of electricity for pain relief can be traced back to Egyptian medicine some 4500 years ago. They used electric fish to treat painful conditions. In Greek medicine, doctors used electric torpedo fish to treat headaches and arthritis (400 BC).

Electrotherapy was revived in modern times after Drs. Ronald Melzack and Patrick Wall proposed their Gate Control theory of pain in 1965 (see Chapter 3). This theory stated that the input of pain signals from the fine nerve fibers (such as C fibers or A-δ fibers) is controlled and modified in the spinal cord by the signals from the large nerve fibers (such as A-β fibers) before the pain signals reach the brain. The spinal cord functions like a gate in that it can be open or closed to the incoming pain signals. For example, if a person hits his finger with a hammer, the C nerve fibers in the finger start to fire pain signals to the brain through the spinal cord, so the brain perceives the finger pain. Then the person might rub or scratch the painful finger. By doing this, the large, low-threshold A-β fibers are activated. Their signals travel faster than those of the fine C nerve fibers, and activate the spinal cord to block the pain signals of the C nerve fibers. This is a simplified picture of the Gate Control theory. A recent study using the techniques of molecular biology has supported the concept that endorphins in the spinal cord exert a strong inhibitory effect on incoming pain signals.[2]

When Dr. Patrick Wall, an expert in pain and spinal cord physiology at St. Thomas's Hospital Medical School in London, and Dr. William Sweet, chief of neurosurgery at Harvard Medical School, realized that the large A-β fibers can be easily activated by electrical stimuli, they developed in 1967 an apparatus for TENS. They placed electrodes on the surface of the skin and used high-frequency electrical stimulation (50 to 100 Hz) to relieve chronic neurogenic pain. Today, battery-operated, solid-state TENS apparatuses are popular medical devices for the treatment of many painful conditions, and are used also by physical therapists and patients themselves.

In the late 1960s, Chinese doctors also started to combine the use of electrical stimulation with acupuncture after some successful experiments with acupuncture anesthesia. Their electrical acupuncture devices were designed to apply electric current to needles inserted into acupoints. As China was isolated from the rest of the world at that time, their development of electrical acupuncture is probably independent of the invention of TENS by Drs. Wall and Sweet.

In the early 1970s, Hans Kosterlitz and his student John Hughes were studying the action of narcotics in the University of Aberdeen in Scotland. They discovered that the brain makes its own natural narcotics, which they named endorphins, from "endogenous morphine." At almost the same time, Sol Snyder and his student Candace Pert at Johns Hopkins University in Baltimore confirmed that the body makes endorphins, which counteract pain among other physical functions.

These discoveries supported the possible endorphin mechanisms of acupuncture needling and TENS. Today we understand that endorphins can be stimulated in many different ways, including acupuncture needling, TENS, psychological process, chiropractic manipulations, exercise, and massage. In addition to counteracting pain, endorphins also have other physiologic functions such as rebalancing the cardiovascular system (bringing blood pressure to normal), hormonal secretions, defense immune activities, and so forth. In general, endorphins naturally normalize the body's function and bring a slight feeling of euphoria.

Four different endorphins, β-endorphin, enkephalin, dynorphin, and endomorphin, have so far been identified. Which of the four endorphins are stimulated depends on the frequency of electrical stimulation, and this frequency-dependence is a valuable feature of the clinical use of EA and TENS.

The research done in the past 2 decades has clearly laid down the guidelines of how to use TENS or EA to achieve maximal pain relief. Here we will discuss only what is needed for clinical use of TENS or EA. We will not go into physiologic details such as the involvement of calcium channels, antibody reactions, or different receptors. Readers who are interested in knowing more about EA and TENS may refer to the relevant published information.

FREQUENCY-DEPENDENT RELEASE OF ENDORPHINS BY PERIPHERAL ELECTRICAL STIMULATION AND THE ANTIENDORPHIN FEEDBACK INTERACTION

The stimulation of EA and TENS is transmitted by A-β and A-δ nerve fibers. Since the parameters of the type of stimulation used with EA and TENS can be reliably and precisely calibrated, it is possible to identify the physiological effects of peripheral electrical stimulation at different frequencies. This frequency-dependent nature of endorphin release has been confirmed in both laboratory animals and human subjects.[3]

Enkephalin and endomorphin are mostly released at 2 Hz, whereas dynorphin release is triggered during 100 Hz stimulation. The release of β-endorphin is triggered at a rate of 2 Hz then gradually decreases as the frequency is increased.

It has been shown that if the stimulation alternates between 2 and 100 Hz, the full release of all four endorphins is achieved, which induces synergistic analgesic effects.[4]

In addition to opioid peptides, other neurochemical analgesic factors are also triggered by peripheral electrical stimulation. Midbrain monoamines such as serotonin and norepinephrine have been confirmed to play a role in EA analgesia.[5,6] Recently it was discovered that brain-derived neurotrophic factor (BDNF) is released by 100 Hz stimulation in bursts, but not by constant 100 Hz stimulation.[7] BDNF has been shown to reverse the dying of neurons in animals.[8]

Part of the brain (ventral periaqueductal gray [vPAG]) reacts to both low frequency (2 Hz) and high frequency (100 Hz), but other parts react to only one frequency: the arcuate nucleus of the hypothalamus (ARH) to low frequency and the parabrachial nucleus (PBN) to high frequency.

The body's wisdom in ensuring the survival mechanism is always ahead of human intelligence. The release of natural endorphins to reduce the body's pain and stress is a natural physiologic process, but we try to use the electrical stimulation to change this physiological process into a pharmacologic process. Our body has a built-in mechanism to prevent overuse of its natural narcotics (endorphins): the release of antiendorphin peptides through negative feedback. Data from animals show that the analgesic effect of endorphins declines when EA stimulation is prolonged for more than 3 hours due to the release of antiendorphin antagonists (antiopioid peptides).[9]

Low-frequency stimulation (2 to 15 Hz), triggers the release of endomorphin, enkephalin, and most β-endorphins, but these frequencies also cause the release of their antagonist peptides, substance P (SP), angiotensin II (AII), and cholesystokinin octapeptide (CCK-8). High-frequency (100 Hz) stimulation significantly increases the release of antagonists AII and CCK-8.[1]

Attention should be paid to the interesting and clinically meaningful fact that low-frequency stimulation (2 Hz) only marginally induces the release of CCK-8 and SP, 50% less than with high-frequency stimulation. It is not difficult to draw the conclusion that high-frequency stimulation releases more antiopioid peptides than low-frequency stimulation because the brain perceives high frequencies (100 Hz) as a more artificial and alien modality than low frequencies (2 to 15 Hz). From birth, low-frequency peripheral electrical stimulation is a common experience to the baby's brain because touch, pressure, rubbing, needling, cuts, and minor injury all transmit low-frequency electrical impulses to the brain by means of the peripheral nerve receptors.

All the laboratory and clinical experimental data indicate that to elicit the maximal release of central opioid peptides (endorphins), electrical stimulation should alternate between 2 Hz and 100 Hz to achieve the synergistic effect of TENS and EA analgesia.[1]

TECHNICAL PARAMETERS OF TENS AND EA

The purpose of electrical analgesia is to electrically depolarize the nerve endings to produce nerve impulses to the brain through the spinal cord. With a modern EA or TENS apparatus the stimulation parameters can be very easily regulated. The prac-

titioner needs to set up (1) frequencies, (2) modes (constant, burst, or alternative, if they are available), and (3) pulse width. All TENS apparatuses have the option of using square wave or biphasic current (Box 15-1).

Voltage

The voltage must be sufficient to overcome the electrical resistance of the tissues in order to generate a current that will depolarize the nerve endings but cause no discomfort to the patient. Dry human skin has a resistance of 2000 ohms, and an inserted needle reduces the resistance to 600 ohms. Skin on a tender point has a resistance between 600 and 2000 ohms, depending on the sensitivity and extent of the tender point. Up to 20V is considered a safe voltage that produces a tolerable current.[10]

Current

The current should be strong enough to generate electrical impulses at the nerve endings while not causing discomfort to the patient. Theoretically the most effective intensity of current should be just below the pain threshold. Whereas the pain threshold is almost the same in every patient, pain tolerance varies dramatically from person to person. The effective but acceptable range of current is 10 to 50 mA, depending on personal tolerance.

Wave Form

Omura suggested that a square wave produces the optimal depolarization,[11] so almost all modern TENS apparatuses output square waves.

Box 15-1

Parameters of Electrical Stimulation Using TENS or EA

Voltage: Up to 20 V
Current: 10-50 mA
Wave-form: Square wave
Pulse width: 0.05-0.5 ms
Polarity: Biphasic
Frequency: Low: 2-4 Hz; medium: 15-20 Hz; high: 100 Hz

Modified from White A: Electroacupuncture and acupuncture analgesia. In Filshie J, White A, editors: *Medical acupuncture: a Western scientific approach,* New York, 1998, Churchill Livingstone, p 157.

Pulse Width

A pulse width of less than 0.05 ms is insufficient to depolarize nerve endings, and widths greater than 0.5 ms are more likely to stimulate C fibers and cause pain. The greater the pulse width, the smaller the current required.

Polarity

Theoretically a unipolar current carries the risk of causing ionization between the needle and the tissues. The ionization leads to electrolysis of the needle, the formation of hydrochloric acid, and local tissue necrosis from electrolysis. The modern apparatus generates a biphasic wave: the initial square wave is followed by a negative pulse, produced by the discharge of a capacitor. There is no risk of electrolysis when using surface electrodes or disposable needles with biphasic current.

Frequency

It is suggested that low or medium frequency (2 to 4 Hz or 15 to 20 Hz, respectively) and high frequency (100 Hz) be used alternately to achieve the maximal synergistic effect of CNS opioid peptides with the least release of antiopioid antagonists (e.g., CCK-8, SP, AII).

Modes

Burst stimulation is more effective for endorphin release.

ACUPOINT SELECTION FOR TENS OR EA USING THE INTEGRATIVE NEUROMUSCULAR ACUPOINT SYSTEM

Proper acupoint selection can greatly enhance the efficacy of TENS and EA treatments. Skin resistance is lower when an acupoint becomes tender, that is, when nerve endings and/or other soft tissues become sensitized. Like the manual needling of tender acupoints, direct electrical stimulation accelerates the desensitization of the sensitized or inflamed nerve endings and other soft tissues.

The Integrative Neuromuscular Acupoint System (INMAS) provides guidance for selecting the highly effective therapeutic acupoints, especially for neuromuscular pain in the lower back, buttocks, and lower and upper limbs, because all 24 HAs usually show a notable degree of tenderness in

more than 80% of people. In cases of acute pain, most of the acute tender points appear around the regional HAs.

Here are a few examples of acupoint selection for TENS and EA. For treating lower back pain, the pair of acupoints can be H15 and H16, H14 and H16, or H14 and H18, depending on whether the pain is located in the lumbar, sacral, or iliotibial region. For treating shoulder pain, the pair of acupoints can be H3 and H8, or H13 and H8, and other pairs of tender acupoints localized around the glenohumeral joint. For leg pain, the pair of acupoints can be H11 and H10, H4 and H6, or H24 and H6, depending on the painful muscles involved.

The general principle of acupoint selection is that the current should travel through the painful muscles or tissues.

CAUTION AND CONTRAINDICATIONS WHEN USING TENS AND EA

A few safety guidelines should be kept in mind when using TENS and EA.

The Heart

TENS and EA should not cross the thorax because of the theoretical danger of interfering with the heart's conducting tissues. If the patient has a cardiac pacemaker, TENS or EA current will change the rhythmic activity of the pacemaker. In general, we do not use TENS or PENS in patients with pacemakers.

The Neck

We do not suggest using TENS or EA on the neck. TENS or EA stimulation on the back of the neck may cause mechanical damage to the neck. The neck facets are much more liable to mechanical injuries, and the vibration generated by the TENS and EA stimulation may mechanically damage the facet structures. In addition, external electrical current should not be used in the area of the medulla oblongata (the brainstem) to avoid the theoretical risk of interfering with cardiovascular and respiratory function.

Do not stimulate above the anterior part of the neck. Pressure from muscle contraction or stimulation of the nerves of the carotid sinus may cause hypotension-induced fainting (syncope). If a person happens to have a supersensitive carotid sinus, the stimulation may cause temporary or permanent cessation of the heart beat. Stimulation of the nerves of the larynx could produce laryngeal spasm.

The Lung

PENS type stimulation should not be used in the chest or upper back area so as to avoid pneumothorax.

The Face

We suggest using only surface electrodes on the face because PENS stimulation may cause bruising or discomfort on the face, especially in female patients.

Local Contraindications

TENS and PENS produce a stimulating current and physical vibration that have some effect on the physical condition of the skin and tissues. It is wise to adhere to the following rules:

1. Do not place electrodes on inflamed, infected, swollen, or otherwise unhealthy skin.
2. Do not stimulate over a pregnant uterus.
3. To avoid sudden unexpected discomfort or excessive pain, the TENS or EA apparatus should be switched off and the intensity set to zero before attaching the electrodes to the patient. The intensity must be increased only slowly because the thresholds for sensation and pain are close together.

ELECTROACUPUNCTURE AND MANUAL ACUPUNCTURE

Both EA and manual acupuncture (MA) activate the self-healing potential of our body. Maintenance of body homeostasis requires the integrated coordination of every physiologic system, but there are four that play the leading role in linking all the systems together to sustain life: the nervous system, immune system, endocrine system, and cardiovascular system.

EA with its strong and continuous electrical stimuli and muscular vibration activates all these systems. For example, EA stimulation of the central nervous system triggers neurochemical releases such as endorphins and serotonin in the spinal cord and the brain, and activates systemic and local blood circulation. The local muscular vibration created by EA relaxes the muscles and improves regional blood circulation.

EA has been extensively used for pain management since the late 1970s after TENS was invented, and it was particularly popular in the early 1980s. The parameters of EA stimulation can be precisely controlled, recorded, and reproduced, and this is why EA has been extensively studied in laboratory research. Using genetically and developmentally standardized laboratory animals, sufficient neurophysiological data have been obtained in both animal and human subjects to support the clinical application of EA over the past 2 decades.

The essential mechanism of EA is the electrical stimulation of A-β nerve fibers with varying frequencies to induce the release of different CNS opioid peptides, which relieve pain and other physiological stress to achieve self-healing. The secondary mechanism of EA is the rhythmic physical vibration of the muscles, which helps to relax tightness and improve blood circulation, which accelerates self-healing.

Some kind of MA stimulation has been used in Egyptian, Greek, Chinese, and other folk medicines for more than 3500 years. Before metal needles were available, ancient healers used sharpened stones, bamboo needles, and broken porcelain to pierce or puncture the tissues to effect healing. It can be imagined that early acupuncture "needling" created much more severe lesions and possible scars. The modern acupuncture needle creates an elegant and less painful lesion without scar formation while it can reach much deeper to relax muscular contracture.

The essential mechanism of MA consists of the needling and the tiny needle-induced lesion in the tissues that stimulates A-δ and C nerve fibers. MA and its lesions are interpreted by the body as foreign invaders and thus induce a series of physiologic processes including the release of CNS opioid peptides and an antiinflammatory reaction. MA produces a weaker electrical stimuli to the central nervous system than does EA, but the needling directly desensitizes the damaged peripheral nerve endings and other soft tissues by activating a local immune reaction and the process of tissue regeneration. MA-induced lesions break and dissolve histologic contracture of the muscles, which helps to improve blood circulation.

Low-frequency EA (2 to 4 Hz) has a mechanism that is closer to MA. So some researchers refer to low-frequency EA stimulation as acupuncture-like stimulation. More research data are needed to investigate the therapeutic potential and differences between the working mechanisms of EA and MA.

When we look at the history of EA and MA, it is obvious that stimulation by accidentally produced lesions similar to those used in acupuncture has been an indispensable part of our built-in survival mechanisms in both phylogenetic evolution (evolution of the species) and ontogenetic development (our personal development from a newborn baby to senior adult). In our daily life, we are often exposed to numerous kinds of tiny lesions and injuries. Without self-healing mechanisms, we would not survive even a minor injury. Our body has developed self-protective mechanisms to exploit the effect of these small lesions and injuries to promote healing. Manual acupuncture uses the same lesion-induced self-healing mechanisms that have been genetically programmed into the body's survival strategy; therefore MA treatments can be repeated as often as needed without causing physiologic adaptation that might reduce efficacy after repeated treatments.

Compared with MA, EA with its well-controlled parameters and frequencies is a new type of stimulation that is not genetically programmed into the body's survival strategy. Prolonged electrical stimulation of the nervous system to release opioid peptides will be balanced by the release of antiopioid peptides. Thus, long-term application of EA results in reduced effectiveness due to the physiologic adaptability of the central nervous system to external stimulation.

Pain can be caused by psychological factors, biochemical processes, and structural abnormalities. Biochemical processes include the chemicals released from injured tissues such as prostaglandin or substance P that irritate the nerves and cause pain. Structural abnormalities happen when muscle contracture is formed within the muscles or a vertebral disk is ruptured. EA stimulation using alternating frequencies with the resulting synergistic release of opioid peptides will combat the biochemical process of pain production. MA does not induce release of the whole spectrum of opioid peptides as EA does, but it triggers other defense reactions and healing mechanisms such as the antiinflammatory reaction and the structural breaking of mild muscle contractures. It is possible that EA will provide better results in treating drug addiction. Both EA and MA have limited efficacy with psychogenic pain, although the opioid peptides (endorphins) do have a mild effect of euphoria.

EA and MA target different nerve fibers. Needling mechanically stimulates the A-δ and possibly C nerve fibers, while EA stimulates the vibration-sensitive A-β nerve fiber (Types II and III) as described by Drs. Wall and Sweet. Clinically this suggests that EA may play a role in the gate control mechanism by blocking pain signals from A-δ and C fibers. MA needling may activate local physiologic mechanisms to desensitize painful A-δ and C fibers.

As a result of extensive clinical observation, Dr. John W. Thompson, a physician and clinical pharmacologist in the University of Newcastle, England, noticed that "A striking and puzzling difference between analgesia produced by TENS and acupuncture (needling) is the duration of pain relief. Whereas TENS usually produces analgesia for minutes or hours, acupuncture can, and usually does, produce analgesia for days or weeks (after a course of acupuncture). The mechanisms discussed above (the author is referring to the CNS neural pathways and the production of opioid peptides) cannot account for the prolonged analgesia commonly seen after acupuncture (needling), so additional mechanisms must be involved."[12]

Dr. Anthony Campbell of the Royal London Homoeopathic Hospital also indicated that "It is important to make sure that the patient...realizes that the pain may well return soon after the (TENS) machine is switched off. This is not, however, invariably the case; in some fortunate people relief of pain may last up to 10 hours."[13]

In Chapter 6 we introduced the quantitative method to classify the patients into four groups: A, B, C, and D. Each group responds to manual acupuncture differently. Our clinical experience indicates that excellent therapeutic results can be achieved in group A patients (28%) by either MA or EA. In general, the observations of Drs. Thompson and Campbell match the results seen most commonly in patients of groups B and C (34% and 30%, respectively).

SUMMARY

With an understanding of both the similarity and the differences between EA and MA it is obvious that they will co-exist in the practice of pain management. They are, in fact, complementary to each other in our clinical practice. We also believe that more research is needed to explore the potential applications of both EA and MA.

References

1. Han J-S: Acupuncture: neuropeptide release produced by electrical stimulation of different frequencies, *Trends Neurosci* 26(1):17-22, 2003.
2. Cheng HYM: DREAM is a critical transcriptional repressor for pain modulation, *Cell* 108:31-43, 2002
3. Han J-S et al: Effects of low- and high-frequency TENS on met-enkephalin-Arg-Phe and dynorphin: an immunoreactivity in human lumbar cerebrospinal fluid, *Pain* 47: 295-298, 1991.

4. Chen XH et al: Optimal conditions for eliciting maximal electoacupuncture analgesia with dense and disperse mode stimulation, *Am J Acupunct* 22:47-53, 1994.

5. Zao FY, Han JS: Acupuncture analgesia in impacted last molar extraction: effect of clomipramine and pargyline. In *The neurochemical basis of pain relief by acupuncture: a collection of papers 1973-1989,* Beijing, 1989, Beijing Medical Science, pp 96-97.

6. Mayer DJ, Watkins LR: Multiple endogenous opiate and nonopiate analgesia systems. In Kruger L, editor: *Advances in pain research and therapy*, vol 6, New York, 1984, Raven, pp 253-276.

7. Gartner A, Staiger V: Neurotrophin release from hippocampal neurons evoked by long term potentiation-inducing electrical stimulation patterns, *Proc Natl Acad Sci* U S A 99:6386-6391, 2002.

8. Ma Y-T, Hsie T, Frost D: Brain-derived neurotrophic factor (BDNF) reduces the death of retinal ganglionic neurons in rat, *J Neurosci* 18(6):2097-2107, March 1998.

9. Han J-S: Opioid and antiopioid peptides: a model of Yin-yang balance in acupuncture mechanism of pain modulation. In Stux G, Hammerschlag R, editors: *Clinical acupuncture scientific basis,* Berlin, 2001, Springer, p 56.

10. White A: Electroacupuncture and acupuncture analgesia. In Filshie J, White A, editors: *Medical acupuncture: a Western scientific approach*, Edinburgh, 1998, Churchill Livingstone, p 157.

11. Omura Y: Basic electrical parameters for safe and effective electro-therapeutics (electro-acupuncture, TES, TENMS (or TEMS), TENS and electro-magnetic field stimulation with or without drug field) for pain, neuromuscular skeletal problems, and circulatory disturbances, *Acupuncture and Electro-Therapeutics Research,* 12:201-225, 1987.

12. Thompson JW: Transcutaneous electrical nerve stimulation (TENS). In Filshie J, White A, editors: *Medical acupuncture: a Western scientific approach*, Edinburgh, 1998, Churchill Livingstone, p 190.

13. Campbell A: Methods of acupuncture. In Filshie J, White A, editors: *Medical acupuncture: a Western scientific approach*, Edinburgh, 1998, Churchill Livingstone, p 31.

CHAPTER 16

Using the Integrative Neuromuscular Acupoint System for Acupoint Injection Therapy

INTRODUCTION

The purpose of this chapter is to present the Integrative Neuromuscular Acupoint System (INMAS) to healthcare professionals who have already used injection therapy for pain management.

In the late 1960s, traditional Chinese medicine (TCM) was experiencing an extraordinary period of development, and the leading direction of research in the field, sponsored by the Chinese government, was the integration of TCM with modern medicine. Many new methods were explored to improve the effectiveness of traditional needling and were referred to as "innovative needling-method therapy" (*xin zhen liao fa*). These new techniques included electrical acupuncture, scalp acupuncture, acupoint implant therapy (surgically implanting foreign material at the acupoints), acupoint tissue extraction therapy (surgically removing fatty tissue from the acupoints), and acupoint injection therapy. In addition, practitioners of Chinese folk medicine were using more than 80 types of needling methods such as eye, nose, wrist-and-ankle needling, and so on.

For injection therapy the Chinese doctors injected about 1cc of a vitamin solution (but not vitamin C, which creates a very painful reaction), and various Chinese herbal extracts at the location of acupoints, and they claimed very good therapeutic results. Like acupuncture anesthesia, this was developed as a move toward the integration of traditional Chinese and modern medicine.

In the United States, Dr. Janet Travell, without previous knowledge of Chinese acupuncture, discovered and published the patterns of pain trigger points in 32 skeletal muscles in 1952.[1] The locations of these trigger points basically matched most acupoint locations in the ancient Chinese system. Dr. Travell injected anesthetics (0.5% procaine in physiologic saline) into these trigger points to treat myofascial pain symptoms such as lower back pain. Today the solutions used for injection may include isotonic saline, procaine, lidocaine, Botulinum toxin A (BTA), corticosteroids, and other longer-acting local anesthetics. Some of these injected solutions have some myotoxic effects.

Both the innovative Chinese acupoint injection method and Dr. Travell's system have their merits. INMAS is a simple and comprehensive method that integrates the Chinese acupuncture channel (meridian) system with Western neuromuscular understanding. All the 20 (or 21) injectable homeostatic acupoints (HAs) that are specified in INMAS match the major acupoints of the ancient 10 channels (meridians) (large intestine, small intestine, stomach, gallbladder, urinary bladder, liver, kidney, lung, spleen, and governor) as well as the major trigger points of the modern neuromuscular system.

THE BENEFITS OF INMAS FOR ACUPOINT INJECTION THERAPY

The Chinese acupoint injection system is based on the traditional concept of *yin-yang* balance and "channel (meridian) theory," whereas Dr. Travell's system focuses on intramuscular trigger points whose locations are based on modern pathology, anatomy, and physiology. INMAS combines the benefits of both because the majority of the 24 HA points are at the same time major channel (meridian) points and trigger points.

Of the 24 HAs that are specified in INMAS all but three are suitable for injection therapy, the exceptions being the facial HAs (H2 great auricular, H19 infraorbital, and H23 supraorbital), with H3 spinal accessory being a unique case requiring special caution on account of the lungs beneath. Note also that:

1. Symmetrical points are injected to prevent spasm in the antagonistic muscles
2. Distal points are injected for treatment of referred pain

INMAS AND CHRONIC MYOFASCIAL PAIN

The area to be injected should contain no damaged tissue, swelling, bruises, or scar tissue. Chronic myofascial pain usually develops around one or more HAs, and the location of these is a guide to the location of the other secondary tender points. Some of the HAs may also be related to referred pain.

For example, in patients with lower back pain, all the 7 HAs associated with the lumbosacral plexus may be tender: H14 superior cluneal, H15 posterior cutaneous of L2, H16 inferior gluteal, H22 posterior cutaneous of L5, H18 iliotibial, H11 lateral popliteal, and H10 sural. In addition to these major points, secondary tender points can develop around:

1. H15, if the pain is in iliopsoas, the lower part of latissimus dorsi, or multifidus in the L2 region
2. H22, if the pain is related to sacroiliac (SI) joints, L4 and L5 region, or multifidus in the S1 region
3. H16, if the pain is felt in the gluteal region in gluteus maximus or piriformis
4. H14, if the pain is felt in the iliotibial band, gluteus minimus, or medius
5. H18, if the pain is palpable in the iliotibial band down to the knee
6. H11 and H10 if the pain is felt in the leg

The HAs specified by INMAS can serve as a map for finding the secondary tender points because the INMAS system traces the interaction between the major nerve trunks and the major muscles of the neuromuscular system.

INMAS AND ACUTE MYOFASCIAL PAIN

Acute pain is a localized symptom, and wherever it occurs some tender HAs can be found around the painful area. Injection can be applied to the painful muscle(s) and the neighboring HAs.

If acute pain is accompanied by tissue injury, swelling, or ecchymosis (bruising), we suggest that injection should not be made into the injured tissue, but acupuncture needles can be used to reduce swelling and bruising, and to promote tissue repair.

TECHNICAL CONSIDERATIONS OF INJECTION THERAPY

Both acupuncture needling and injection share the same mechanism, which is to create healing-promoting lesions and a harmless temporary foreign body–immune reaction to treat myofascial pain. Injection needles are thicker than acupuncture needles so some technical safety factors should be taken into consideration.

Skin Cleaning

Injection needles make large lesions, so an aseptic area of skin should be carefully prepared for injection. Any common antiseptic can be used for cleaning the skin. Avoid any inflamed, swollen, or infected skin.

Bleeding

Injection may cause more bleeding than do the fine needles used in acupuncture. To avoid excessive capillary bleeding, patients can be advised to take vitamin C to decrease capillary fragility for 1 week before the injection. Patients also should not take any blood-thinning drugs such as aspirin for 3 days before the injection.

Needle Sizes

The purpose of the injection is to stretch the contracture inside the muscles, so the needles should be long enough to reach the depth where the contracture is situated. Thinner needles are less painful to patients, but they are liable to bend inside the muscles. Deep, thick muscles may unexpectedly contract and cause the needle to detach from the syringe if it is not firmly held. A large-diameter needle gives a better sense of tissue penetration and is therefore easier for the practitioner to use; however, the needling is more painful, so the practitioner has to find the appropriate diameter and length to suit the patient's level of tolerance.

Injection Volume

The process of injection physically pushes the muscle tissue aside to stretch the contracted muscle fibers. The needling itself first breaks some muscle contracture and stretches the contracted muscle fibers, then the hydraulic tension of the injected liquid reinforces the muscle stretching. A large volume of injected liquid may create excessive tissue lesions and increase the chance of liquid being unintentionally forced into a blood vessel, and clinical experience shows that a volume less than 1 cc (1 ml) is both safe and effective, and reaches the right compromise between tissue healing and tissue destruction.

Commonly Used Solutions for Injection Therapy

Since the late 1960s Chinese doctors have used vitamins B1, B6, and B12 for injection into acupoints. U.S. doctors use isotonic saline; local anesthetics such as procaine, lidocaine, and other long-acting anesthetics; corticosteroids; BTA; and epinephrine. Some of these substances are more myotoxic than others.

Isotonic saline can be injected into the HAs for pain relief. A controlled, double-blind comparison between isotonic saline and a myotoxic, long-acting anesthetic (0.5% mepivacaine) showed that isotonic saline offered the same or even better efficacy than mepivacaine.[2]

Procaine is the least myotoxic among the local anesthetics and is hydrolyzed in the blood. A 1% solution is suitable for injection therapy. This anesthetic blocks nerve conduction by binding to the calcium sites of the cellular membrane of the neuron.

A 1% solution of lidocaine is also used for injection. This anesthetic is longer-acting than procaine but more toxic because it is fat-soluble and is metabolized primarily in the liver.

Corticosteroids are antiinflammatory agents. There is no known controlled study on the effectiveness of steroid injection in comparison with other injected substances, but repeated injections of steroids should be avoided due to known side effects such as atrophy of skin and subcutaneous tissue.

Patients should be told that they may experience loss of sensation for up to 30 minutes after injection.

In general, procaine and lidocaine are the least myotoxic when used at 1% or lower concentrations. Solutions stronger than 1% become significantly myotoxic. Dr. Travell recommended a procaine concentration of 0.5% in physiologic saline, and she found that higher concentrations gave no additional pain relief.[3] Longer-acting anesthetics are more myotoxic without appreciable clinical advantage in treating myofascial pain. Local anesthetics at a lower concentration (0.25%) will selectively block small fibers, while higher concentrations will also block the larger A-δ (IIIb and IIIa) fibers.[4]

Local anesthetics definitely reduce the sensation of soreness and other discomfort immediately after injection. However, evidence shows that the efficacy of injection therapy in pain relief does not depend on any specific properties that these injected substances may possess, but rather on the stimulation effect of the needling used for their injection.[5]

Postinjection Maintenance

After injection the patients should not physically overload the injected muscles for a few days. Mild physical exercise such as walking would be appropriate for the first 3 days.

Avoiding Reactions to Needling

As with acupuncture, injection may cause a harmless but alarming reaction like a short syncope. This is completely preventable. The practitioner should inform patients that they should not be hungry or overfull at the beginning of treatment. It is better to eat no more than a light snack 1 hour before the treatment. If patients are physically exhausted, sweating excessively, very cold, or nervous, they should rest to regain their normal condition before having injections. Finally, patients should be positioned comfortably and securely. We suggest using a recumbent posture (supine, prone, or on the side). If the sitting position has to be used, patients should be well secured so that they will not fall if there is a syncope.

Syncope is most often seen in healthy male patients in their twenties, or female patients from 20 to 50 years of age, usually with lower blood pressure (110/70 or lower).

HISTOPATHOLOGIC EFFECT OF INJECTION THERAPY

A classic experiment using intramuscular injection in rats showed that injection of low volumes (1 cc or less) and low concentration (1% or less) caused only occasional, minor damage to muscle fibers. A temporary inflammatory reaction developed in 24 to 72 hours: a mild infiltration of neutrophils, lymphocytes, and macrophages was observed during this time. The damaged fibers was eventually phagocytized. No changes could be detected beyond 7 days.[6] These established data match our clinical observations.

SUMMARY

INMAS provides a map for finding the most effective points for intramuscular injection for both chronic and acute myofascial pain. In addition, it is an easy and reliable procedure for restoring homeostasis, or *yin-yang* balance, which helps to restore general health as well as give local pain relief.

References

1. Travell J, Rinzler SH: The myofascial genesis of pain, *Postgrad Med* 11:425-434, 1952.
2. Frost FA, Jessen B, Siggard-Anderson J: A control, double-blind comparison of mepivacaine injection versus saline injection for myofascial pain, *Lancet* 1:499-501, 1980.
3. Travell J: Temporomandibular joint pain referred from muscles of the head and neck, *J Prosthet Dent* 10:745-763, 1960.
4. Bekkering R, van Bussel R: Segmental acupuncture. In Filshie J, White A, editors: *Medical acupuncture: a Western scientific approach*, Edinburgh, 1998, Churchill Livingstone, p 109.
5. Baldry P: Trigger point acupuncture. In Filshie J, White A, editors: *Medical acupuncture: a Western scientific approach*, Edinburgh, 1998, Churchill Livingstone, p 39.
6. Pissolato P, Mannheimer W: *Histopathologic effects of local anesthetic drugs and related substances,* Springfield, Ill, 1961, Charles C. Thomas, pp 40, 41, 60, and 71.

CHAPTER 17

Case Studies

INTRODUCTION

The cases presented here illustrate two principles:
1. Applying the quantitative acupuncture evaluation (QAE) method to predict the result and duration of treatment
2. Applying and individualizing the standardized Integrative Neuromuscular Acupoint System (INMAS) protocol to each particular patient and symptom

Quantitative Acupuncture Evaluation

The principle of QAE is discussed in detail in Chapter 6 and we provide only a summary here.

Quantitative evaluation is based on the following factors:

1. The homeostatic status of a person is the same as the self-healing potential of that person in acupuncture therapy
2. The number of tender (passive) points in the body is an indicator of the healing potential—the more tender points, the lower the expected healing potential
3. As homeostasis declines, tender points appear in a predictable sequence in predictable anatomic locations

We selected 16 acupoints as evaluation points: palpating 4 points on the deep radial nerve on both arms and 4 points on the saphenous nerve on both legs enables us to divide patients into four groups: A, B, C, and D (Table 17-1).

Practitioners should understand that there is no drastic pathological difference between patients in groups A and B, and within each group there are differences between patients. For example, some group B patients may need 6 to 8 treatments, whereas others may need 8 to 10 treatments. Furthermore, the self-healing capability of some group A patients may be very close to that of some group B patients. For example, it is possible that some group A patients may need 7 to 8 treatments, whereas some group B patients may need only 5 to 6 treatments.

Standardized but Individualized INMAS Protocol

The INMAS treatment protocol ensures that every patient receives appropriately standardized treatment that is also adjusted to the patient's personal condition. The INMAS protocol is described in detail in Chapter 5 and we provide only a summary here.

INMAS comprises three types of acupoint: homeostatic acupoints (HAs), symptomatic acupoints (SAs), and paravertebral acupoints (PAs). The HAs form the standardized part of the protocol and the SAs and PAs are used to adjust the protocol to each patient's individual condition. For safety reasons, all patients are treated in recumbent positions: prone, supine, or on one side. All or some of the HAs available in the selected position are needled. The determination of whether to needle all or only some HAs depends on the patient's needle tolerance and health. Fewer HAs will be used if the patient is less tolerant to needles, or is very weak and lacks sufficient energy to support the self-healing of a large number of needle-induced lesions. However fewer needles will also be appropriate for a patient who is very healthy, since in such a case a small number of needles will be sufficient for effective treatment. Weaker patients may feel very tired for a day or two after treatment.

About 5 to 10 SAs are commonly used for each treatment. The practitioner should palpate the symptomatic area carefully to find the most tender points.

PAs and SAs should be in the same segment. For example, PAs along C5-T1 are used for symptoms on the arm, whereas PAs along L3-L5 are used for knee pain.

The principles of quantitative evaluation and individualization of the standardized INMAS

Table 17-1				
Quantitative Evaluation of Patients with Soft Tissue Pain				

The Number of Passive Diagnostic Points (H1-1, -2, -3, -4 and H4-1, -2, -3, -4)	Less than 4	4-8	8-12	12-16
Group classification	A	B	C	D
Average number of treatments needed	4	8	16	More than 16
Duration of pain relief	More than 1 yr	Months *and* more than 1 yr (average 5±1 months)	Weeks to months	Days to weeks

Modified from *Anatomical acupuncture*, San Antonio, 1997, Antarctic Press, p. 226.

protocol are depicted in every case presented below. All of these cases involved real patients but their names have been changed to protect their privacy.

NECK AND BACK PAIN

Group A: Excellent Results

Case 1: Lower Back Pain JK, a 42-year-old man, is a manager in a construction company. He is physically active and enjoys outdoor activities such as boating and hiking. One-and-a-half years ago, JK felt lower back pain after moving heavy furniture. After this episode, he was in constant pain that became more severe when he would sit down for about 30 minutes to work on his computer. The pain was more tolerable in the morning when he got up but sometimes became severe in the evening. He visited a chiropractor and several massage therapists, and obtained some relief for a short period following each treatment. A CT scan did not show any detectable problems.

Before the furniture-moving episode, JK occasionally felt soreness and stiffness in the lower back for a few days after heavy work. He had not had any accidents or severe injuries except for slightly hurting his biceps while doing weight lifting 6 years previously.

Quantitative evaluation placed JK in group A. Visual evaluation showed that his right shoulder was about 1 inch lower than his left. During physical examination, the right acupoints H14, H15, H16, and H22 were very tender upon palpation. The skin around right H15 was shiny, suggesting some swelling and inflammation. The impression was that the pain was caused by lumbar muscle strain. Considering that the pain had persisted for one and a half years, the prognosis was that it would take 4 to

8 treatments to achieve optimal recovery of the lumbar muscles for this group A individual.

Treatment Plan Treatments were administered in the prone position. The acupoints selected were:

HAs: all of the HAs accessible to this position.
SAs: lumbar HAs are in fact SAs in this case.
PAs: lumbar HAs are in fact PAs in this case.

Treatments were scheduled every 5 days. After the second treatment, JK felt much better and his lumbar muscles were much more relaxed. After the fourth treatment, JK felt almost no pain. He was told not to resume his strenuous exercise routine because his injured muscles were still weak. After the sixth treatment, JK cancelled the remaining two treatments because he felt pain-free and returned to his usual physical activities.

At present, JK has resumed his vigorous lifestyle, coming to our clinic about once a month for maintenance treatments, which prevent his back and neck muscles from becoming tight and sore.

Case 2: Lower Back and Neck Pain AB is a 20-year-old male bluegrass guitarist and a sophomore at a university. He came to the clinic with complaints of severe lower back pain, which he experienced after performing in the national bluegrass contest several days prior to visiting the clinic.

AB is fit and healthy and has no previous physical injuries. Quantitative evaluation placed him in group A. Visual examination showed that his left shoulder was higher than his right. Upon palpation, acupoints on the left of the neck and the left shoulder area (H7, H3, H13, and H8) were more tender than acupoints on the right side. Left lumbar acupoints (H14, H15, and H16) were sore upon palpation. The impression was that the pain in the lower back and neck was of an acute nature. The prognosis was that pain relief could be achieved within four treatments.

Treatment Plan Treatments were done in the prone position. The acupoints selected were:

HAs: all accessible HAs in this position.
SAs: two tender points on left lateral neck, and two points on right lateral neck.
PAs: three points along T1-T3.

Treatments were scheduled every 3 days. Immediately after the first treatment, AB felt much more relaxed, his left shoulder moved lower, and his lower back pain subsided. The following day AB felt much better, the pain still lingered but was less disturbing. Two days after the second treatment, AB felt no pain and was able to continue to perform with his band.

Case 3: Lower Back Pain YS was referred to the clinic by a local spine surgeon. She is 70 years old, in good health, active, and a world traveler. Three months prior to visiting the clinic she experienced lower back pain; she felt better after taking Advil but the pain would soon come back. She felt better in the morning but the pain became more severe as she engaged in her daily routine. At the same time she was experiencing a swelling of the left hypochondrium. Her medical doctor did not detect any abnormal condition in the spine.

YV was a smoker for more than 30 years but had quit 20 years previously. She had three children. At 40 years of age she had a left ovariotomy; at 50 she experienced mild whiplash from a low-speed car accident; at 55 she was hospitalized for lower back pain but was discharged without surgery. She adhered to a healthy low-carbohydrate and low-fat diet and prior to the current back pain she used to walk 3 to 4 miles a day.

YS is a healthy individual with only a few tender points on the body. Quantitative evaluation placed YS in group A. Visual examination showed that her left shoulder was a little lower than her right. Palpation revealed no tender points on the neck but very tender left lumbar acupoints (H14 and H15). The impression was that YS had lumbar muscle strain. The prognosis was that four to six acupuncture treatments would be needed.

Treatment Plan Prone position:

HAs: lumbar HAs (H14, H15, H16, H22).
SAs: lumbar HAs are SAs in this case.

PAs: considering that the swollen left hypochondrium was on dermatomes T6-T10, four needles on each side along T6-T10 were used.

Supine position:

SAs: 15 small needles (15 mm in length) were inserted into the swollen skin

Treatments were administered every 4 days. After the second treatment, YS felt much better. After the fourth treatment, YS felt no pain and no swelling and discontinued the treatments, although she continues to come in periodically for maintenance treatments.

Case 4: Neck Pain Caused by Whiplash from a Car Accident JL is a 17-year-old male high school senior who experienced whiplash after his car was hit from behind. One day after the accident he experienced neck and upper back pain. He hoped that the pain would resolve itself but after the pain had continued for 2 months his mother brought him to the clinic.

JL is healthy, without any previous medical problems. Quantitative evaluation placed him in group A. Upon palpation, his neck muscles on the sides and back were very tender, especially at the levels of C1-C2 and C4-C5. Also the muscles along T1-T10 were painful to palpation. The lumbar acupoints H15 and H22 were tender because the lower back muscles were also sensitive. Since the muscle pain extended from the cervical spine down to the sacral spine, the prognosis was that eight acupuncture treatments would be needed.

Treatment Plan The treatments were administered in the prone position. The acupoints selected were:

HAs: neck (H7), shoulder (H3, H7, H13 and H8) and lumbar (H14, H15, H16, and H22).
SAs: two needles were inserted into each side of the cervical spine at C4-C5 level where the most tender points were palpated.
PAs: two needles were inserted on both sides of C5; five needles were inserted on each side along T1 to T8.

Treatments were administered every 4 days. JL felt sore one day after the first treatment but felt much better the next day. After the fifth treatment, the pain in the neck, upper back, and lower back completely disappeared.

Group B: Good Results

Case 5: Lower Back Pain DS is a 36-year-old female school teacher. She experienced lower back pain about 5 months before coming to the clinic. The CT scan showed severe degenerative changes in the vertebrae L4-L5-S1. Two months prior to her visit she had received steroid injections but they did not provide relief. She does not have a history of injury or accident and lives a sedentary lifestyle.

Quantitative evaluation placed her in group B. Upon palpation, her lumbar acupoints H14, H15, H16, and H22 were tender and the area along L4-S4 was very painful. The neck and shoulder acupoints were also sensitive. Given that DS is a group B patient, the prognosis was that she would need about eight treatments to achieve stable relief.

Treatment Plan Treatments were administered in the prone position. The acupoints selected were:

HAs: neck (H7), shoulder (H3, H7, H13, and H8) and lumbar (H14, H15, H16, and H22).
SAs: four needles were inserted into each side along L4-S4.
PAs: none because PAs along L4-S4 are in fact SAs.

Treatments were repeated every 4 to 5 days. After three treatments, DS felt that the pain was starting to subside. After the sixth treatment, she did not feel any pain and left for a 2-week vacation. After coming back from vacation, she felt some pain when working in the kitchen (she is a tall woman and the sink seems to have been too low for her) and resumed treatments. After a total of eight treatments, she did not feel any pain. One year later, DS is still pain free.

Case 6: Neck Pain RF is a 62-year old retired accountant. He experienced neck pain for at least 3 years prior to coming to the clinic. He had a very limited range of motion in the neck and always had to turn his whole body in order to look to the side. RF took prescribed pain medications but the pain came back when he stopped taking the pills and it was recommended that he "learn to live with the pain." He has arthritis on C5. An MRI of the lumbar spine showed a large prolapsed disk herniation to the left of midline at L4-L5 associated with retrolisthesis at that level. In addition, he experienced pain on both IT bands.

Twenty years ago his car was rear ended in a car accident at a speed of 10 mph and he was diagnosed with whiplash. After the accident he started to experience neck pain. At the time of his first acupuncture appointment, he had been in pain for 3 years. He has asthma and uses a steroid inhalant in small dosages every morning. He is a little underweight but maintains a good appetite.

Quantitative evaluation placed RF in group B. Upon palpation, he had tender muscles in the back and on both sides of the neck from C1 to C7 and tender lumbar and leg acupoints (H14, H15, H16, H22, H18, H11, and H10). The prognosis was that 8 to 12 treatments would be needed.

Treatment Plan Treatments were administered in the prone position. The selected acupoints were:

HAs: neck (H7), shoulder (H3, H7, H13, and H8), lumbar (H14, H15, H16, and H22) and leg (H18, H11 and H10).
SAs: three needles were inserted into each side of the cervical spine at C3, C5, and C6 levels where the most tender points were palpated.
PAs: two needles were inserted on both sides of C5.

Treatments were repeated every 5 days. Routine neck exercises were suggested. After the fourth treatment, RF felt sufficiently better to go on a long strenuous hike in the mountains, which required frequent head movement. The next day after the hike, RF experienced severe pain and came to the clinic for an emergency treatment. After six treatments, his lower back and leg pain were gone and his neck pain was subsiding.

During subsequent treatments, the leg acupoints were no longer used. After the twelfth treatment, RF did not feel any more neck pain even after going for a long hike, and he could rotate his head more than 60 degrees to both sides without turning his body. RF decided to continue acupuncture treatments to improve the range of motion of his neck and for general maintenance.

Case 7: Lower Back Pain BG is a 52-year-old banker. He had experienced lower back stiffness, especially in the morning, for 30 years prior to presenting at the clinic. He runs three times a week for about 2 miles and is an avid golfer. Six months before his first appointment, his back stiffness became painful. Medical evaluation revealed disk degeneration at L4-L5.

BG had no previous medical problems. Quantitative evaluation placed him in group B. Upon palpation, his left lumbar muscles were more sensitive than those on the right, and the left lumbar acupoints (H15, H14, H22, and H16) were tender, especially H22. The neck area was healthy, without any tender points. Given the foregoing, treatments were concentrated on the lower back. The back pain was treatable because of its acute nature. The prognosis was that about eight treatments should be enough to reduce the present pain and, given 30-years-worth of lower back stiffness, about four more treatments would be needed to prevent lower back pain in the future. Thus, the prognosis was that initially eight treatments would be necessary.

Treatment Plan Treatments were administered in the prone position. The acupoints selected were:

> HAs: neck (H7), shoulder (H3, H7, H13 and H8), lumbar (H14, H15, H16, and H22), and leg HAs (H18, H11 and H10).
> SAs: three needles were inserted into each side of levels L4-S1 where the most tender points were palpated.
> PAs: none because PAs and SAs are the same in this case.

Treatments were repeated every 5 days. After the third treatment, BG no longer felt pain but he continued the treatments to reduce the morning stiffness of his lower back. BG comes for treatment once a month to prevent lower back pain and to improve his golf game due to better muscular coordination.

Case 8: Neck Pain

CH is a 55-year-old business manager. For 20 years she experienced tight shoulder muscles, especially the trapezius muscle. Six months prior to presenting to the clinic she felt neck pain that restricted her head rotation to the right. Medical evaluation suggested facet arthritis of C4-C5 and disk C4-C5 herniation. Her family physician prescribed steroid medication for 3 months. The medication did not relieve her pain but she experienced vasoconstriction in the skin area left to C7-T1, puffiness in the face, and left shoulder and arm pain.

CH is generally healthy. She has three children and had a hysterectomy at the age of 30. Fourteen years ago, she sustained whiplash from a car accident and experienced neck pain one hour after the accident. She continued to walk 3 miles a day even with the recent constant neck pain.

Quantitative evaluation placed CH in group B. Upon palpation, her neck muscles, especially the left side, were found to be very tender and warmer than normal, suggesting inflammation. Also tender were her shoulder and arm acupoints (H2, H7, H3, H13, H8, H9, H1, and H12) and the lumbar acupoints (H14, H15, and H16). Considering the severe neck pain as the results of arthritis and disk

herniation, the prognosis was that 8 to 16 treatments would be needed.

Treatment Plan Treatments were administered in the prone position. The acupoints selected were:

> HAs: neck (H7), shoulder (H3, H7, H13, and H8), arm (H9, H1, and H12), and lumbar (H14, for two months, H15, H16, and H22).
> SAs: three needles were inserted into each side of the cervical spine at C3, C5, and C6, where the most tender areas were detected.
> PAs: two needles are inserted on both sides at C5 and C6.

Treatments were administered every 4 to 5 days. CH experienced improvement after the fifth treatment. After the seventh treatment, she went on vacation and to her surprise did not feel any neck, shoulder, or arm pain during the vacation. She continued to receive preventive acupuncture therapy treatments weekly until the twelfth treatment and was advised to continue acupuncture treatments once a month for 6 months.

Case 9: Lower Back Pain

YM is a 43-year-old computer engineer. He had suffered lower back pain for 2 years prior to presenting at the clinic. Medical evaluation revealed disk herniation at L4-L5. YM felt back pain whenever he stood or sat. At night he felt better only when sleeping on his side in the fetal position. His neurosurgeon advised him that he should delay surgery for several more years, until the disk herniation would become severe enough to justify it.

YM had no previous medical problems. Qualitative evaluation placed him in group B. Upon palpation, slightly tender HAs were found in the neck and shoulder areas and his left lumbar muscles were more sensitive than those on the right. The most tender tissue palpated was in the lumbosacral region left of L4 and S4. All of the lumbar acupoints (H15, H22, H14, and H16) also were very tender, especially on the left side. Considering the herniation of disks L4-L5 and the nature of this patient's work, which required many hours in front of the computer, the prognosis was that eight treatments, with subsequent maintenance treatments, would be needed.

Treatment Plan Treatments were administered in the prone position. The acupoints selected were:

> HAs: neck (H7), shoulder (H3, H7, H13, and H8), lumbar (H14, H15, H16, and H22), and leg (H18, H11, and H10).

SAs: three needles were inserted into each side at the L3-S2 levels, where the most tender areas were palpated.
PAs: none, because PAs and SAs are the same in this case.

Treatments were administered once a week. After the fourth treatment, YM did not feel pain, only a tightness on the left side. Considering the L4-L5 herniation, YM decided to continue receiving maintenance treatments every 2 weeks. At present, YM has been receiving treatments at the clinic for 3 years. He feels slight pain sometimes after a long working day but the pain disappears after a maintenance treatment.

Case 10: Neck and Lower Back Pain CG is a 55-year-old dentist. She had no history of pain problems during her 20 years of practice, until a sudden onset of neck and lower back pain about 5 months before she presented to the clinic. After the onset, she continued to work for 2 months but eventually was no longer able to tolerate the pain and had to leave her practice. An MRI did not reveal any problems.

Fifteen years ago CG experienced minor whiplash from a low-speed car accident; three years ago she tore her right ACL ligament and underwent corrective surgery. CG started menopause at the age of 51.

Qualitative evaluation placed CG in group B. Upon palpation, all of her neck and shoulder acupoints (H2, H7, H3, H13, and H8) were very tender and the lateral sides and back of the neck were very painful. All the back and leg acupoints (H15, H22, H14, H16, H18, H11, and H10) were tender, and swelling skin was observed on the lumbar area. Considering the extensive pain in both neck and lower back, the prognosis was that 8 to 16 treatments were needed.

Treatment Plan Treatments were administered in the prone position. The acupoints selected were:

HAs: neck (H7), shoulder (H3, H7, H13, and H8), lumbar (H14, H15, H16, and H22), and leg (H18, H11, and H10).
SAs: two needles were inserted into each lateral side of the neck where the most tender areas were palpated. There were no SAs in the lumbar area because HAs are both PAs and SAs in this case.
PAs: one needle was inserted on both sides of C4 level because these areas were more tender than other areas on the neck. There were no PAs in the lumbar area because HAs are both PAs and SAs in this case.

Treatments were administered twice a week for the first 2 weeks and then once a week. Prior to each treatment, the neck was carefully palpated to identify the new SAs and the treatment was adjusted accordingly. The lower back acupoints remained unchanged. CG felt improvement in both the neck and the lower back after the fourth treatment. After the seventh treatment, she no longer felt pain in the neck and felt only a slight pain in the lower back, and resumed her work as a dentist. Because of her busy medical practice, CG comes once a week for treatment to prevent recurrence of the lower back, neck, and shoulder pain.

Group C: Average Results

Case 11: Lower Back Pain LR is a 40-year-old housewife. She presented with severe lower back pain that she had felt all day long for many months. At night she could not sleep on her back. An MRI showed that she had a severe disk herniation at the L4-L5 level. LR's spine surgeon told her that she needed immediate surgery or her pain would not only disable her but would cause further nerve degeneration. LR came to our clinic to find an alternative approach.

After reading her medical evaluation, we could not make any promises in this case, but did our best to treat her for 1 month. We told her that she should consider surgery if no progress was achieved after this time. LR has high blood pressure, which is controlled by medication, and occasionally she experiences cramping pain during the first day of her menses. Quantitative evaluation placed LR in group C.

Upon palpation, her lumbar acupoints were very tender (H15, H22, H14, H16), especially the left H22. The left leg acupoints (H18, H11, H10, and H6) were more sensitive than those on the right. Neck and shoulder acupoints were tender but not as sensitive as lumbar and leg acupoints. LR has low tolerance to the pain of needling so we had to design treatments that used a minimal number of points. Due to the severity of the symptoms, her poor health, and low tolerance to needling, the patient was not given any prognosis, but she decided to commit to the treatments in any case.

Treatment Plan Treatments were administered in the prone position. The acupoints selected were:

HAs: lumbar (H14, H15, H16, and H22) and leg (H18, H11, and H10).
SAs: two needles were inserted into each lateral side of L5 and S2 because this area was very tender.

PAs: no PAs were used, because PAs are SAs in this case.

Treatments were administered twice a week for 4 weeks and then once weekly. The same treatment was used each time. After the fourth treatment, LR felt better and decided to continue receiving treatments in order to avoid surgery. She experienced severe pain after the fifth treatment because of the onset of her menses. After the eighth treatment she felt more than 50% pain relief. We continued to use the same procedure for each treatment. After the sixteenth treatment, she felt very little pain and could walk and do most household chores with little pain. After the 24th treatment, she did not feel pain anymore, only occasional discomfort in the lumbar area. Whenever she experienced discomfort, she came for one or two sessions.

Case 12: Neck/Hip Pain (Whiplash/Arthritis)

AA is a successful 52-year-old businesswoman. She was involved in three car accidents that left her with severe neck pain. Her whole body was very weak. If she lay in the prone position for more than 10 minutes she would experience unbearable pain. Sitting for more than 15 minutes also caused her pain because of arthritis in her hip. She experienced pain while walking even a short distance. She had steroid injections, which helped for a short time. Surgery for neck pain was recommended.

Quantitative evaluation placed AA in group C. Upon palpation, all of her neck muscles on the lateral sides and back were very tender; the right shoulder muscles and the muscles right to the region of T1-T7 were also tender. AA has arthritis in the right hip, which causes pain in her right hip and leg. Based on her medical history, the prognosis was that more than 16 treatments were needed.

Treatment Plan   Treatments were administered in the prone position. Since AA could lie prone for only 10 minutes because of neck pain, we focused on the neck first. The acupoints selected were:

HAs: neck (H7), shoulder (H3, H7, H13, and H8), lumbar (H14, H15, H16, and H22), and leg (H18, H10).
SAs: one needle was inserted into each lateral side of the neck where the most tender areas were palpated.
PAs: two needles were inserted on both sides of C3 and C5 level because these areas were more tender than other areas on the neck. Three needles are used on each side along T1-T5.

Treatments were repeated twice a week. After the sixth session, AA felt less neck pain and was able to lie prone for 20 minutes.

Starting from the seventh session, we continued to repeat the same treatment plan but also added two needles on the right hip and two needles on the right IT band where very tender areas were palpated. We continued administering these treatments twice a week. AA was getting stronger and reported a reduction in the pain level. After receiving treatments for 2 months, AA felt very little occasional pain in the neck, hip, and leg and could walk for 40 minutes every day, which accelerated her recovery. After 3 months of treatments, her neck pain was completely gone, and she felt only some hip and leg discomfort if she walked for more than 2 hours.

Case 13: Lower Back Pain

BM, a 74-year-old woman, complained of chronic lower back pain. BM used to run a farm with her late husband and continued to run the family business. She had had 16 surgeries including four on her lower back. The most recent lower back surgery was 2 years ago for L2-L3 disk herniation. After a short relief, her lower back pain had returned and she was recommended to have no more lower back surgery.

BM looked strong for her age, but had had several strokes and atrial fibrillation. She told us that she had lumbar spinal stenosis at L2-L4 and foraminal stenosis at L4-S1. Scars from the previous four surgeries were observed on her lower back. Because of the multiple lower back surgeries and stenoses, it was difficult to estimate how many treatments, if any, could benefit this patient. However, BM insisted on starting acupuncture treatment. She told us, "Please take me, I am a fighter."

Quantitative evaluation placed BM in group C but close to D. She was placed in group C due to her strong willpower and determination to regain her normal life ("I will do everything needed. I am a fighter."). Upon palpation, her lower back was sore on both sides along L1-S2; all of the lumbar and leg acupoints (H15, H22, H14, H16, H18, H11, and H10) were tender; and there were secondary tender acupoints appearing around some of the primary acupoints. (At present it is not clear how multiple surgeries change the physiology of acupoints.)

Treatment Plan   BM could not lie prone because of her shoulder pain. Thus, treatments were administered when BM was lying on her left side. The acupoints selected were:

HAs: lumbar (bilateral H15, H16 and H22, right H14), and right leg (H18, H11, and H10).

SAs: two needles were inserted into each lateral side of the L5 and S2 because these two points were more sensitive upon palpation.
PAs: PAs were not needed because lumbar HAs are PAs and SAs in this case.

Treatments were administered once a week. After the fourth treatment, BM felt better and was able to walk without a walker. After 12 treatments, BM reported that she experienced more than 70% pain relief. She still felt pain but was able to do many things, including gardening, that she was not able to do before the acupuncture treatment. Encouraged by the results, BM continues to receive treatments once every 2 weeks.

Group D: Low Responders

Case 14: Lower Back Pain RM is an 85-year-old woman who used to run a construction business with her late husband. She presented to the clinic with such severe lower back pain that she could not walk upright and had to lie in bed most of the time.

She has arthritis in most of her fingers and toes. These affected joints were swollen. She used to be a very strong and healthy woman but now the lower back pain was practically disabling her. Quantitative evaluation showed that RM belongs to group D. As a friend of BM of the previous case, she was encouraged by BM's example, and was very hopeful and optimistic. RM was determined to follow the treatment regimen, had a strong support group at home, and was not willing to let the pain control her any more.

Upon palpation, her body had many tender acupoints, especially on the lower back area, and every lumbar acupoint was a tender area. Our prognosis was that she needed more than 16 treatments and that she should use transcutaneous electrical nerve stimulation (TENS) to treat herself at home for 20 minutes every day. Fortunately, RM has a granddaughter who is a massage therapist. We suggested that RM should receive light massage three times a week and acupuncture treatments once weekly.

Treatment Plan Treatments were administered in the prone position. The acupoints selected were:

HAs: neck (H7), shoulder (H3, H7, H13, and H8), lumbar (H14, H15, H16, and H22), and leg (H18, H11, and H10).
SAs: two needles were inserted into each lateral side of the L5 and S2 because these two points were more sensitive upon palpation.

PAs: PAs were not needed because lumbar HAs are PAs and SAs in this case.

Treatments were repeated weekly, with the locations of SAs periodically changed according to the tenderness of the points in the lumbosacral region. After the first month, RM started to feel improvement. Two months later, she felt some pain but her back became more flexible and she could walk 30 minutes a day with only a little pain. She received a total of 18 treatments in our clinic. Five months later she informed us that she was taking all her children and grandchildren on a boat cruise to Alaska.

Case 15: Lower Back Pain KK is a 69-year-old businessman who appeared very tall and emaciated. He presented to the clinic for severe lower back and right leg pain. The pain was more prominent on the right side, especially exactly on the right buttock muscle gluteus maximus where H16 inferior gluteal is located. The pain radiated to the lateral side on the IT band and front thigh. Sometimes he felt pain in both thighs.

A computed axial tomography (CAT) scan showed multilevel degenerative and postoperative changes in this patient who had undergone a wide laminectomy between the L1-2 disk space and the L3-4 disk space. There was also a large disk herniation with material prolapsing behind the posterior lower half of the L3 vertebral body. The disk herniation to the left of midline appeared to be causing a mass effect on at least one root that passed over it. There was also evidence of a possible arachnoiditis, particularly to the right of midline at the L2-3 disk space level and at the L3-4 disk space level and a small neuroma at the L3-4 level.

KK used to be physically fit and active, a mountain climber. Four years ago, he started to feel lower back pain and some signs of Parkinson's disease. He had lower back surgery 15 months ago but it did not help. He received one steroid injection, which reduced the pain for only 1 week. He was taking about twenty different drugs daily for various reasons. His muscles were weak because he could not exercise sufficiently.

Quantitative evaluation placed KK in group D. We warned KK that his case was not easy and that he should make a commitment to work with us for a while. He would also have to regularly use TENS, receive massages, and walk with a walker for at least 30 minutes daily.

We used the INMAS protocol with minor adjustment of the SAs according to his pain during every session. KK received two treatments a week for the first 2 weeks, then one session a week. He felt some improvement after each treatment, but the pain would come back the following day. After the eighth session, KK decided to stop acupuncture treatment and to have another surgery.

Some possible reasons why treatment was not successful were that KK was too weak to follow the home routine; his family and friends did not believe in acupuncture and thus did not adequately support him; and only a few treatments were delivered. It is also possible that acupuncture simply does not work in his case.

NECK AND UPPER LIMB PAIN

Case 16: Neck and Upper Limb Pain   ML is a 42-year-old artist. He presented to the clinic with right shoulder and arm pain. He had a tingling sensation radiating from the right shoulder down to the tip of the right index finger. He had felt occasional tingling sensations for 1 year, but the tingling had become constant about 1 month previously. He had not consulted his medical doctor.

ML had bursitis in the same shoulder 20 years ago. He quit smoking 5 years ago. Also 5 years ago he was involved in a car accident that resulted in chronic neck pain.

ML is a healthy man and quantitative evaluation placed him in group B. Upon palpation, his neck and shoulder acupoints were sore (H7, H3, H13, H8), especially on the right side. The right arm acupoints H9 and H1 were also painful upon palpation, as were the lower back acupoints (H15, H22, H14, and H16). Acupoints on the right side of his body were more sore than those on the left. Sensitive points had appeared on the shoulder around H3 on the trapezius muscle, teres minor and major muscles, deltoid muscle, and the tendons of both heads of the biceps. ML's pain was considered chronic because it lasted for more than 1 year. However, given that the patient was healthy the prognosis was that about eight treatments would be needed.

Treatment Plan   Prone position. The acupoints selected were:

HAs: neck and shoulder (H7, H3, H13, and H8), lower back (H15, H22, H14, and H16).
SAs: tender points on both lateral sides of the neck, palpable tender points close to the attachment to the humerus on the muscles supraspinatus, latissimus dorsi, teres major and minor. A few tender points were selected from these locations in every session.

PAs: three needles on each side along C5-T1.

Supine position. The acupoints selected were:

HAs: upper limb (H9, H1, and H12).
SAs: tender points on the deltoid muscles and biceps, especially the tendons of both heads of the biceps.

Both prone and supine positions were used in every session to desensitize all the affected muscles and soft tissues. Treatments were administered once a week. ML felt better after the second treatment. After six treatments, ML felt no more pain and tingling.

Case 17: Neck, Shoulder, and Upper Limb and Lower Back Pain   TB is a 34-year-old financier who works long hours in front of a computer. For 3 months prior to presenting to the clinic she experienced pain on the right side of the neck, in the right elbow, and in the right wrist while she was working. She was referred to the clinic by a spine surgeon.

TB suffered lower back pain 8 or 9 months previously. Physical therapy and chiropractic manipulation reduced the lower back pain but now the pain had come back and spread to the neck, shoulder, elbow, and wrist. In the last 15 years, she had three car accidents; two of them left her with whiplash and one caused a minor concussion. She used to be physically active until 3 months previously when severe pain greatly reduced her physical activity.

TB has no other medical problems. Quantitative evaluation placed her in group B. Upon palpation, her neck, right shoulder, and right arm muscles were very tender and her lower back acupoints also were very tender. The prognosis was eight treatments.

Treatment Plan   Prone position. The acupoints selected were:

HAs: neck and shoulder (H7, H3, H13, and H8), lower back (H15, H22, H14, and H16).
SAs: tender points on both lateral sides of the neck, tender points palpable close to attachment of the humerus on the muscles supraspinatus, latissimus dorsi, teres major and minor. A few tender points were selected from these locations in every session.
PAs: three needles on each side along C5-T1.

Supine position. The acupoints selected were:

HAs: upper limb (H9, H1, and H12).

SAs: tender points on the deltoid muscles, biceps, and muscles of the forearm extensors and flexors, especially the tender points right on the top of the carpal tunnel (palm side, between the base of the metacarpal and the wrist crease). During each session, one or two tender SAs on each part of the right upper limb were selected.

Both prone and supine positions were used in every session. Treatments were administered twice a week for the first 2 weeks then once a week. TB felt better after the fourth treatment. After six treatments, TB felt a drastic reduction in all of her neck, shoulder, arm, and lower back pain. TB received a total of nine treatments to obtain total relief from her pain symptoms.

Case 18: Finger Pain from Mountain Climbing

MT, a 32-year-old avid mountain climber, presented to the clinic for finger pain. During the previous 4 weeks he experienced sharp pain in the right middle finger when he grasped a rock during climbing.

MT is very healthy and quantitative evaluation placed him in group A. Physical examination revealed a tender area that was palpable on lateral sides of the joint between the proximal and middle phalanges. The pain was possibly caused by inflammation of the tendon of flexor digitorum superficialis. Usually tendinitis is caused by the tight muscle. We suggested that MT stop climbing until the injured tendon was completely healed. The prognosis was six treatments (between four and eight treatments).

Treatment Plan   Treatments were administered in the supine position. Local symptomatic treatment can provide complete healing of an acute inflammation. The SAs selected were:

1. Two small needles were inserted on each side of the joint between proximal and middle phalanges of the right middle finger.
2. Five tender points were palpated on the flexor muscles of the right forearm and were deeply needled.

Treatments were repeated once every 5 days. Finger pain was reduced upon palpation after the second treatment. After four treatments the pain was completely gone. MT waited for another 2 weeks before starting to climb again.

Case 19: Rotator Cuff Injury

AS is a 42-year-old social worker. She came to the clinic with a left rotator cuff injury. Three weeks previously she felt pain on the left shoulder after exercising in the gym. Her doctor diagnosed the shoulder pain as a rotator cuff injury, but no further medical evaluation was ordered. AS was prescribed an antiinflammatory drug, which she preferred not to take.

AS is athletically active and has no previous injuries. Quantitative evaluation placed her in group B. Upon palpation, tender points were found in the left lateral side of the neck, on the trapezius, the muscles of the scapula, the deltoid, and the pectoralis major and minor, especially on the front of the head of the humerus. Lumbar acupoints were also tender. Without data from a medical evaluation, such as magnetic resonance imaging (MRI), we could not assess the injury, but we were able to reduce pain and inflammation. The prognosis was that six to eight treatments would be needed.

Treatment Plan   The patient was positioned on the right side, so that both the front and back of the left shoulder were accessible. Treatments focused on the shoulder, neck, and lower back. The acupoints selected were:

HAs: neck (left H7), shoulder (left H3, H13, H8, and H17), lower back (H15, H22, left H14, and left H16).
SAs: the shoulder area was carefully palpated, especially on the head of the humerus, and five to eight tender points were selected to needle.
PAs: three needles on each side along C5-T1.

Treatments were administered once every 5 days, with the same protocol being used for every session. After seven treatments, AS felt completely pain-free.

HIP, LOWER LIMB AND FOOT PAIN.

Case 20: Foot Fasciitis

ST is a 37-year-old businessman. He had experienced pain on the sole and lateral side of the right foot for almost 1 year prior to presenting at the clinic. ST could not walk for more than 30 minutes because of debilitating pain in the right foot.

Thirteen months before presenting at the clinic, ST had surgery on the tendon of the right peroneus longus because he had torn the tendon during a basketball game. After the surgery ST began to feel foot pain.

ST is healthy and used to be athletic, but could not exercise since the foot problem. Qualitative analysis placed ST in group A. Palpation showed that the pain might have been caused by an inflammation of the plantar fascia (fasciitis). To supplement the acupuncture treatments, we suggested that ST wear an orthopedic shoe as often as possible. Considering the prior surgical intervention, the prognosis was that 8 to 12 treatments would be needed.

Treatment Plan   Treatments were administered in the prone position. The acupoints selected were:

> HAs: lumbar and leg (H15, H22, H15, H16, H18, H11, and H10).
> SAs: three to five needles were inserted on the painful area on the sole and lateral side of the right foot. The needles were inserted all the way to the bone.
> PAs: two needles were inserted on both sides of L5-S1, where tender points were detected.

Treatments were performed twice weekly for the first 2 weeks, then once a week. The same treatment was used each time. ST started to wear an orthopedic shoe and felt better after the third treatment. After nine treatments, he did not feel foot pain even when wearing a normal shoe. At this point ST discontinued his treatments. One month later, he told us that his foot felt normal and he started to play basketball again, but with caution.

Case 21: Pain in the Achilles Tendon   MR is a 48-year-old schoolteacher who played tennis 2 to 3 times a week. Six months ago, he heard a snapping noise on the left Achilles tendon during a tennis game. The next day he experienced pain in the Achilles tendon and found that the middle portion of the tendon was swollen. He was prescribed a nonsteroidal antiinflammatory drug by his medical doctor, learned stretching exercises from his physical therapist, and visited a massage therapist. The pain became more severe and he walked with a limp. He decided to try acupuncture.

MR is a healthy man without any history of previous injuries. Because quantitative evaluation placed MR in group A, we thought it possible to achieve healing through symptomatic treatment. Since there had been an insufficient blood supply to the Achilles tendon, the prognosis was that about eight sessions would be needed because tendinitis in a physically active person takes longer to heal than do muscular disorders.

Treatment Plan   Treatments were administered in the prone position. The acupoints selected were:

> HAs: all lumbar and leg HAs (H15, H22, H14, H16, H18, and H11).

SAs: H10 and the two tender points that were palpated around it; four to six needles were inserted into the swollen part of the Achilles tendon.
PAs: two needles were inserted on both sides of L5-S1, where nerve fibers are sent to the Achilles tendon.

The treatment was repeated every 5 days. After three treatments, MR felt significant pain relief. After seven treatments, the pain was completely gone, although the injured portion of the tendon was still slightly enlarged. MR gradually resumed his exercise routine without feeling any pain.

Case 22: Bursitis   KR, a physical therapist, just turned 26. She likes skiing and hiking during weekends. For the last 3 months, she experienced lower back pain, which was relieved after physical therapy. However, after some time she felt the pain again, around the attachment area of the left hamstring muscles. She felt the pain if she sat or walked for more than 1 hour. She told us that she believed the pain was caused by bursitis.

KR is healthy and has no previous injuries. Quantitative evaluation placed her in group B. During physical evaluation, pain was felt upon pressure on the left proximal attachment of the hamstring muscles. Upon palpation, the left lumbar and leg HAs were more tender than the right ones. Since KR's pain was acute, the prognosis was that four to eight treatments would be needed to achieve healing.

Treatment Plan   Prone position. The acupoints selected were:

> HAs: lumbar and leg (H15, H22, H14, H16, H18, H11, and H10).
> SAs: four to five needles were inserted into the tender attachment area of the hamstring muscles.
> PAs: two needles were inserted on both sides along L5-S2.

Supine position. The acupoints selected were:

> HAs: leg (H4, H24, H6, and H5).
> SAs: the medial, anterior, and lateral thigh areas were palpated to find tender points. One to three tender points were selected for needling in each session.

Treatments were administered once every 4 to 5 days. After five treatments, KR felt complete relief from the bursitis.

Case 23: Knee Pain   YY is a 49-year-old research scientist. He came to the clinic complaining of right knee pain, which he had felt for 2 weeks. The knee pain partially disabled him—he could walk with a tolerable level of pain on flat ground but could not climb stairs.

YY is healthy, living a sedentary lifestyle, although he walks about 2 miles a day. He had no previous medical problems. Quantitative evaluation placed him in group B. Since YY did not have a knee injury or arthritis, the knee pain was mostly caused by the tightening of the thigh muscles, which pull on the knee tendons. Upon palpation, the adductor muscles on the medial side of the thigh, and the lower part of sartorius, harbored several tender points. The area just below the medial condyle of the tibia was also very sensitive. Given that the pain was acute and that YY had no other medical problems, the prognosis was that four to eight treatments would be sufficient to achieve pain relief.

Treatment Plan   Prone position. The acupoints selected were:

HAs: lumbar and leg (H15, H22, H14, H16, H18, H11, and H10).
SAs: no SAs in this position.
PAs: two needles were inserted on both sides along L2-L5 (in addition to H22).

Supine position. The acupoints selected were:

HAs: leg (H4, H24, H6, and H5).
SAs: the medial, anterior, and lateral thigh areas were palpated to find tender points, and one to three tender points were selected for needling in each session. One needle was inserted into the dimple area on each side of the patellar tendon. The area around the medial condyle of the tibia was palpated and one to two points were selected for needling in each session.

Treatment was administered every 5 days. YY felt complete pain relief after the second session. He came for the third session and then discontinued the treatments. Four months later, the knee pain returned. He received two more treatments and the pain was completely relieved.

Case 24: Hip Pain   RV is a 66-year-old retired office manager who came to the clinic for right hip pain. She has arthritis on the right hip, which makes walking very difficult, so she walks very little. Both of her legs were swollen.

RV was taking medications for a cardiovascular problem (aneurysm) and high blood pressure. She also experienced some difficulty breathing. She had smoked for 30 years and quit 10 years previously. Quantitative evaluation placed RV in group C. Upon palpation, her hip area, especially around the greater trochanter, was very sore and resistant to touch. Considering the nature of the hip pain and RV's general health, our prognosis was that she would need long-term treatment.

Treatment Plan   RV cannot lie prone, so treatments were administered with the patient lying on her left side. In this position, the posterior, lateral, and anterior sides of the hip are accessible.

HAs: lumbar (H15, H14, H22, H16 [right], H18 [right], and H10 [right]).
SAs: Five to six needles were inserted around the greater trochanter where the area was tender.
PAs: Five needles were inserted on each side of the thoracic spine along T1-T7. These needles help to improve shortness of breath.

For swollen legs, RV resumed the supine position. A cushion was propped behind the knee to raise the knee. H24, H6, and H5 were needled on both sides.

This treatment plan was repeated weekly. The swelling of the legs improved with each treatment, and the hip pain was gradually reduced to a tolerable level of soreness. RV started to walk more with the help of a cane or walker. The shortness of breath also was improving with each treatment, although it would get worse with weather changes. RV's hip was becoming stronger after 10 treatments, allowing her to take increasingly longer walks, although the hip soreness persists. She continues to come for a treatment from time to time, whenever she feels she needs one.

SHINGLES

Case 25: Shingles   YZ is a 26-year-old graduate student. Five days before presenting to the clinic she felt itching in the left hypochondrium and lumbar region and the next day shiny blisters appeared on the skin. She felt excruciating burning pain in the infected area. She took Advil to reduce the pain but obtained little relief.

YZ is healthy and has no previous medical problems. Quantitative evaluation placed her in group B. Given that her shingle eruption was acute, our prognosis was that eight treatments would be needed.

Treatment Plan   Treatments were administered with the patient lying on her right side. The acupoints selected were:

HAs: shoulder and neck (H7 [left], H3 [left], and H8 [left]), left arm (H9, H1, and H12), lumbar (H15, H22, H14, and H16 [left]).
SAs: no SAs at this stage.
PAs: the infected dermatomes are supplied by spinal nerves T7-T10; thus, five needles were inserted on each side along spine T7-T10.

This treatment plan was repeated for every session. Treatments were administered every day for 5 days.

From the sixth treatment, in addition to the above HAs and PAs, 25 to 30 small needles (15 mm in length) were inserted into the infected skin. This treatment was repeated once every other day. After the eighth treatment, YZ felt recovered but continued for two more sessions.

The efficacy of acupuncture in treating post-herpetic neuralgia is very controversial. The basic mechanism of acupuncture therapy should here be mentioned again: acupuncture does not target particular symptoms but just activates the healing potential of the body. The efficacy of acupuncture treatments for postherpetic neuralgia (shingles) or trigeminal neuralgia mostly depends on the healing capacity of the body. In the case presented above, YZ is young and healthy, so recovery was expected. In cases with low self-healing potential, such as patients of group D, acupuncture efficacy drops as the number of passive acupoints in the body increases. This is why acupuncture, in cases of postherpetic neuralgia, offers good healing for some but little or no results for others.

HEADACHE

Case 26: Headache   NH is a 46-year-old lawyer. She had experienced headaches for 5 years, mostly with pain in the left temple or behind the left eye. The headaches were not severe but persistent. She did not visit her family physician for the headaches but diagnosed them herself as tension headaches. An ophthalmologist examined her eyes and did not find any abnormalities. She tried homeopathic medications and chiropractic manipulation, which did not provide relief. Massage provided some relief for 1 or 2 days.

NH works very hard. She gets up at 5 AM and goes to bed at 9 PM. She practices yoga every day and exercises twice a week in a gym. She has no history of previous injuries but had a urethra surgery 30 years ago. Quantitative evaluation placed NH in group B. Visual examination showed that her left shoulder was higher than her right, and she said that it had been this way for years. Upon palpation, HAs on the neck, shoulder, and lower back were very sore, especially on the left side. Given that the headache was chronic because it had persisted for 5 years, the prognosis was that at least eight treatments were needed to provide pain relief that might last for months.

Treatment Plan   Treatments were administered in the prone position. The acupoints selected were:

HAs: neck (H7); shoulder (H3, H13, and H8), lumbar (H15, H22, H14, and H18).
SAs: one needle was inserted into each lateral side of the neck where the most tender spot was palpated. Two to three tender points were identified and needled around H3. One tender point on the muscle supraspinatus was needled.
PAs: two needles were inserted into each side along C5-T1; three needles were inserted into each side along T2-T7.

Treatments were repeated every 4 to 5 days. NH felt increasingly better with each treatment. After six treatments she felt no pain for an entire week. After the eighth session, she decided to stop treatments. She came back about 2 months later because she started to experience headaches again due to a stressful project. We repeated the same treatment plan for another four sessions. We believe that as long as her left shoulder is higher than the right, headaches can be triggered by any stressful situation or by cumulative daily stress.

Case 27: Headache   CC is a 31-year-old homemaker. She had experienced a severe headache one to three times a week on the left half of the skull for almost 6 years. This headache is often accompanied by nausea and stomach upsets. She does not take any pain medication because it irritates her stomach.

CC had a car accident 7 years ago, which resulted in severe lower back and neck pain for several months. CC also suffered from severe constipation. She ate vegetables, meats, and beans but had bowel movements about once or twice a week.

Quantitative evaluation placed CC in group C. Upon palpation, tender acupoints were found around every HA. We believed that her headache was related to her homeostatic condition and suggested that she drink fresh vegetable juice several times a day to cure the constipation. Our prognosis was that she needed 2 to 3 months of acupuncture treatments.

Treatment Plan Prone position. The acupoints selected were:

HAs: all HAs accessible in this position.
SAs: one or two needles were inserted on each lateral side of the neck during each session according to the palpated tender points.
PAs: no PAs were selected because there were no local somatic symptoms.

Supine position. The acupoints selected were:

HAs: all HAs accessible in this position.
SAs: one needle was inserted bilaterally into the point about 2 inches lateral to the umbilicus. These two points, Stomach 25 in the classic acupuncture system, may help to relieve constipation.

Each session included treatments in both the prone and supine positions. Treatments were administered once every week. After the fourth treatment, CC experienced headaches less frequently. She drank juice regularly and had more frequent bowel movements. After the eighth treatment she went on vacation for 2 weeks and did not experience a headache. She continued with four more treatments after returning from vacation. Because CC belonged to group C, we warned her that her headache may recur after a while and that she should continue with maintenance treatments once every 2 weeks to stabilize her improvement. We also advised her that special attention should be paid to maintaining regular bowel movements.

NON-PAIN SYMPTOMS

Please note that the prediction of non-pain symptoms is less reliable than pain symptoms, and therefore the prediction is omitted in these cases.

Case 28: Bell's Palsy (1) Bell's palsy is the paralysis of the muscles on one side of the face caused by neuropathy of the facial nerve. It can result from injury to the facial nerve, tumor, in rare cases, or unknown causes. The symptom is often no more than a temporary condition for a few days or weeks. However, it is not uncommon to see patients who take months or longer to

recover if there is no treatment. If the symptom lasts too long, branches of the facial nerve can degenerate.

Acupuncture therapy will accelerate the healing process. However, if paralysis has persisted for a long time, acupuncture can do little or nothing.

RS is a 27-year-old computer programmer. Six months prior to presenting to the clinic he was involved in an accident that caused pain on the C5-C7 level. One week later he suddenly had paralysis on the left side of the face: the left corner of his mouth was sagging; the left eye could not be closed; and it was difficult to drink, chew, and swallow. This paralysis had persisted for 6 months without any improvement.

RS is healthy and exercises in a gym everyday. He has no previous medical problems.

Quantitative evaluation placed him in group B. However, since the palsy had lasted for 6 months, recovery was expected to be slow.

Treatment Plan Prone position. The acupoints selected were:

HAs: all HAs accessible in this position.
SAs: no SAs were selected.
PAs: two needles were inserted on each side along C5-C7.

Supine position. The acupoints selected were:

HAs: facial and arm (H2, H23, H19, H9, H1, and H12). Leg HAs were not selected because of no symptoms in those areas.
SAs: on the affected facial muscles except orbicularis oculi: zygomaticus major and minor, orbicularis oris, levators labii.

The treatment plan was repeated every session twice weekly for the first 2 weeks, and then once a week. After six treatments, RS felt that the muscles were strong enough to bring up the drooping mouth corner and that eating and drinking had become easier. RS had a total of 16 treatments over 3 months, at the end of which the facial paralysis was no longer noticeable, although the left eye still did not close well at night. Subsequently, RS came to treatment irregularly and 4 months later the muscle orbicularis oculi could blink and close.

Case 29: Bell's Palsy (2) AS, a 65-year-old woman, came to the clinic with Bell's palsy. She retired from her job in a bank 5 years previously. She started to have shingles on the left foot, leg, and hip. One month later, in the morning, she suddenly felt paralysis on the left side of the face. She was told that the paralysis would resolve itself in a few days. She waited for 2 months and still did not experience any improvement.

She has a complicated medical history. Thirty five years ago she broke two left ribs and damaged her neck (whiplash) in a car accident. Thirty years ago a complete hysterectomy was performed. She got hepatitis C from a blood transfusion. Ten years ago she had surgery on both wrists for carpal tunnel syndrome. She takes medication to control diabetes and occasionally experiences migraine headaches. She has a rotator cuff tear so she cannot lie in the prone position.

Quantitative evaluation placed AS in group C, very close to group D. Our prognosis was that her health and energy might not be able to sustain intensive acupuncture treatment and thus the treatment process might take longer.

Treatment Plan   Treatments were administered in the supine position because AS can only lie on her back. The acupoints selected were:

HAs: facial and arm (H2, H23, H19, H9, H1, and H12), leg (H4, H6, and H24).
SAs: on the affected facial muscles except orbicularis oculi.

The treatment plan was repeated in every session. AS received treatments once a week. After 10 treatments, she felt that the muscles were strong enough to bring up the drooping mouth corner and that eating and drinking had become easier. RS received a total of 16 treatments in 4 months. At the end of the treatments her facial paralysis was no longer noticeable but the left eye still did not close well at night and she needed to use eye drops to keep her eye moist.

One year later, AS felt a sharp pain for a few hours in the right shoulder area and experienced paralysis on the right side of her face the next morning. This time she received a total of eight treatments to bring the paralytic muscles back to normal.

Case 30: Sinusitis   NC is a 22-year-old student of architecture who came to the clinic with very painful chronic sinusitis. Her medical doctors suggested surgery. She recently had an ear infection and she thought it was caused by the sinusitis.

NC is reasonably healthy but has had chronic sinusitis and bronchitis since childhood. She is allergic to milk. Quantitative evaluation placed NC in group B.

Treatment Plan   Prone position. Acupoints selected were:

HAs: all HAs accessible in this position.
SAs: no SAs.
PAs: five needles on each side along T1-T7 for bronchitis.

Supine position. Acupoints selected were:

HAs: all HAs accessible in this position.
SAs: one needle was inserted into the nasion (midline between the eyes), and 1 needle on each ala nasi of the nose.

This treatment plan was repeated once every week. Immediately after the first treatment, NC said she felt better. After three treatments, she felt a significant improvement. Since her sinusitis was not related to the seasons (allergies), NC decided to come for an additional four treatments to stabilize the result. The additional treatments were administered once every 2 weeks.

Case 31: Urticaria or Neurodermatitis   KV just turned 48 and is an office manager. She experienced itchy and burning red wheals over her entire body 1 hour after she had finished working in her garden, where she was doing yard work under the sun for 3 hours.

KV is healthy and athletic. She had experienced similar urticaria two to three times many years ago but not in the previous 5 years. Quantitative evaluation placed KV in group B.

Treatment Plan   Prone position. The acupoints selected were:

HAs: all HAs accessible in this position.
SAs: no SAs were selected at this stage. Her problem was not pain related.
PAs: five needles were used on each side of the thoracic spine along T1-T7.

Supine position. The acupoints selected were:

HAs: all HAs accessible in this position.

The treatment plan was repeated once every day for 2 days. Most skin wheals subsided after the third treatment except the skin on the medial sides of the thigh and on the cubital fossa. After the third treatment the same needling was repeated with the addition of 5 to 10 needles inserted into the itchy skin on the medial thighs and cubital fossae. After the fifth treatment, the skin completely cleared up and the itching stopped.

Neurodermatitis can be treated in the same way. Apply needles to the following acupoints:

HAs: all HAs over the body.

SAs: insert several needles in itchy areas.

PAs: PAs are selected according to the dermatome relationship with SAs. For example, if itchy skin is located on the arms, PAs along C5-T1 should be selected. If itching appears on the lower limb, S1-S4 should be used.

Acronyms and Abbreviations

Clinical Acupuncture

INMAS:	Integrative Neuromuscular Acupoint System
HAs:	Homeostatic acupoints
PAs:	Paravertebral acupoints
SAs:	Symptomatic acupoints
PHP:	Prone homeostatic protocol
cPHP:	Complete PHP
rPHP:	Reduced PHP
SHP:	Supine homeostatic protocol
cSHP:	Complete SHP
rSHP:	Reduced SHP
QAE:	Quantitative acupuncture evaluation

Basic Neuroanatomy and Neurophysiology

Ach:	Acetylcholine
ANS:	Autonomic nervous system
BS-HPA axis:	Broad-sense HPA axis
CNS:	Central nervous system
fMRI:	Functional magnetic resonance imaging
HAP axis:	Hypothalamic-autonomic-parasympathetic axis (vagus nerve outflow)
HAS axis:	Hypothalamic-autonomic-sympathetic nervous system
HPA axis:	Hypothalamus-pituitary-adrenal axis
IL-1β:	Interleukin-1β
NE:	Norepinephrine
PET:	Positron emission tomography
PNS:	Peripheral nervous system
TNF-α:	Tumor necrosis factor-α

Cross Reference Between 24 Homeostatic Acupoints and Their Corresponding Meridian Nomenclature

Location	Homeostatic Acupoint	Corresponding Meridian Nomenclature	
Head and neck	H2 great auricular	SJ 17	Yifeng
	H7 greater occipital	B 10	Tianzhu
	H19 infraorbital	S 2	Sibai
	H23 supraorbital	B 2	Zanzhu
Shoulder	H3 spinal accessory	G 21	Jianjing
	H8 suprascapular	SI 11	Tianzong
	H13 dorsal scapular	SI 14	Jianwaishu
	H17 lateral pectoral	S 15	Wuyi
Upper limb	H1 deep radial	LI 10	Shousanli
	H9 lateral antebrachial cutaneous	LI 11	Quchi
	H12 superficial radial	LI 4	Hegu
Torso	H14 superior cluneal	(No corresponding name)	
	H15 posterior cutaneous of L2	B 23	Shenshu
	H20 spinous process of T7	Du 9	Zhiyang
	H21 posterior cutaneous of T6	B 16	Dushu
	H22 posterior cutaneous of L5	B 26	Guanyuanshu
Lower limb	H4 saphenous	Liv 8	Ququan
	H5 deep peroneal	Liv 3	Taichong
	H6 tibial	Sp 6	Sanyinjiao
	H10 sural	B 57	Chengshan
	H11 lateral popliteal	B 39	Weiyang
	H16 inferior gluteal	Extra 34	Huanzhong
	H18 iliotibial	G 31	Fengshi
	H24 common peroneal	G 34	Yanglingquan

Traditional names of the acupoints are from Chen X, editor: *Chinese acupuncture and moxibustion*, Beijing, 1997, Foreign Language Press. The anatomic location of each homeostatic acupoint (HA) may vary slightly from person to person due to individual anatomic variation. Therefore manual palpation of each HA is necessary in clinical practice.

INDEX

Page references followed by "f" indicate figures, by "t" indicate tables, and by "b" indicate boxes.

Supraorbital point (H23)
  clinical notes for, 57
  location of, 54f
  neuroanatomy of, 57, 58f
Suprascapular nerve, 64
Suprascapular point (H8)
  clinical notes for, 64
  location of, 55f, 142f
  neuroanatomy of, 63f, 64
Sural nerve, 66
Sural point (H10)
  location of, 55f
  neuroanatomy of, 66
Swimming, 135
Sympathetic nervous system, 5-7
  acupuncture effect on, 7
  course of, 8f
  function of, 6
  general plan of, 9f
  in spinal sensitization, 68-69
  of upper limb, 150-151
Symptomatic acupoints
  description of, general, 53
  in individualized protocol, 91-92
  for non-pain symptoms, 215-216
  physical properties of, 19-20
  spinal mechanisms of, 68-69, 69f, 70f
  treatment protocol for, 69-71
Synapse, 5f
Syncope, 85-86, 86f
Systemic model, 19-20
Systemic pain-related disorders, 209-214
  complex regional pain syndrome as, 213-214
  headache as, 209-211
  shingles as, 211-212
  temporomandibular joint disorders as, 212
  trigeminal neuralgia as, 211

T

Talofibular ligament, 205f
Temporomandibular joint disorders, 212
  H19 infraorbital acupoint for, 57
Tender points
  in INMAS, 52-56
  peripheral *vs.* spinal nerve in, 69-70
  significance of, 15
Tendinitis, 125, 126f
  bicipital, 176
  of elbow, 176-177
    symptomatic point location for, 91-92
  of rotator cuff, 174-176
    case study of, 247
  in sports medicine, 225
Tendons
  in back pain, 125, 126f
  calcaneal, 206
Tennis, 135
Tennis elbow, 176-177
  symptomatic point location for, 91-92
Tenosynovitis, 179
TENS (transcutaneous electrical nerve stimulation), 227-231

TENS (transcutaneous electrical nerve stimulation) *(Continued)*
  acupoint selection in, 230
  contraindications for, 230
  technical parameters of, 229b, 229-230
Thalamus, 38
Thigh. *See also* Lower extremity
  muscles of, 187-189, 190t-191t
    adductors, 192f
    flexors, 189f
    hamstrings, 192f
    transverse section for, 193f
  treatment protocol for, 207f, 207-208, 208f
Thoracic outlet syndrome, 179
Thoracic spine
  structure of, 113-114
    vertebral body in, 114f
  T6 level of, H21 acupoint on
    location of, 55f
    neuroanatomy of, 67
  T7 level of, H20 acupoint on
    clinical notes for, 67
    location of, 55f
    neuroanatomy of, 67
Tibia, 184-185, 186f
Tibial nerve, 66
  distribution of, 191, 199f
Tibial point (H6)
  clinical notes for, 66
  location of, 54f
  neuroanatomy of, 66
Tic douloureux, 211
TMJ, 212
Transcutaneous electrical nerve stimulation (TENS), 227-231
  acupoint selection in, 230
  contraindications for, 230-231
  technical parameters of, 229b, 229-230
Travell, Janet, 234, 236
Trigeminal nerve (V)
  acupoints on, 60
  anatomical location of, 6f
  importance of, 3
Trigeminal neuralgia, 211
Trigger points
  attachment, 1
  central, 1
  definition of, 1
  vs. acupoints, 17
  histopathic characteristics of, 20-21, 21f
  injection therapy for, 234
Trochanteric bursitis, 196

U

Ulcers, 217-218
  tender points in, 53
Ulnar nerve, 149
  entrapment of, 179
  innervation of, 149t
Unusual symptoms, 220
Upper extremity, 145-182
  arm
    muscles in, 161, 161t-162t

Upper extremity *(Continued)*
    nerves in, 148f, 162, 162t
    vessels in, 148f
  bones of, 146, 146f
  brachial plexus, 146-151
    divisions of, 147f
    infraclavicular branches of, 148-150, 149t, 150t
    supraclavicular branches of, 147-148
    sympathetic supply in, 150t, 150-151
  case study for, 246-247
  elbow joints, 162-164, 163f, 164f
  forearm, 164-166
    extensors in, 165-166, 170t, 171f, 172f
    flexors in, 164-165, 165t, 166f, 167, 167t, 167f
  hand, 170-173, 173f, 174f
  homeostatic acupoints on
    neuroanatomy of, 60-64, 61f-63f
  introduction to, 145-146
  pain in, 173-180
    from joint and bone, 179-180
    from nerve lesion, 177-179
      carpal tunnel syndrome in, 177-179, 178f
      tenosynovitis, 179
      ulnar nerve entrapment in, 179
    from soft tissue, 173-177
      bicipital tendinitis in, 176
      epicondylitis in, 176-177
      frozen shoulder in, 176
      general considerations for, 173-174
      olecranon bursitis in, 177
      rotator cuff tendinopathy in, 174-176
      subacromial bursitis in, 176
  shoulder, 151-156
    acromioclavicular joint in, 153-154, 154f
    bicipital-humeral joint in, 155-156
    glenohumeral joint in, 151-153, 152f, 153t, 153f
    movement in, 156t, 156-158
    humeral, 158, 160f
    scapular, 157, 157t, 157f-160f
    pain locations in, 158, 161
    scapulothoracic joint in, 155, 156f
    sternoclavicular joint in, 154-155, 155f
  treatment protocol for, 180, 181f, 182f
  wrist complex, 166-170, 173f-175f
Urticaria, 218
  case study for, 252-253

V

Vagus nerve
  anatomical location of, 6f
  stimulation of, 42, 43f, 45
Vasovagal reaction, 86